Socio-Demographic Factors and Cancer Research

Socio-Demographic Factors and Cancer Research

Guest Editors

Mitchell S. Fourman

Amanda N. Goldin

MDPI

Basel • Beijing • Wuhan • Barcelona • Belgrade • Novi Sad • Cluj • Manchester

Guest Editors
Mitchell S. Fourman
Department of Orthopedic Surgery
Albert Einstein College of Medicine
Bronx
USA

Amanda N. Goldin
Department of Orthopaedic Surgery
University of California
Irvine School of Medicine
Orange
USA

Editorial Office
MDPI AG
Grosspeteranlage 5
4052 Basel, Switzerland

This is a reprint of the Special Issue, published open access by the journal *Cancers* (ISSN 2072-6694), freely accessible at: https://www.mdpi.com/journal/cancers/special_issues/8K9PDOICO4.

For citation purposes, cite each article independently as indicated on the article page online and as indicated below:

Lastname, A.A.; Lastname, B.B. Article Title. *Journal Name* **Year**, *Volume Number*, Page Range.

ISBN 978-3-7258-6197-2 (Hbk)
ISBN 978-3-7258-6198-9 (PDF)
https://doi.org/10.3390/books978-3-7258-6198-9

Contents

About the Editors vii

Preface ix

Nóra Kovács and Orsolya Varga
Socioeconomic and Healthcare Indicators and Colorectal Cancer Burden: Analysis of Eurostat and Global Burden of Disease Study 2021 Data
Reprinted from: *Cancers* **2025**, *17*, 2075, https://doi.org/10.3390/cancers17132075 1

Kella L. Vangsness, Ronald M. Cornely, Andre-Philippe Sam, Naikhoba C. O. Munabi, Michael Chu, Mouchammed Agko, et al.
Barriers to Post-Mastectomy Breast Reconstruction: A Comprehensive Retrospective Study
Reprinted from: *Cancers* **2025**, *17*, 2002, https://doi.org/10.3390/cancers17122002 12

Emerson Delacroix, Sarah Austin, John D. Rice, Elena Martinez Stoffel, Erika Koeppe, Jennifer J. Griggs and Ken Resnicow
Clinician Recommendation for Hereditary Genetic Testing in Participants at Increased Risk for Hereditary Cancer
Reprinted from: *Cancers* **2025**, *17*, 1994, https://doi.org/10.3390/cancers17121994 25

Mitesh Rajpurohit, Mojgan Golzy, Nai-Wei Chen, Katie S. Murray and Geoffrey Rosen
Relationship Among Body Mass Index, Survival, Cancer Treatment and Health-Related Quality of Life Among Older Patients with Bladder Cancer
Reprinted from: *Cancers* **2025**, *17*, 1200, https://doi.org/10.3390/cancers17071200 37

Daniel Heilig, Ákos Szabó, Petra Fadgyas-Freyler and Judit Simon
The Impact of Homelessness on Lung Cancer Survival and Healthcare Utilization in the Hungarian Universal Healthcare System
Reprinted from: *Cancers* **2025**, *17*, 1158, https://doi.org/10.3390/cancers17071158 51

Ronit Pinchas-Mizrachi and Dan Bouhnik
A Retrospective Analysis of Breast Cancer Mortality among Jewish and Muslim Arab Women in Israel: The Role of Sociodemographic Factors
Reprinted from: *Cancers* **2024**, *16*, 2763, https://doi.org/10.3390/cancers16152763 64

Rafael De la Garza Ramos, Jessica Ryvlin, Ali Haider Bangash, Mousa K. Hamad, Mitchell S. Fourman, John H. Shin, et al.
Predictors of Clavien–Dindo Grade III–IV or Grade V Complications after Metastatic Spinal Tumor Surgery: An Analysis of Sociodemographic, Socioeconomic, Clinical, Oncologic, and Operative Parameters
Reprinted from: *Cancers* **2024**, *16*, 2741, https://doi.org/10.3390/cancers16152741 74

Nicola Gentili, William Balzi, Flavia Foca, Valentina Danesi, Mattia Altini, Angelo Delmonte, et al.
Healthcare Costs and Resource Utilisation of Italian Metastatic Non-Small Cell Lung Cancer Patients
Reprinted from: *Cancers* **2024**, *16*, 592, https://doi.org/10.3390/cancers16030592 85

Hadiza Galadima, Rexford Anson-Dwamena, Ashley Johnson, Ghalib Bello, Georges Adunlin and James Blando
Machine Learning as a Tool for Early Detection: A Focus on Late-Stage Colorectal Cancer across Socioeconomic Spectrums
Reprinted from: *Cancers* **2024**, *16*, 540, https://doi.org/10.3390/cancers16030540 100

Courtney M. Vaughn and Bradley V. Vaughn
Sleep and Cancer
Reprinted from: *Cancers* **2025**, *17*, 911, https://doi.org/10.3390/cancers17060911 . . . . **121**

Anabela Amarelo, Marisa Mota, Bruno Amarelo, Marta Campos Ferreira and Carla Sílvia Fernandes
Technological Resources for Physical Rehabilitation in Cancer Patients Undergoing Chemotherapy: A Scoping Review
Reprinted from: *Cancers* **2024**, *16*, 3949, https://doi.org/10.3390/cancers16233949 . . . . **147**

Helena Fiats Ribeiro, Fernando Castilho Pelloso, Beatriz Sousa da Fonseca, Camila Wohlenberg Camparoto, Maria Dalva de Barros Carvalho, Vlaudimir Dias Marques, et al.
Racial and Socioeconomic Disparity in Breast Cancer Mortality: A Systematic Review and Meta-Analysis
Reprinted from: *Cancers* **2025**, *17*, 1641, https://doi.org/10.3390/cancers17101641 . . . . **171**

About the Editors

Mitchell S. Fourman

Mitchell S. Fourman, is an attending physician and Assistant Professor of Orthopedic Surgery at Montefiore-Einstein. Dr. Fourman's clinical focus is the orthopaedic oncology and spine surgery. His interests include spinal deformity, adult degenerative spine pathology, metastatic cancer to the spine, primary spine tumours, and Scheuermann's kyphosis. He also studies multiple aspects of adult spinal deformity in collaboration with the International Spine Study Group (ISSG). He has won several awards for his research, including the Philip D. Wilson Award for Excellence in Orthopaedic Surgery Research at Hospital for Special Surgery during his fellowship.

Amanda N. Goldin

Amanda N. Goldin, MD, FAAOS, is an ABOS board-certified orthopaedic surgeon who specializes in the surgical treatment of musculoskeletal tumors. She is an attending orthopaedic surgeon in the Department of Orthopaedic Surgery at the University of California, Irvine, and also works with the Chao Family Comprehensive Cancer Center, an NCI-designated cancer center. Dr. Goldin treats both adult and pediatric patients with tumors of the extremities and pelvis. Her clinical interests include the management of bone and soft tissue sarcomas, skeletal metastatic disease, benign bone and soft tissue tumors, limb salvage and reconstruction following oncologic surgery, and socioeconomic disparities in medicine and surgery. She completed her residency in orthopaedic surgery at the University of California, San Diego, followed by fellowship training in musculoskeletal oncology at Vanderbilt University Medical Center, one of the busiest sarcoma centers in the United States. Dr. Goldin is actively involved in clinical care, research, and medical education, and is committed to providing compassionate, transparent, and evidence-based care to her patients.

Preface

It is well established that socioeconomic factors influence cancer treatment outcomes, even when optimal therapies are employed. These contributors are often modifiable and community/culture-dependent, warranting focused research.

This Reprint aims to address the specific socioeconomic factors that influence the care of individuals with a broad spectrum of cancers, with a focus on both global and region-specific factors. It also seeks to further understand the influence that these socioeconomic factors have on the provision and outcomes of cancer care.

Mitchell S. Fourman and Amanda N. Goldin
Guest Editors

cancers

MDPI

Article

Socioeconomic and Healthcare Indicators and Colorectal Cancer Burden: Analysis of Eurostat and Global Burden of Disease Study 2021 Data

Nóra Kovács [1,*] and Orsolya Varga [1,2]

[1] Department of Public Health and Epidemiology, Faculty of Medicine, University of Debrecen, 4028 Debrecen, Hungary; varga.orsolya@med.unideb.hu
[2] Syreon Research Institute, 1142 Budapest, Hungary
* Correspondence: kovacs.nora@med.unideb.hu

Simple Summary: Colorectal cancer (CRC) remains a major health and economic challenge across the European Union (EU). This study aimed to examine trends and inequalities in CRC burden and to explore its association with country-level socioeconomic and healthcare indicators across 24 EU member states. CRC burden was measured using age-standardized mortality, years lived with disability (YLD), years of life lost (YLL), and disability-adjusted life years (DALY) rates, which were obtained from the Global Burden of Disease Study 2021. Socioeconomic and healthcare data were collected from Eurostat between 2005 and 2021. While inequality in YLD rate decreased, disparities in mortality, YLL, and DALY rates increased. Higher numbers of physicians and higher education levels were linked to lower CRC burden, while a greater income inequality was linked to higher burden. These findings emphasize the importance of expanding screening programs, improving healthcare capacity, and reducing social inequalities to address CRC disparities in the EU.

Abstract: Background/Objectives: Colorectal cancer (CRC) is a leading cause of cancer-related morbidity and mortality worldwide, posing a substantial health and economic burden. Despite advances in screening and treatment, significant socioeconomic and healthcare-related disparities persist across European Union (EU) member states. This study aims to identify trends and inequality in CRC burden over time and to explore the relationship between country-level socioeconomic and healthcare indicators and CRC burden across EU member states. **Methods:** Age-standardized mortality, years lived with disability (YLD), years of life lost (YLL), and disability-adjusted life years (DALY) rates were extracted from Global Burden of Diseases Study 2021 for 24 EU countries. Socioeconomic and healthcare indicators were extracted from Eurostat between 2005 and 2021. The Gini index was calculated to evaluate CRC-related health inequality, and generalized linear mixed models were used to assess the link between indicators and disease burden. **Results:** The Gini index for age-standardized YLDs declined from 0.19 to 0.12 between 1990 and 2021, while inequality in YLL (from 0.11 to 0.16), DALY (from 0.11 to 0.15), and mortality rates (from 0.12 to 0.14) increased. The number of practicing physicians ($p < 0.05$) and higher levels of education ($p < 0.001$) were related to lower death, DALY, YLD, and YLL rates. Conversely, greater income inequality was linked to higher mortality, DALY, and YLL rates ($p < 0.05$). **Conclusions:** Our findings underscore that, in addition to expanding organized screening programs, enhancing physician availability and addressing socioeconomic inequalities are essential for reducing the burden of CRC.

Keywords: healthcare indicators; disease burden; colorectal cancer; inequality; Gini index

1. Introduction

Colorectal cancer (CRC) is a major global public health concern, ranking as the third most common cancer worldwide. In 2020, there were over 1.9 million new cases and approximately 930,000 deaths attributed to CRC, highlighting its substantial contribution to global morbidity and mortality [1,2].

Within the European Union (EU), it accounted for 11.6% of all cancer deaths in 2021 [3]. According to the Global Burden of Disease Study 2021, CRC was responsible for more than 175,000 deaths and over 3.3 million disability-adjusted life years (DALYs) across EU member states, with considerable variation across countries [2,4].

In 2018, the economic burden of colorectal cancer in the European Union was estimated at €19 billion (€12.2 billion for colon and €6.8 billion for rectum cancers), covering direct healthcare, informal care, and indirect costs. Informal care and indirect costs combined were closely equal to direct costs, demonstrating the broader social impact of the disease [5].

CRC disproportionately impacts individuals from low socioeconomic backgrounds and certain racial minorities, partly due to greater exposure to risk factors like poor diet, inactivity, and reduced access to preventive measures such as chemoprevention [6]. Screening programs have contributed substantially to the reduction in CRC incidence and mortality rates across many European countries over the past two decades, particularly in countries where long-standing screening programs are in place (e.g., Austria, the Czech Republic, and Germany) [7]. However, participation remains suboptimal, and significant socioeconomic inequalities persist. Numerous studies have shown that individuals from lower social groups are considerably less likely to participate in CRC screening [8,9]. These disparities, however, are not limited to screening but extend to treatment access, survival, and overall mortality. Previous studies found that patients with low SES are more likely to experience delays in treatment [10] and are less likely to receive surgery and adjuvant therapies [11], which in turn negatively impacts prognosis and survival [11–13].

Healthcare system capacity is also a key determinant of colorectal cancer burden in terms of access to screening, early diagnosis, availability of treatment, and follow-up care. A recent meta-analysis found that regions with limited healthcare resources (including a shortage of medical specialists) experience longer diagnostic intervals [14]. All of these factors are critical for improving patient outcomes and reducing mortality [15–17].

While individual-level CRC disparities are well documented, comparative EU-wide studies on CRC burden remain limited. To address this gap, the present study aimed to explore how selected socioeconomic and healthcare indicators are related to CRC burden across EU member states by linking data from the Global Burden of Disease Study (GBD) 2021 with publicly available datasets from the Statistical Office of the European Union (Eurostat).

2. Materials and Methods

2.1. Study Design and Data Sources

Data for this study were obtained from two publicly available databases. Age-standardized disease burden data for colon and rectum cancer were retrieved from the Global Health Data Exchange (GHDx), while healthcare and socioeconomic indicators for EU member states were sourced from the Eurostat database. Data were obtained for 24 of the 27 EU member states. Greece, Portugal, and Slovakia were excluded because data on the number of practicing physicians were not available for these countries during the study period.

The Global Burden of Disease (GBD) 2021 study provides comprehensive estimates for 371 diseases and injuries, 88 risk factors by sex and age across 204 countries and territories [18]. GBD 2021 provides annual estimates between 1990 and 2021 available through the publicly accessible GHDx platform (http://ghdx.healthdata.org/gbd-results-tool (accessed on 10 May 2025)).

Data from 24 EU member states were collected using the GBD 2021 database. We utilized age-standardized rates of death, disability-adjusted life years (DALYs), years lived with disability (YLDs), and years of life lost (YLLs) associated with colon and rectum cancer at European Union and national levels. All rates were expressed per 100,000 population. Age-standardized rates were used to ensure comparability over time and between populations, given the demographic shifts in population growth and aging. YLL represents the years of life lost due to a specific cause when compared to the standard life expectancy. YLD refers to the years lived with any disability, weighted by the severity of the health condition. The DALY was used to measure the total burden of chronic diseases by summing YLD and YLL values [19,20]. The detailed methodology for calculating age-standardized rates and DALYs can be found in GBD publications [21].

The Eurostat database provides statistics for European Union member states using various data sources, including the European Union Statistics on Income and Living Conditions (EU-SILC), which has provided annually updated and comparable cross-country data on income, poverty, social exclusion, and living conditions since 2003. Relevant indicators related to healthcare and socioeconomic status were selected for analysis. The following indicators were extracted from the Eurostat database for 24 EU member states, covering the period 2005–2021 based on data availability: healthcare indicators included current healthcare expenditure in percentage of gross domestic product (GDP), number of hospital beds, and practicing physicians; socioeconomic indicators included income inequality, unemployment rate, and proportion of population with tertiary education. The definitions of each indicator are available in Supplementary File.

2.2. Statistical Analysis

The data on Eurostat indicators were available for limited period, and the trend analysis of country-specific age-standardized rates was conducted using the Joinpoint regression analysis during 2005–2021. The average annual percent change (AAPC) was calculated with log-transformation and automatic selection of the best fitting model. All Joinpoint analyses were performed using Joinpoint Regression Program (Version 5.4.0—16 April 2025, Statistical Methodology and Applications Branch, Surveillance Research Program, National Cancer Institute) [22].

We used the Gini index to assess the CRC-associated health inequality across 24 member states over time from 1990 to 2021. The Gini index is a measure of inequality, calculated based on the Lorenz curve. The Lorenz curve shows the cumulative proportion of the population ranked by health, as well as a cumulative proportion of health variable within the population. A hypothetical diagonal line at 45° is drawn to represent a perfect distribution of health within the population. The Gini coefficient measures deviation from an equal distribution and is calculated based on the area between the 45° line and the Lorenz curve. This coefficient ranges from 0 (perfect equality) to 1 (total inequality), with a higher value indicating greater inequality [23,24]. In this study, the health measures used to calculate the Gini index were the annual age-standardized death, DALY, YLD, and YLL rates of CRC for each country.

Generalized linear mixed model (GLMM) with a gamma distribution and log link function, including a random intercept for country, was used to account for repeated measures across countries. Model fit was assessed using likelihood ratio (LR) tests, the Akaike Information Criterion (AIC), and Bayesian Information Criterion (BIC). Results of GLMM models are reported as β coefficients with corresponding 95% confidence intervals.

Statistical analyses were conducted using STATA IC version 13.0 (Stata Corp., College Station, TX, USA). The Gini index was calculated using the ineqdeco package. A p-value of less than 0.05 was considered statistically significant.

3. Results

The overall age-standardized mortality rate across all EU-27 countries has changed from 22.91 (95% UI: 21.44–23.83) to 17.12 per 100,000 (95% UI: 15.52–18.23) from 1990 to 2021. The age-standardized DALY rate has decreased from 503.53 (95% uncertainty interval (UI): 480.39–520.57) in 1990 to 370.57 per 100,000 (95% UI: 344.49–391.88) in 2021. The trend of age-standardized YLL rate showed a similar pattern to the DALY trend; the rate decreased from 484.93 (95% UI: 462.99–500.61) to 348.94 per 100,000 (95% UI: 324.09–368.44). In contrast, age-standardized YLD showed a slight increase from 18.59 (95% UI: 13.93–23.84) to 21.63 per 100,000 (95% UI: 16.06–28.18) between 1990 and 2021.

Figure 1 presents the country-specific average AAPC restricted to the period 2005–2021. The results of the Joinpoint regression indicated that most EU member states experienced significant declines in DALY, mortality rates, and YLL and YLD rates between the study period (2005–2021). Bulgaria and Romania were the only two countries where all four health outcomes increased over the period. The highest improvements were observed in age-standardized YLL rates with average AAPCs in the 1.12% to −3.12% range (Figure 1).

According to the Gini index, health inequality was observed across 24 EU member states (Figure 2). Between 1990 and 2021, the Gini index for age-standardized YLDs in EU member states declined from 0.19 to 0.12. In contrast, inequality in YLL increased from 0.11 to 0.16 over the same period. Inequality for the age-standardized DALY rate showed a similar upward trend, rising from 0.11 in 1990 to 0.15 in 2021. The Gini index for age-standardized death rate increased slightly from 0.12 to 0.14 during the investigated period (Figure 2).

As reported in Table 1, greater number of practicing physicians was related to lower death ($\beta = -0.036$, $p = 0.022$), DALY ($\beta = -0.035$, $p = 0.019$), YLD ($\beta = -0.060$, $p < 0.001$) and YLL ($\beta = -0.034$, $p = 0.022$) rates. In contrast, health expenditure in share of GDP and hospital bed availability showed no significant relationship in any model (Table 1).

Among socioeconomic indicators, a higher education attainment was significantly linked to lower disease burden across all four health outcomes (age-standardized death rate: $\beta = -0.009$, $p < 0.001$, DALY rates ($\beta = -0.009$, $p < 0.001$), YLD rates ($\beta = -0.008$, $p < 0.001$) and YLL rates ($\beta = -0.009$, $p < 0.001$). Income inequality was positively related to higher death ($\beta = 0.015$, $p = 0.035$), DALY ($\beta = 0.019$, $p = 0.005$), and YLL ($\beta = 0.019$, $p = 0.004$) rates, but not to YLD. The unemployment rate was not a significant factor in any of the models (Table 1).

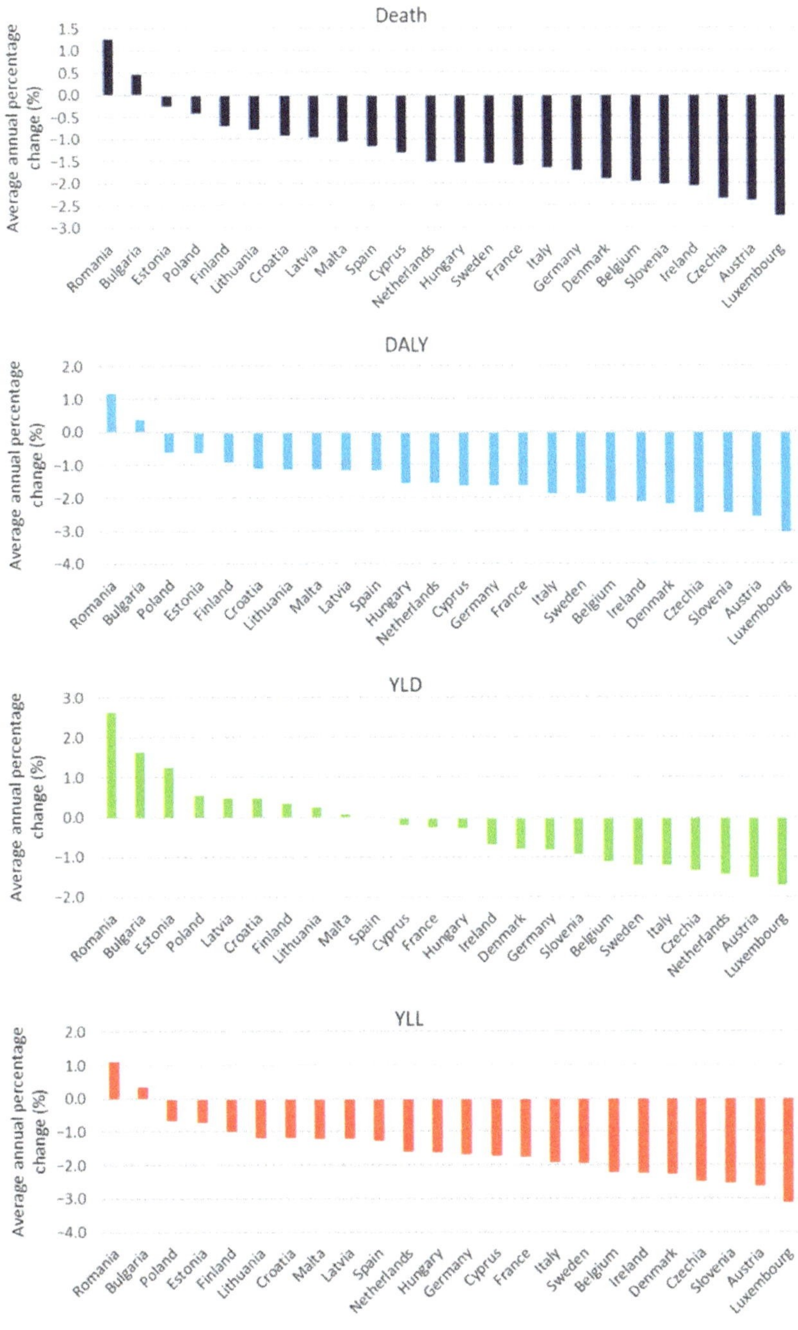

Figure 1. Average annual percent change (AAPC) of age-standardized death, DALY, YLD, and YLL rates in 24 EU member states for the period of 2005–2021.

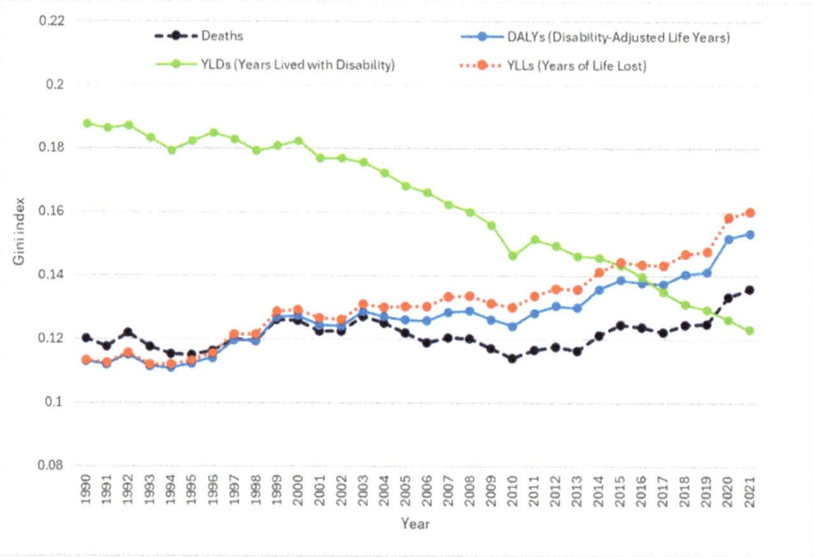

Figure 2. Trends in Gini index of age-standardized death, DALY, YLD, and YLL rates in 24 European Union member states, 1990–2021.

Table 1. Mixed-effect GLM model for age-standardized death, DALY, YLD, and YLL rates in 24 EU member states.

	Death		DALY		YLD		YLL	
	β (95% CI)	*p*-Value	β (95% CI)	*p*-Value	β (95% CI)	*p*-Value	β (95% CI)	*p*-Value
Healthcare indicators								
Current healthcare expenditure in share of GDP (%)	−0.004 (−0.012, 0.004)	0.283	−0.005 (−0.013, 0.003)	0.195	−0.007 (−0.016, 0.002)	0.132	−0.005 (−0.012, 0.003)	0.224
Practicing physicians (per 1000)	−0.036 (−0.066, −0.005)	**0.022**	−0.035 (−0.064, −0.006)	**0.019**	−0.060 (−0.094, −0.026)	**<0.001**	−0.034 (−0.063, −0.005)	**0.022**
Hospital bed (per 1000)	−0.009 (−0.024, 0.005)	0.193	−0.002 (−0.016, 0.011)	0.762	−0.011 (−0.027, 0.005)	0.186	−0.001 (−0.015, 0.012)	0.847
Socioeconomic indicators								
Proportion of population with tertiary education (%)	−0.009 (−0.012, −0.006)	**<0.001**	−0.009 (−0.012, −0.006)	**<0.001**	−0.008 (−0.012, −0.005)	**<0.001**	−0.009 (−0.012, −0.006)	**<0.001**
Income inequality	0.015 (0.001, 0.029)	**0.035**	0.019 (0.006, 0.032)	**0.005**	0.014 (−0.001, 0.030)	0.068	0.019 (0.006, 0.033)	**0.004**
Unemployment rate (%)	−0.000 (−0.002, 0.002)	0.920	−0.000 (−0.002, 0.002)	0.723	0.000 (−0.002, 0.003)	0.775	−0.000 (−0.002, 0.002)	0.638
Intercept	12.430 (5.785, 19.076)	**<0.001**	17.175 (10.840, 23.509)	**<0.001**	−10.866 (−18.317, −3.415)	**0.004**	18.550 (12.190, 24.911)	**<0.001**
Country intercept	0.038 (0.022, 0.068)	**<0.001**	0.043 (0.024, 0.077)	**<0.001**	0.072 (0.040, 0.129)	**<0.001**	0.042 (0.023, 0.074)	**<0.001**

All models adjusted for year (2005–2021) and included a country-level random intercept. DALY: disability-adjusted life years, YLD: years lived with disability, YLL: years of life lost, CI: confidence interval, GDP: gross domestic product. Significant results are shown in bold.

4. Discussion

Our study showed that colorectal cancer burden has decreased across EU member states in recent decades. This improvement is driven mainly by the widespread implementation of organized screening programs, which enable cancers to be detected and treated at an earlier stage of the disease [7]. A recent population-based study of nine European countries reported that screen-detected cancer cases were diagnosed at a more favorable stage than those detected otherwise [25]. Another study found that a 1% rise in screening uptake corresponds to a 2.9% decrease in late-stage incidence rate, which highlights the crucial role of screening in preventing advanced-stage diagnoses [26]. At the same time, advances in treatment, including improved surgical techniques and more effective radiotherapy and chemotherapy regimens, targeted therapies, immunotherapy, and better palliative care, have extended survival and quality of life for CRC patients [27–29].

Trend analysis revealed that the improving trend was observed in almost all investigated member states, whereas Bulgaria and Romania were outliers with worsening trends across all burden metrics. In these countries, the unfavorable colorectal cancer outcomes largely stem from the lack of a national, population-based screening program [30], high prevalence of cancer-related risk factors [30,31], and limited access to services due to a shortage of specialist health professionals [30,31].

Country-level differences in CRC burden may reflect variation in healthcare system models, which influence access, equity, and efficiency in cancer prevention and treatment. Additionally, disparities in national policies on CRC screening, health spending priorities, and the strength of primary care infrastructure likely contribute to the observed cross-country heterogeneity [15].

The observed rise in age-standardized YLD reflects the growing population of CRC survivors living with a wide range of long-term physical [32–36] and psychological [35,37] morbidities, which have been described as the survivorship burden in cancer survivors. This trend highlights the need to develop comprehensive survivorship care models focusing on physical rehabilitation, mental health support, and long-term follow-up to improve functional outcomes and quality of life for survivors [35,37].

The inequality analysis revealed that, while disparities in the burden of CRC have decreased in terms of YLD, widening inequalities were observed for mortality, YLL, and DALY over the past decades. These findings indicate that differences in the overall disease burden have not yet been eliminated. The reduction in YLD-related inequality may reflect improvements in equitable access to survivorship care and rehabilitation services across Europe. In contrast, the increasing inequalities in mortality, YLL, and DALYs likely reflect uneven distribution of advancements in early detection, timely diagnosis, and access to effective treatments. Persistent disparities by socioeconomic status remain a major public health challenge in addressing the CRC burden [11].

The observed inverse relationship between physician density and CRC burden is consistent with previous findings that greater availability of physicians (both GPs and specialists) significantly improves CRC outcomes through earlier diagnosis [26,38]. For example, a recent spatial analysis demonstrated that regions with higher primary care physician density experience significantly lower rates of late-stage CRC incidence and mortality [26]. These findings indicate that policy efforts should focus on regions with lower ratios of physicians to population to ensure more equitable access to care.

The strong, consistent link between higher educational attainment and CRC burden suggests that education may serve as a proxy for health literacy, which in turn may influence participation in screening programs [39]. Moreover, low health literacy is not only associated with reduced screening uptake but also linked to a significantly higher incidence of postoperative complications, longer hospital stays, greater hospital charges [40], and poorer quality of life [41] among CRC cancer survivors. Our findings confirm that inadequate education (health literacy) level contributes to the disproportionate burden of CRC faced by socioeconomically disadvantaged populations.

We found a positive link between income inequality and CRC mortality, DALY, and YLL, which reflects that regions with larger income disparities suffer from poorer cancer survival. This finding is consistent with existing literature, including a meta-analysis, which demonstrated that people living in regions with high income inequality exhibit an elevated risk for premature mortality, independent of their socioeconomic status [42]. Moreover, a nationwide Swedish register-based study of colon and rectal cancer patients documented pronounced income-related disparities in life-years lost [43].

The lack of a significant relationship between overall health expenditure as a share of GDP or hospital bed availability and CRC burden highlights the pivotal role of socioeconomic determinants. Recent research revealed that even in regions with high hospital bed density, deprivation-related disparities in CRC detection persist, suggesting that hospital bed availability cannot fully eliminate health disparities due to socioeconomic deprivation [44].

Thus, the major policy implication of this study is that policymakers should invest in expanding access to CRC screening programs and improving early detection in countries with weaker health system performance, particularly those with low healthcare spending and high out-of-pocket costs. Systematic monitoring of CRC screening campaigns is also essential to understand their effectiveness and to inform future optimization efforts [45–47]. Additionally, targeted interventions are needed to address CRC disparities among populations with lower socioeconomic status by integrating social protection mechanisms and subsidizing preventive care. Future research is needed to incorporate data on population-based CRC screening programs in EU countries alongside healthcare and socioeconomic indicators. This could provide valuable insights into the effectiveness of national screening campaigns in different settings.

Strengths and Limitations

One key strength of this study is the use of population-based data to deliver comprehensive estimates of colorectal cancer burden patterns and its relation to healthcare and SES indicators across 24 EU member states. However, several limitations should be acknowledged. First, this ecological study relied on aggregated country-level data, which may hide important subnational heterogeneity in data collection methods, population structure, and lifestyle factors. The health burden may be underestimated because of the hidden morbidity of CRC, particularly in countries with less effective screening programs. Additionally, this study does not account for differences in national healthcare system models (e.g., Bismarckian vs. Beveridge), which may influence the access, delivery, and outcomes of CRC care. Furthermore, the regression analysis was performed for 2005–2021 (due to data availability); extending this period could increase the robustness of the findings. Additional Eurostat indicators with incomplete coverage across countries and years were excluded from the analysis. Despite these limitations, the data sources (Eurostat and GBD) and methodology used in this study were adequate to identify inequalities and trends in CRC burden.

5. Conclusions

Our findings suggest that while years lived with disability have become more equitable, reflecting better survivorship care, inequalities in mortality, YLL, and DALYs persist and are widening. Our findings highlight that, alongside expanding organized screening, strengthening physician supply and reducing socioeconomic inequalities are essential strategies for mitigating the unequal burden of colorectal cancer.

Supplementary Materials: The following supporting information can be downloaded at: https://www.mdpi.com/article/10.3390/cancers17132075/s1, Table S1: Definitions of the socioeconomic and healthcare variables that were used in our study.

Author Contributions: Conceptualization, N.K. and O.V.; Methodology, N.K.; Formal Analysis, N.K.; Data Curation, N.K.; Writing—original draft preparation, N.K.; Writing—review and editing, O.V.; Visualization, N.K.; Supervision, O.V.; Funding acquisition, O.V. All authors have read and agreed to the published version of the manuscript.

Funding: This study was supported in the form of funding by the funder National Research, Development, and Innovation Fund of Hungary (Research Project No. 143383) awarded to Orsolya Varga. The study was also supported by the EKÖP-24-4 University Research Scholarship Program of the Ministry for Culture and Innovation from the source of the National Research, Development and Innovation Fund (EKÖP-24-4-II-DE-88).

Institutional Review Board Statement: Not applicable.

Informed Consent Statement: Not applicable.

Data Availability Statement: Publicly available datasets were analyzed in this study. This data can be found here: http://ghdx.healthdata.org/gbd-results-tool (accessed on 13 May 2025) and https://ec.europa.eu/eurostat/data/database (accessed on 13 May 2025).

Conflicts of Interest: The authors declare no conflicts of interest.

Abbreviations

The following abbreviations are used in this manuscript:

AAPC	average annual percent change
CRC	Colorectal cancer
DALY	Disability-adjusted life years
EU	European Union
GBD	Global Burden of Disease
DALY	Disability-adjusted life years
YLD	Years lived with disability
YLL	Years of life lost

References

1. Morgan, E.; Arnold, M.; Gini, A.; Lorenzoni, V.; Cabasag, C.J.; Laversanne, M.; Vignat, J.; Ferlay, J.; Murphy, N.; Bray, F. Global Burden of Colorectal Cancer in 2020 and 2040: Incidence and Mortality Estimates from GLOBOCAN. *Gut* **2023**, *72*, 338–344. [CrossRef]
2. Sung, H.; Ferlay, J.; Siegel, R.L.; Laversanne, M.; Soerjomataram, I.; Jemal, A.; Bray, F. Global Cancer Statistics 2020: GLOBOCAN Estimates of Incidence and Mortality Worldwide for 36 Cancers in 185 Countries. *CA A Cancer J. Clin.* **2021**, *71*, 209–249. [CrossRef] [PubMed]
3. Cancer Statistics—Specific Cancers. Available online: https://ec.europa.eu/eurostat/statistics-explained/index.php?title=Cancer_statistics_-_specific_cancers (accessed on 21 May 2025).
4. Global Burden of Disease Collaborative Network. *Global Burden of Disease Study 2021 (GBD 2021) Results*; Institute for Health Metrics and Evaluation (IHME): Seattle, WA, USA, 2021.
5. Hofmarcher, T.; Lindgren, P. *The Cost of Cancers of the Digestive System in Europe*; IHE Report: Lund, Sweden, 2020.
6. Carethers, J.M.; Doubeni, C.A. Causes of Socioeconomic Disparities in Colorectal Cancer and Intervention Framework and Strategies. *Gastroenterology* **2020**, *158*, 354–367. [CrossRef] [PubMed]
7. Cardoso, R.; Guo, F.; Heisser, T.; Hackl, M.; Ihle, P.; Schutter, H.D.; Damme, N.V.; Valerianova, Z.; Atanasov, T.; Májek, O.; et al. Colorectal Cancer Incidence, Mortality, and Stage Distribution in European Countries in the Colorectal Cancer Screening Era: An International Population-Based Study. *Lancet Oncol.* **2021**, *22*, 1002–1013. [CrossRef]

8. Ola, I.; Cardoso, R.; Hoffmeister, M.; Brenner, H. Utilization of Colorectal Cancer Screening Tests across European Countries: A Cross-Sectional Analysis of the European Health Interview Survey 2018-2020. *Lancet Reg. Health Eur.* **2024**, *41*, 100920. [CrossRef] [PubMed]
9. Bozhar, H.; McKee, M.; Spadea, T.; Veerus, P.; Heinävaara, S.; Anttila, A.; Senore, C.; Zielonke, N.; de Kok, I.M.C.M.; van Ravesteyn, N.T.; et al. Socio-Economic Inequality of Utilization of Cancer Testing in Europe: A Cross-Sectional Study. *Prev. Med. Rep.* **2022**, *26*, 101733. [CrossRef]
10. Hayes, L.; Adams, J.; McCallum, I.; Forrest, L.; Hidajat, M.; White, M.; Sharp, L. Age-Related and Socioeconomic Inequalities in Timeliness of Referral and Start of Treatment in Colorectal Cancer: A Population-Based Analysis. *J. Epidemiol. Community Health* **2021**, *75*, 1–9. [CrossRef]
11. Aarts, M.J.; Lemmens, V.E.P.P.; Louwman, M.W.J.; Kunst, A.E.; Coebergh, J.W.W. Socioeconomic Status and Changing Inequalities in Colorectal Cancer? A Review of the Associations with Risk, Treatment and Outcome. *Eur. J. Cancer* **2010**, *46*, 2681–2695. [CrossRef]
12. Feller, A.; Schmidlin, K.; Bordoni, A.; Bouchardy, C.; Bulliard, J.; Camey, B.; Konzelmann, I.; Maspoli, M.; Wanner, M.; Zwahlen, M.; et al. Socioeconomic and Demographic Inequalities in Stage at Diagnosis and Survival among Colorectal Cancer Patients: Evidence from a Swiss Population-based Study. *Cancer Med.* **2018**, *7*, 1498–1510. [CrossRef]
13. Jansen, L.; Behrens, G.; Finke, I.; Maier, W.; Gerken, M.; Pritzkuleit, R.; Holleczek, B.; Brenner, H. Area-Based Socioeconomic Inequalities in Colorectal Cancer Survival in Germany: Investigation Based on Population-Based Clinical Cancer Registration. *Front. Oncol.* **2020**, *10*, 857. [CrossRef]
14. Ungvari, Z.; Fekete, M.; Fekete, J.T.; Lehoczki, A.; Buda, A.; Munkácsy, G.; Varga, P.; Ungvari, A.; Győrffy, B. Treatment Delay Significantly Increases Mortality in Colorectal Cancer: A Meta-Analysis. *GeroScience* **2025**. [CrossRef] [PubMed]
15. Hollis, R.H.; Chu, D.I. Healthcare Disparities and Colorectal Cancer. *Surg. Oncol. Clin. N. Am.* **2022**, *31*, 157–169. [CrossRef]
16. Lejeune, C.; Sassi, F.; Ellis, L.; Godward, S.; Mak, V.; Day, M.; Rachet, B. Socio-Economic Disparities in Access to Treatment and Their Impact on Colorectal Cancer Survival. *Int. J. Epidemiol.* **2010**, *39*, 710–717. [CrossRef] [PubMed]
17. Campbell, N.C.; Elliott, A.M.; Sharp, L.; Ritchie, L.D.; Cassidy, J.; Little, J. Rural and Urban Differences in Stage at Diagnosis of Colorectal and Lung Cancers. *Br. J. Cancer* **2001**, *84*, 910–914. [CrossRef] [PubMed]
18. Naghavi, M.; Ong, K.L.; Aali, A.; Ababneh, H.S.; Abate, Y.H.; Abbafati, C.; Abbasgholizadeh, R.; Abbasian, M.; Abbasi-Kangevari, M.; Abbastabar, H.; et al. Global Burden of 288 Causes of Death and Life Expectancy Decomposition in 204 Countries and Territories and 811 Subnational Locations, 1990–2021: A Systematic Analysis for the Global Burden of Disease Study 2021. *Lancet* **2024**, *403*, 2100–2132. [CrossRef]
19. Kim, Y.-E.; Jung, Y.-S.; Ock, M.; Yoon, S.-J. DALY Estimation Approaches: Understanding and Using the Incidence-Based Approach and the Prevalence-Based Approach. *J. Prev. Med. Public Health* **2022**, *55*, 10–18. [CrossRef]
20. Ferrari, A.J.; Santomauro, D.F.; Aali, A.; Abate, Y.H.; Abbafati, C.; Abbastabar, H.; ElHafeez, S.A.; Abdelmasseh, M.; Abd-Elsalam, S.; Abdollahi, A.; et al. Global Incidence, Prevalence, Years Lived with Disability (YLDs), Disability-Adjusted Life-Years (DALYs), and Healthy Life Expectancy (HALE) for 371 Diseases and Injuries in 204 Countries and Territories and 811 Subnational Locations, 1990–2021: A Systematic Analysis for the Global Burden of Disease Study 2021. *Lancet* **2024**, *403*, 2133–2161. [CrossRef]
21. World Health Organization. *Department of Data and Analytics Division of Data, Analytics and Delivery for Impact WHO Methods and Data Sources for Global Burden of Disease Estimates 2000–2019*; WHO: Geneva, Switzerland, 2020.
22. National Cancer Institute. Surveillance Research Program, Statistical Methodology and Applications Branch. In *Joinpoint Regression Program, Version 5.4.0.0—April 2025*; National Cancer Institute: Bethesda, MD, USA, 2025.
23. Bleichrodt, H.; van Doorslaer, E. A Welfare Economics Foundation for Health Inequality Measurement. *J. Health Econ.* **2006**, *25*, 945–957. [CrossRef]
24. Pan American Health Organization. Measuring Health Inequalities: Gini Coefficient and Concentration Index. *Epidemiol. Bull.* **2001**, *22*, 3–4.
25. Cardoso, R.; Guo, F.; Heisser, T.; De Schutter, H.; Van Damme, N.; Nilbert, M.C.; Tybjerg, A.J.; Bouvier, A.-M.; Bouvier, V.; Launoy, G.; et al. Proportion and Stage Distribution of Screen-Detected and Non-Screen-Detected Colorectal Cancer in Nine European Countries: An International, Population-Based Study. *Lancet Gastroenterol. Hepatol.* **2022**, *7*, 711–723. [CrossRef]
26. Draganic, D.; Wangen, K.R. Spatial Analysis of Colorectal Cancer Outcomes: Investigating the Impact of Place-Specific Factors Using Causal Inference Methods for Spatial Data. *J. Public Health* **2025**, fdaf044. [CrossRef]
27. Sharma, R.; Abbasi-Kangevari, M.; Abd-Rabu, R.; Abidi, H.; Abu-Gharbieh, E.; Acuna, J.M.; Adhikari, S.; Advani, S.M.; Afzal, M.S.; Meybodi, M.A.; et al. Global, Regional, and National Burden of Colorectal Cancer and Its Risk Factors, 1990–2019: A Systematic Analysis for the Global Burden of Disease Study 2019. *Lancet Gastroenterol. Hepatol.* **2022**, *7*, 627–647. [CrossRef] [PubMed]
28. Van Cutsem, E.; Cervantes, A.; Adam, R.; Sobrero, A.; Van Krieken, J.H.; Aderka, D.; Aranda Aguilar, E.; Bardelli, A.; Benson, A.; Bodoky, G.; et al. ESMO Consensus Guidelines for the Management of Patients with Metastatic Colorectal Cancer. *Ann. Oncol.* **2016**, *27*, 1386–1422. [CrossRef] [PubMed]

29. Dekker, E.; Tanis, P.J.; Vleugels, J.L.A.; Kasi, P.M.; Wallace, M.B. Colorectal Cancer. *Lancet* **2019**, *394*, 1467–1480. [CrossRef] [PubMed]
30. OECD. *EU Country Cancer Profile: Bulgaria 2023, EU Country Cancer Profiles*; OECD Publishing: Paris, France, 2023.
31. OECD. *EU Country Cancer Profile: Romania 2023, EU Country Cancer Profiles*; OECD Publishing: Paris, France, 2023.
32. O'Gorman, C.; Stack, J.; O'Ceilleachair, A.; Denieffe, S.; Gooney, M.; McKnight, M.; Sharp, L. Colorectal Cancer Survivors: An Investigation of Symptom Burden and Influencing Factors. *BMC Cancer* **2018**, *18*, 1022. [CrossRef]
33. Nikoletti, S.; Young, J.; Levitt, M.; King, M.; Chidlow, C.; Hollingsworth, S. Bowel Problems, Self-Care Practices, and Information Needs of Colorectal Cancer Survivors at 6 to 24 Months after Sphincter-Saving Surgery. *Cancer Nurs.* **2008**, *31*, 389–398. [CrossRef]
34. Yabroff, K.R.; Lawrence, W.F.; Clauser, S.; Davis, W.W.; Brown, M.L. Burden of Illness in Cancer Survivors: Findings From a Population-Based National Sample. *JNCI J. Natl. Cancer Inst.* **2004**, *96*, 1322–1330. [CrossRef]
35. Santin, O.; Murray, L.; Prue, G.; Gavin, A.; Gormley, G.; Donnelly, M. Self-Reported Psychosocial Needs and Health-Related Quality of Life of Colorectal Cancer Survivors. *Eur. J. Oncol. Nurs.* **2015**, *19*, 336–342. [CrossRef]
36. Walling, A.M.; Weeks, J.C.; Kahn, K.L.; Tisnado, D.; Keating, N.L.; Dy, S.M.; Arora, N.K.; Mack, J.W.; Pantoja, P.M.; Malin, J.L. Symptom Prevalence in Lung and Colorectal Cancer Patients. *J Pain Symptom Manag.* **2015**, *49*, 192–202. [CrossRef]
37. Wu, H.-S.; Harden, J.K. Symptom Burden and Quality of Life in Survivorship: A Review of the Literature. *Cancer Nurs.* **2015**, *38*, E29. [CrossRef]
38. Ananthakrishnan, A.N.; Hoffmann, R.G.; Saeian, K. Higher Physician Density Is Associated with Lower Incidence of Late-Stage Colorectal Cancer. *J. Gen. Intern. Med.* **2010**, *25*, 1164–1171. [CrossRef] [PubMed]
39. van der Heide, I.; Uiters, E.; Jantine Schuit, A.; Rademakers, J.; Fransen, M. Health Literacy and Informed Decision Making Regarding Colorectal Cancer Screening: A Systematic Review. *Eur. J. Public Health* **2015**, *25*, 575–582. [CrossRef]
40. Qin, P.-P.; Jin, J.-Y.; Min, S.; Wang, W.-J.; Shen, Y.-W. Association Between Health Literacy and Enhanced Recovery After Surgery Protocol Adherence and Postoperative Outcomes Among Patients Undergoing Colorectal Cancer Surgery: A Prospective Cohort Study. *Anesth. Analg.* **2022**, *134*, 330. [CrossRef]
41. Husson, O.; Mols, F.; Fransen, M.P.; van de Poll-Franse, L.V.; Ezendam, N.P.M. Low Subjective Health Literacy Is Associated with Adverse Health Behaviors and Worse Health-Related Quality of Life among Colorectal Cancer Survivors: Results from the Profiles Registry. *Psycho-Oncol.* **2015**, *24*, 478–486. [CrossRef] [PubMed]
42. Kondo, N.; Sembajwe, G.; Kawachi, I.; Van Dam, R.M.; Subramanian, S.V.; Yamagata, Z. Income Inequality, Mortality, and Self Rated Health: Meta-Analysis of Multilevel Studies. *BMJ* **2009**, *339*, b4471. [CrossRef] [PubMed]
43. Syriopoulou, E.; Osterman, E.; Miething, A.; Nordenvall, C.; Andersson, T.M.-L. Income Disparities in Loss in Life Expectancy after Colon and Rectal Cancers: A Swedish Register-Based Study. *J. Epidemiol. Community Health* **2024**, *78*, 402–408. [CrossRef]
44. Shibata, T.; Shinjo, D.; Fushimi, K. The Impact of Deprivation on Colorectal Cancer-stage Distribution in a Setting with High Hospital Bed Density: A Japanese Multilevel Study. *Cancer Med.* **2024**, *13*, e70042. [CrossRef]
45. Lee, H.J.; Lee, K.; Kim, B.C.; Jun, J.K.; Choi, K.S.; Suh, M. Effectiveness of the Korean National Cancer Screening Program in Reducing Colorectal Cancer Mortality. *Cancers* **2024**, *16*, 4278. [CrossRef]
46. Zorzi, M.; Hassan, C.; Selby, K.; Rugge, M. Do Not Leave FIT Positives Alone! *Off. J. Am. Coll. Gastroenterol. ACG* **2018**, *113*, 913. [CrossRef]
47. Tinmouth, J.; Lansdorp-Vogelaar, I.; Allison, J.E. Faecal Immunochemical Tests versus Guaiac Faecal Occult Blood Tests: What Clinicians and Colorectal Cancer Screening Programme Organisers Need to Know. *Gut* **2015**, *64*, 1327–1337. [CrossRef]

cancers

MDPI

Article

Barriers to Post-Mastectomy Breast Reconstruction: A Comprehensive Retrospective Study

Kella L. Vangsness [1,*], Ronald M. Cornely [2], Andre-Philippe Sam [3], Naikhoba C. O. Munabi [4], Michael Chu [5], Mouchammed Agko [6], Jeff Chang [6] and Antoine L. Carre [6]

1 Community Memorial Hospital System, Ventura, CA 93036, USA
2 Emory University, Atlanta, GA 30322, USA
3 Riverside School of Medicine, University of California, Riverside, CA 92507, USA
4 Department of Plastic and Reconstructive Surgery, Columbia University, New York, NY 10032, USA
5 Department of Plastic & Reconstructive Surgery, Kaiser Permanente, Los Angeles, CA 90034, USA
6 Department of Plastic & Reconstructive Surgery, City of Hope, Duarte, CA 90034, USA
* Correspondence: kvangsness@cmhshealth.org

Simple Summary: Many demographics affect post-mastectomy reconstruction care, including an older age, lower income, care at a public hospital, rural care, and non-White race. This data is significant because it identifies vulnerable populations and factors impeding breast reconstruction despite multiple federal regulations in place.

Abstract: Background and Objectives: Breast reconstruction following mastectomy improves quality of life and psychosocial outcomes, yet it is not consistently performed despite multiple federal mandates. Current data shows decreased reconstruction in minority races, those with a low socioeconomic status, and those holding public health insurance. Many barriers remain misunderstood or unstudied. This study examines barriers to post-mastectomy breast reconstruction to promote a supportive clinical climate by addressing multifactorial obstacles to equitable access to care. Materials and Methods: The California Cancer Registry Data Surveillance, Epidemiology, and End Results (SEER) database and California Health and Human Services Agency Cancer Surgeries Database (2013–2021 and 2000–2021, respectively) were used in this retrospective observational study on mastectomy with immediate breast reconstruction (IBR), delayed breast reconstruction (DBR), or mastectomy only (MO) rates. Data were collected on age, sex, race, insurance type, hospital type, socioeconomic status, and residence. Pearson's chi-square analysis was performed. Results: We found that 168,494 mastectomy and reconstruction surgeries were performed (82.36% MO, 7% IBR, 10.6% DBR). The 40–49 age group received significantly less MO (38.1%) compared to the 70–74 age group (94.8%, (p = <0.001). Significantly more reconstruction was carried out in patients with private, HMO, or PPO insurance (IBR 75.86%, DBR 75.32%, p = <0.001). Almost all breast surgeries were in urban areas as opposed to rural/isolated rural areas (96.02% vs. 1.55%, p = <0.001). There was no significant difference between races. Of all surgeries, 7.46% were completed in a cancer center with significantly higher rates of IBR. LA County, San Luis Obispo/Ventura County, and Northern CA had significantly more MO than other regions (p = <0.001). Conclusions: Reconstruction rates after mastectomy are low, with only 17.64% of patients undergoing reconstruction. Nationally, 70.5% of patients received MO, with 29.6% undergoing reconstruction. Significant factors positively contributing to reconstruction were private insurance, high SES, cancer center care, and urban residency. Identified barriers include public health insurance enrollment, rural or non-urban residence, older age, low SES, and non-white race/ethnicity, indicating potential monetary influences on care.

Keywords: breast reconstruction; barriers; mastectomy; plastic surgery; breast cancer

1. Introduction

Breast reconstruction for post-mastectomy cancer patients is not consistently performed as part of routine care despite a 13% average lifetime risk of breast cancer (one in eight women [1]), and proven psychosocial, physical, and quality-of-life benefits [2–5]. Current surgical breast cancer options include removal of the whole breast or a portion of it, with improved quality of life and major psychological benefits if reconstructive efforts are undertaken [6]. Reconstructive options include immediate breast reconstruction (IBR) with autologous tissue replacement or implant-based interventions, or delayed breast reconstruction (DBR), which takes place further along in the treatment course. IBR is associated with fewer operations and potential improved psychosocial benefits [3], but carries higher complication rates compared to DBR. Radiation therapy [3] and tumor characteristics [7] are major determinants in IBR, both of which significantly reduce reconstructive rates.

Between 1998 and 2015, only 5.2% of patients who underwent a mastectomy would go on to receive IBR [8]. In attempts to improve outcomes, the Women's Health and Cancer Rights Act of 1997 [9] was instituted to require coverage for breast reconstruction following mastectomy. It stipulated that coverage was to include all stages of reconstruction to match breasts in shape, size, and form, as well as prostheses and procedural complications. The Patient Protection and Affordable Care Act of 2010 [10] required that from then on all women undergoing mastectomy would be referred to a plastic surgeon [10]. This continues to be supported by the American College of Surgeons and National Accreditation Program for Breast Cancer. Specific religious sponsored health plans and Medicaid do not cover costs; however, Medicare may cover reconstructive procedures if deemed medically necessary by the surgeon. Rates have since improved, and as of 2013, the rate of all reconstruction types was 17% nationally [11], with states varying between 17% and 35% [3,12–14]. Over this same time period, IBR rates grew as the desired reconstruction option from 6.3% in 1996 to 16.8% in 2015 [8].

Reports vary [15], but they indicate that DBR may impact body image and reduce overall quality of life [3,16] when compared to immediate reconstruction [8]. Delayed or absent reconstruction may increase physical health risks such as chronic pain and long-term musculoskeletal strain from uneven weight distribution following unilateral mastectomy [2]. These physical and psychological challenges are further exacerbated by socioeconomic and healthcare disparities, which disproportionately impact underserved populations [17,18].

Negatively contributing factors in the current literature are identified as a minority race and ethnicity [6,19,20], geography, public health insurance type [19,21], income <USD 38,000 a year [19], hospital type [22], older age, increased number of comorbidities [23], treatment type [7,24], and patient lack of awareness of options [7] or preference to forgo or delay reconstruction [25].

Statistically significant findings support racial disparities in breast reconstruction [6,26,27]. White, Non-Hispanic White, and Caucasian patients have been found to be statistically significantly more likely to receive mastectomies [14,28] when compared to African American [29], Asian [28,29], Latina [6,19,20], American Indian, and Alaska Native patients [14]. African American women are also less likely to receive breast reconstruction than Caucasian and Asian women [14,24], while Alaska Natives are the least likely to receive breast reconstruction out of all racial groups, with higher rates of treatment delays [14].

Geographic barriers have also been observed when comparing the eastern US region to the western and southern regions, the relative distances to surgery centers, the plastic surgeon density, and the presence of a non-academic or cancer center [6,26,27].

Additionally, patient preferences for a reconstructive approach may influence reconstruction rates. Bailey et al. found that amongst 134 patients who underwent MO procedures, 38 (28%) declined a plastic surgeon referral, 37 (28%) were not IBR candidates, and 29 (22%) underwent delayed reconstruction [25]. An additional 21 (16%) were seen by a plastic surgeon but declined reconstruction, 3 (2%) were referred but did not attend their appointment, and 6 (4%) had unknown reasons for not undergoing reconstruction [25]. The type of breast cancer treatment also contributes to reconstruction decisions [30]. Notably, adjuvant radiation therapy has been identified as a significant predictor of breast reconstruction among Caucasian women, but not among African American women [18,31].

Despite the available literature outlining barriers to post-mastectomy breast reconstruction, much of the available data is limited, with most focused on racial disparities. Given the paucity of information regarding the impacts of social determinants of health on breast reconstruction, the present literature could benefit from a more comprehensive analysis. This study aims to provide an updated assessment of current barriers to accessing post-mastectomy breast reconstruction.

2. Materials and Methods

2.1. Data Sources

This retrospective descriptive study utilizes the California Cancer Registry Data Surveillance, Epidemiology, and End Results (SEER) database in conjunction with the California Health and Human Services Agency Cancer Surgeries Database (CHHS). The CHHS database was used to collect the number of cancer surgeries performed in California hospitals between 2013 and 2021. Categories included year, county of hospital location, hospital name, type of cancer surgery, and number of cancer surgeries performed in Californian acute care hospitals (ICD9 and ICD-10 codes). Hospitals were also identified and characterized as academic vs. community, private or public, or cancer centers using publicly available data. The SEER 22 "Incidence-SEER Research Data, 17 Registries, Nov 2023 Sub (2000–2021)" registry was used for its national, comprehensive, and cancer-specific population-based data. These databases were selected for their comprehensive population-level data and use in prior high-impact analyses of breast reconstruction barriers [3,20,21].

All data is de-identified within both databases; therefore, no informed consent was required.

2.2. Inclusion Criteria

Inclusion criteria were female patients with a diagnosis of breast cancer who underwent specific procedures during the years 2000–2021. Patient inclusion criteria were eligible patients undergoing breast implant insertion or replacement post-mastectomy (CPT 19340, 19342); the use of tissue expanders with or without implant replacement (CPT 19357, 11971, 11970); revision of the peri-implant capsule, including capsulotomy, capsulectomy, and complete capsulectomy (CPT 19370, 19371); or AlloDerm [LifeCell Corporation, Branchburg, USA] implantation in breast reconstruction (CPT 15777). Patients who received a lumpectomy or breast-conserving surgery were excluded from this study. Collected data included the patient ID, race/ethnicity, age, sex, comorbidities, income/median household income/SES, marital status at diagnosis, rural–urban continuum/county attributes, site-specific surgery, surgery of primary site, year of diagnosis, year of follow-up, first malignancy/sequence number, admission type, insurance type, cancer versus non-cancer center,

American Joint Committee on Cancer staging system, time from diagnosis to treatment, and reporting source.

Site-specific surgery coding for the breast included IDC-0: 174.0–174.6, 174.8–174.9, 175.9. Surgery codes for the primary surgery site were categorized by the type of mastectomy or breast reconstruction. Mastectomy type: 20–24—Breast-conserving or -preserving surgery, 20—Partial mastectomy, less than total mastectomy, 40—Total (simple) mastectomy, 41—Simple bilateral mastectomy, 76—Bilateral mastectomy for single tumor, 43—Simple mastectomy with tissue expanders, 50—Modified radical mastectomy, 60—Radical mastectomy, 71—Extended radical mastectomy, 80—Mastectomy, 90—Breast surgery + pathological specimen, 41, 51, 61, 71—Without removal of uninvolved contralateral breast, 42, 52, 62, 72—With removal of uninvolved contralateral breast. Breast reconstruction types: 30—Subcutaneous mastectomy (nipple-sparing mastectomy), 43, 47, 53, 57, 64, 68—Reconstruction, 44, 48, 54, 58, 65, 69—Tissue, 45, 49, 55, 59, 66, 73—Implant, 46, 56, 63, 67, 74, 75—Combined tissue and implant. Code 90—Death certificate only, unknown if surgery performed.

2.3. Statistical Analysis

The SEER database was used for a detailed analysis of demographics, initial surgery, and reconstruction type, if any. CHHS focused data allowed us to analyze state trends by hospital type, county, and breast surgery type. California's vast socioeconomic landscape allowed for an in-depth view of disparities specific to geography, institutions, and patients. Together, these sources allowed for a robust examination.

Descriptive statistics we analyzed included frequencies and percentages (i.e., distribution) of breast cancer surgeries by year, county, and hospital. Descriptive statistics of the number of surgeries by hospital characteristics were analyzed by stratifying the mean number of surgeries by the categories of interest. An independent sample t-test was applied to determine whether mean differences were statistically significant.

Surgery codes were categorized into three groups: mastectomy only (MO), immediate breast reconstruction (IBR), or delayed breast reconstruction (DBR). Complications were identified as the removal of an intact implant due to reported infection, malposition, capsular contraction (CPT 19328), or ruptured implant (CPT 19330). Data were analyzed using a chi-square test of independence to understand if there were demographic differences between patients across groups. Pearson's chi-squared analysis was performed. A p-value of <0.05 was deemed to be significant.

For age, a mean difference analysis was performed using a one-way analysis of variance to understand if the average ages of patients were statistically significantly different from one another. Age was additionally analyzed by category. Pearson's chi-square test of independence was employed to search for statistically significant differences amongst categorical variables across the three surgical groups, to evaluate if differences occurred by chance.

Descriptive statistics, chi-squared tests, and t-tests were employed where appropriate, and age comparisons were made using a one-way ANOVA aligning with the standard epidemiological methodology and previous retrospective cohort studies. Descriptive and bivariate analyses were chosen to avoid overinterpreting causality or misrepresenting associations without linked data.

Prior work by Lang et al. demonstrates the SEER database's utility in tracking trends and disparities in care, while published work by Sergesketter et al. validates the added benefit of tracking sociodemographic trends utilizing this database [3,20]. SEER-specific characteristics are essential to allow for the analysis of trends over time, particularly in the context of federal and state mandates on breast reconstruction post-mastectomy.

Utilizing sampling data would significantly limit the ability to make conclusions on national reconstruction trends. Albornoz et al. and Sergesketter et al. also demonstrate the utility of SEER in identifying geographic and sociodemographic disparities, which is essential in the present analysis to allow the exploration of barriers to post-mastectomy care [20,21]. The success of prior studies in producing high-impact findings reinforces SEER's reliability, especially given that it is specifically tailored to cancer epidemiology, which aligns with this study's objectives.

3. Results

3.1. California Health and Human Services Agency Cancer Surgeries Database

California is diverse in almost all socioeconomic variables, which allow for the extrapolation of data for a comprehensive assessment of barriers. A total of 243,887 breast surgeries were performed in California between the years 2013 and 2021 in 322 hospitals. Of these surgeries, 168,494 were mastectomy-only, IBR, or DBR, which had rates of 82.36%, 7%, and 10.6%, respectively. Private hospitals comprised 83% (268) and public hospitals 17% (54) of the 322 hospitals examined. The surgeries at private hospitals accounted for 88% of the breast cancer surgeries performed, higher than the expected 83%. Public hospitals accounted for 12% of breast cancer surgeries, lower than the expected 17%. A statistically significant difference was found in the average number of surgeries performed in private (M = 804, SD = 1053.38) vs. public (M = 526, SD = 681.87) hospitals (t (111.13) = 2.46, $p < 0.05$; equal variances were not assumed).

Academic hospitals totaled 14% (44) and community hospitals 86% (278) of the 322 hospitals. The breast cancer surgeries performed at academic hospitals accounted for 28%, higher than the expected 14%. Public hospitals accounted for 72% of breast cancer surgeries, lower than the expected 86%. There was a statistically significant difference in the average number of surgeries performed in academic (M = 1548, SD = 1369.62) vs. community (M = 632, SD = 874.53) hospitals (t (48.70) = 4.30, $p < 0.001$; equal variances were not assumed).

Cancer centers comprised 2.5% (8) and non-cancer centers 97.5% (314) of the 322 hospitals included in the analysis. Cancer center surgeries accounted for 9.4% of all breast cancer surgeries performed, almost four times higher than the expected 2.5%. A statistically significant difference was found in the average number of surgeries performed in cancer centers (M = 2867, SD = 1427.81) vs. non-cancer centers (M = 704, SD = 934.99) (t (7.15) = 4.26, $p < 0.01$; equal variances were not assumed).

Between 2013 and 2021, 243,887 breast surgeries were performed in the state of California. The highest rate of all breast surgeries over this time period was in the counties of Los Angeles (n = 64,662, 26.51%), San Diego (pop. n = 23,399, 9.59%), and Orange (n = 22,007, 9.02%). The populations of these counties were roughly 33 million, 13 million, and 3 million, respectively.

No significant differences were found between racial groups and rates of breast reconstruction in the state of California. Cancer centers had statistically significantly higher rates of IBR (7.64%) compared to other hospital types. Most of the reported reconstruction surgeries in California were completed in urban areas (96.02%) compared to rural locations (1.55%). Only 0.99% of IBR occurred in rural areas. The highest frequency of IBR was in Orange County. The highest mastectomy-only rates occurred in Los Angeles County, San Luis/Obispo/Ventura County, and Northern California.

Many counties had a lower than 0.10% rate of total breast cancer procedures. These were found in the counties of Amador (pop. 40k, n = 33, 0.01%), Calaveras (pop. 45k, n = 64, 0.03%), Del Norte (pop. 27k, n = 75, 0.03%), Inyo (pop. 19k, n = 82, 0.03%), Lake (pop. 68k, n = 44, 0.02%), Lassen (pop. 31k, n = 3, 0.00%), Madera (156k, n = 167, 0.07%),

Plumas (19.5k, $n = 30$, 0.01%), San Benito (64k, $n = 85$, 0.03%), Tehama (65k, $n = 62$, 0.03%), Trinity (pop. 135.k, $n = 6$, 0.00%), and Yuba (pop. 72.5k, $n = 187$, 0.08%).

3.2. *Surveillance, Epidemiology, and End Results (SEER) Database*

SEER-specific database characteristics are essential to the analysis of barriers. Nationally, 29.6% received post-mastectomy breast reconstruction. Within this group that underwent post-mastectomy breast reconstruction, 26.4% received IBR, 3.2% underwent DBR, and 70.5% had MO. Individuals of non-white race/ethnicity had a decreased likelihood of undergoing breast reconstruction. Those who identified as non-Hispanic White individuals were more likely to receive IBR, at a rate of 27.7% (68.7% MO, 27.7% DBR). Hispanic, Black, Asian or Pacific Islander, and American Indian/Alaska Native patients received MO at rates under 80% (73.3%, 74.3%, 75.5%, and 77.1%, respectively).

Of those who received breast reconstruction, the majority underwent IBR as opposed to DBR: Hispanic: 24.4% IBR vs. 2.3% DBR, Black: 23.1% IBR vs. 2.6% DBR, Asian or Pacific Islander: 22.4% IBR vs. 1.9% DBR, and American Indian/Alaska Native: 20.6% IBR vs. 2.4% DBR (Figure 1).

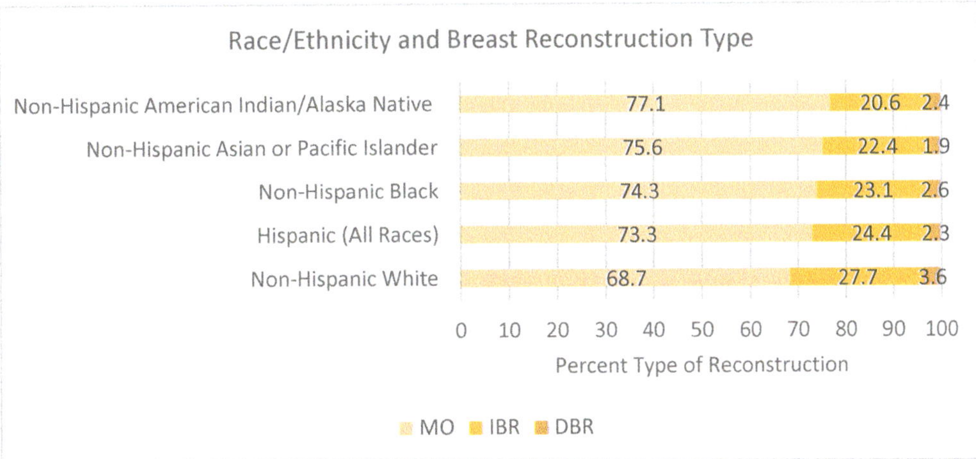

Figure 1. Race/ethnicity and breast reconstruction type.

When examining the state of California within the SEER database specifically, we found that only 17.64% of patients proceeded with any reconstruction after mastectomy, and 82.4% underwent an MO procedure. Of those who underwent reconstruction, 10.6% received DBR and 7% IBR. The reconstruction rate of the 40–49-year-old age group was greater than that of the 70–74-year-old age group and demonstrated a statistically significant difference. However, the 40–49-year-old age group underwent mastectomy only at a rate of 38.1%, compared to 94.8% of those aged 70–74 ($p = <0.001$).

Decreased rates of reconstruction were found in older age (Figure 2). The highest rates of MO were in the 90+ (92.4%), 80–89 (90.9%), 70–79 (84.5%), 60–69 (73.9%), and 50–59 (64.9%) age groups compared to the 20–29 (51.3%), 30–39 (52.4%), and 40–49 (56.1%) age groups. Younger patients were more likely to opt for IBR versus DBR if they did undergo breast reconstruction. Those aged 20–29 underwent IBR at a rate of 45.9% vs. 2.8% DBR, 30–39 IBR 44.9% vs. 2.7%, 40–49 40.8% vs. 3.1%. Rates of IBR decreased as age increased, dropping by almost half between the 70–79 and 80–89 age groups (12.9% and 7.4%, respectively). The group with the lowest rate of any reconstruction type was the 90+-year-old cohort, with 6.4% IBR and 1.2% DBR.

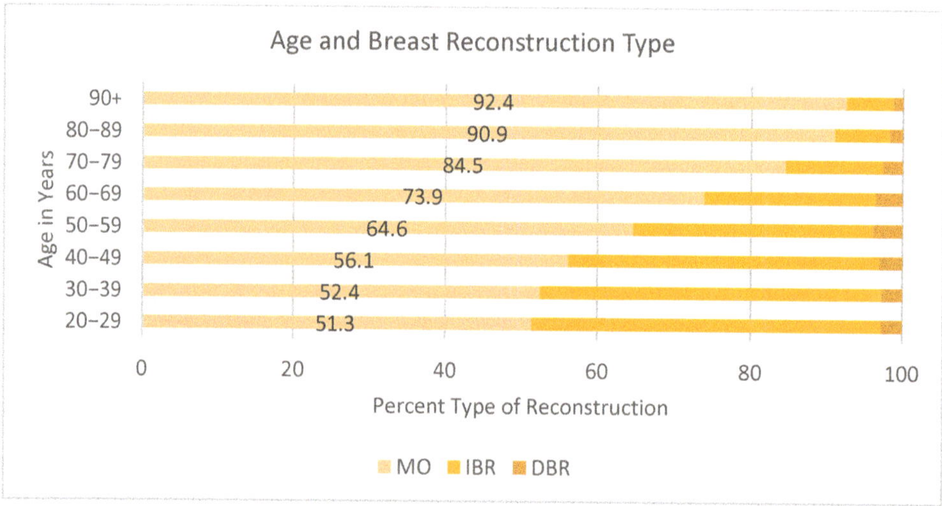

Figure 2. Age and breast reconstruction type.

An income of <USD 70,000 was associated with a decreased likelihood of receiving breast reconstruction (Figure 3). As income increased, so did reconstruction rates for both IBR and DBR. Those earning less than USD 40,000 a year had above 80% MO rates [USD <35k (85.8 % MO, 12.3 % IBR, 1.9 % DBR); USD 35–29k (82.60% MO, 15.6% IBR, 1.8% DBR)]. Between USD 40,000 and USD 64,999, MO rates were between 79.9% and 72.1% and IBR between 18.1% and 24.8%. Once income was greater than USD 70,000, the rate of MO dropped below 70%, and at USD 75,000, IBR was above 31% [USD 70,000–74,999: 67.9% MO, 28.9% IBR, 3.1% DBR; and USD >75k: 65.1% MO, 31.1% IBR, 3.7% DBR].

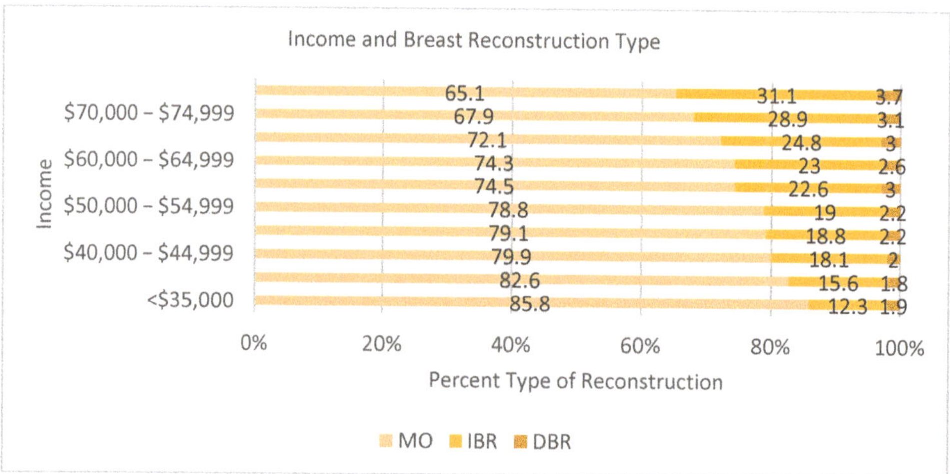

Figure 3. Income and breast reconstruction type.

The insurance type was also examined as a variable. We found that 8% of all MO patients were on public health insurance. In the years examined, 75% of IBR that was performed was covered under private insurance. Significantly more reconstruction was carried out in patients who had private, HMO, or PPO insurance, at rates of IBR at 75.86%

and DBR at 75.32% (p = <0.001), compared to those with government insurance for the elderly or low earning specifically.

Those whose residence was outside of an urban population (<1 million) were less likely to receive breast reconstruction, with an MO reconstruction rate greater than 70% (Figure 4) (81.1% not adjacent to a metropolitan area, 80.4% adjacent to a metropolitan area, 78.8% <250,000 population, 70.8% 250,000 to 1 million population). At a population density of 1 million, the proportion of IBR cases was approximately 30%. However, there were minimal differences between the area of residence and percentage of DBR (3.4% per million people versus 2.1%) when not adjacent to a metropolitan area.

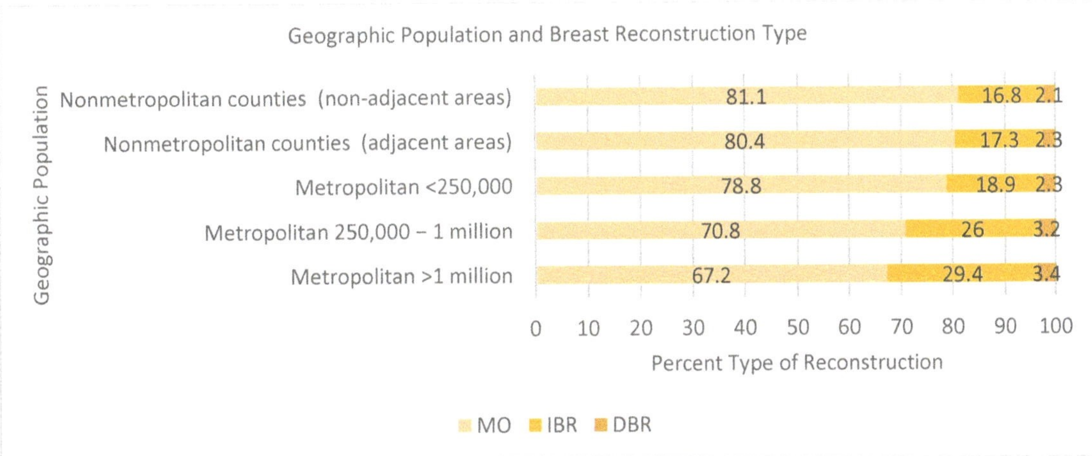

Figure 4. Geographic location population and breast reconstruction type.

4. Discussion

This work has found that the national breast reconstruction rate is currently 29.6%, which is an increase from 11.7% in 1996 and 21.7% in 2008 [3]. Nonetheless, the rate remains relatively stagnant despite multiple federal mandates put into place. This study corroborates previous findings [27] and provides an update on current barriers, which include the insurance type (private vs. public), hospital type, geographic residence, socioeconomic status (SES), and age, as potential areas of future mandate improvements.

Discordant racial data was found when comparing national findings with those specific to California. While national data demonstrates significant racial disparities, no differences were observed in the California-based analysis. Nationally, racial and ethnic minorities experience inequitable access to breast reconstruction due to sociodemographic disparities and implicit biases [30,32]. This study shows that non-Hispanic White women are more likely to undergo mastectomy with immediate breast reconstruction (IBR) than Hispanic, Black, Asian or Pacific Islander, and American Indian/Alaska Native women. Our results are congruent with previous findings by Sergesketter et al. [20], who found racial and ethnically marginalized groups (non-Hispanic Black and Hispanic women) to have a statistically significantly lower likelihoods of undergoing reconstruction post-mastectomy in a national cohort [17]. A systematic review conducted by Doren et al. [32] also found a higher likelihood of undergoing overall reconstruction in those who identified as White compared to Black patients [32].

However, California-specific analyses suggests that the SES, insurance type, and geographic location may play more prominent roles in determining access to breast reconstruction than race. These findings align with the current literature and emphasize the complex interplay of system, physician, and patient-related factors contributing to disparities [33]. The observed disparity in California may be attributable to the state's large and diverse population, varying socioeconomic conditions, and access to healthcare. From this data, we infer that areas with a larger and more diverse population may be better equipped to provide resources that allow for overcoming certain barriers, as demonstrated by race not being included as a barrier in California versus nationally.

Schafer et al. assessed the impact of the Affordable Care Act on racial and ethnic diversity between the years 2005 and 2022 [34]. Prior to federal mandate changes, American Indian or Alaska Native, Asian, and Black or African American individuals underwent less IBR compared to White patients ($p < 0.001$). Hispanic-identifying patients specifically obtained IBR at 28% compared to their White counterparts at 33.4% ($p < 0.001$). In the coming years, the trends did not equalize, and all non-White patients underwent IBR at a lower rate than that of White patients ($p < 0.001$), with Hispanics as the only exception, for whom the IBR rate increased to 53.8% compared to White patients at 47.9% ($p < 0.001$) [35]. Wirth et al. [35] identified persistent racial disparities nationally, particularly for Black women, which was not statistically significant in our California-focused analysis, suggesting that regional healthcare systems may moderate racial disparities. These findings highlight the need for region-specific and demographically informed interventions to improve equitable access to post-mastectomy breast reconstruction.

Patient-specific factors related to SES (e.g., income, occupation, education, and social and cultural capital) were also strongly associated with the variation in reconstruction rates, which supports a more nuanced understanding of access inequity. A higher SES correlated with higher breast reconstruction rates (30% of patients in high-SES groups vs. 10.03% in low-SES groups). Restrepo et al. also identified being White, having a higher income, and having a higher educational background as significant predictors of reconstruction rates, supporting the current study's findings [19]. The insurance type also emerged as a key determinant. Private insurance (HMO/PPO) was associated with significantly higher rates of IBR and DBR compared to public health insurance, suggesting that federal policies—the Cancer Rights Act of 1998 and the Affordable Care Act of 2010—have been ineffective in addressing the reconstructive needs of breast cancer patients.

The geographic location played a major role, with significantly higher reconstruction rates in urban (96.02%) than rural areas (1.55%). Private hospitals had higher reconstructive surgery volumes than public hospitals, with private hospitals performing 88% of reconstructions, versus the expected 83%, and public hospitals performing 12%, versus the expected 17%. The statistically significant differences in reconstruction rates between hospital types support the idea that resource allocation and geographic factors influence the access to reconstructive care. The geographic isolation of rural communities and the relative concentration of hospital resources in urban areas exacerbate these access barriers. The availability of plastic surgeons and specialized facilities (e.g., cancer centers and hospitals) is critical to bridging the equity gap. Wareham et al. found that not only are there fewer breast surgeons than plastic surgeons but also that 14% of breast surgeons did not have a plastic surgeon within a 10-mile distance, though that is a fall from 25% in 2018 [36].

Cancer centers also demonstrated greater surgical volumes (mean = 2867 procedures per institution vs. 704 at non-cancer centers) and significantly higher IBR rates. Despite representing only 2.5% of hospitals in California, cancer centers performed a disproportionately high number of reconstructions and had significantly higher IBR rates (7.64%). Access to specialized care centers may facilitate equitable care for this complex patient population and underscores the critical role of cancer center care.

These findings are consistent with the prior literature, as Albornoz et al. [21] found that reconstruction rates are positively correlated with private hospital systems as well as private insurance carriers. The protective effects of a high SES and private insurance emphasize the role of economic factors in healthcare access, particularly when examined within California.

Older age is also negatively correlated to breast reconstruction of both types, consistent with findings by Cortina et al. [6]. Women are more likely to receive IBR at younger ages, with those aged 70+ receiving the majority of MO. However, likely confounding variables include an increased number of comorbidities, patient education, and personal choice, so limited conclusions can be made.

This study found that 17.64% of patients underwent any type of reconstruction following mastectomy. When comparing delayed versus immediate reconstruction, we found that 10.6% chose delayed and 7% underwent immediate reconstruction. This may provide insight into patient preference, but due to the lack of subjective data, no true causation can be highlighted. However, in a systematic review by Doren et al., the contributors to poor reconstruction rates included issues with individual or community interactions with the healthcare system (54% and 36%, respectively), the sociocultural environment (39%), and individual behavioral factors (31%) [32], allowing some inference to be made, but more objective data and analyses are required. Unmeasured and unexamined barriers remain, such as cultural perceptions, communication gaps, and implicit biases during clinical interactions, which could contribute to the observed disparities in reconstructive access.

Despite a comprehensive analysis, limitations remain. Due to California's unique demographic and healthcare structure, data cannot be generalized to all national regions. Additionally, the absence of qualitative data prevented the exploration of patient-level factors that may influence decision-making, including but not limited to cultural attitudes or provider–patient communication and education. Future studies should integrate patient-reported outcomes, comorbidities, or a mixed-methods approach to overcome our lack of qualitative insights, as noted in the prior literature by Retrouvey et al. and Connors et al. [7,18]. An underrepresentation of rural patients and public hospitals may also skew data, potentially misrepresenting populations and resources. Although the cancer center data is compelling, it may not fully reflect the outcomes at non-specialized facilities where differences in surgeon expertise and available resources can affect results. Furthermore, racial, ethnic, and age disparities may not fully capture nuanced subgroup differences or systemic inequities.

Advocacy and Policy Recommendations

Clinicians, health systems, and governmental entities could consider actionable steps to address these inequities. These may include introducing equity-focused counseling to address health literacy gaps, particularly among historically underserved populations; utilizing interpreters and providing culturally appropriate materials in a range of languages for improved communication and education; ensuring providers' and staffs' continued participation in implicit bias training; standardizing referral protocols based on pre-determined clinical criteria to minimize variability and potential bias in access to plastic surgery consultations; and implementing data-driven interventions by collecting patient-reported information on barriers such as cultural beliefs, mistrust, and financial limitations. These data could inform more tailored support services.

Health systems can play a key role by expanding outreach efforts, redistributing care services, and tracking equity metrics. A recent study by Stankowski et al. found that women with public health insurance and living furthest from a plastic surgeon were less likely to receive reconstruction [37]. Outreach to rural and underserved communities may include establishing mobile health units, satellite clinics, or telemedicine programs staffed by reconstructive specialists. Facilitating the distribution of plastic surgeons within breast cancer centers can also improve the access to timely, integrated care specifically targeting these barriers. Furthermore, tracking reconstructive procedure rates alongside race, ethnicity, insurance status, and geographic data can help systems identify inequitable gaps in care and set measurable goals for improvement.

Government institutions can support equity through policy and funding mechanisms. This includes incentivizing medical practice in underserved areas through loan forgiveness, grants, or reimbursement bonuses for reconstructive plastic surgeons. Operational funding could be directed toward non-urban hospitals to strengthen the reconstructive service infrastructure. In addition, investing in patient navigation programs, transportation assistance, and educational initiatives could help address logistical and informational barriers to care. Policy reforms mandating parity in insurance coverage for reconstruction and streamlining the authorization process may further reduce delays and denials. Lastly, regional collaboration could be promoted by fostering partnerships between high-volume cancer centers and smaller hospitals, improving referral networks and visiting specialists.

By implementing these coordinated strategies, clinicians, health systems, and governmental bodies can work in tandem to reduce disparities and ensure more equitable access to post-mastectomy breast reconstruction for all patients.

Future work could include multi-state studies to validate these findings and examine whether California's lack of racial disparities is replicable elsewhere. This is best carried out with linked or enriched datasets, allowing researchers to perform multivariate analyses, if possible. Incorporating mixed methods or qualitative elements would allow researchers to further investigate the factors influencing patient decision-making, particularly racial minorities, cultural perceptions, provider communication, and awareness of reconstruction options. The goal of identifying disparities in access allows for targeted interventions.

5. Conclusions

Improvements in reconstruction rates after mastectomy are slow, with only 17.64% proceeding with reconstruction. Nationally, 70.5% of patients receive MO and 29.6% undergo reconstruction. Significant factors positively contributing to reconstruction are private insurance, a high SES, cancer center care, and urban residencies. Identified barriers include public health insurance enrollment, rural or non-urban residence, older age, a low SES, and non-white race/ethnicity, possibly indicating monetary influences on care.

Author Contributions: Conceptualization, A.L.C. and K.L.V.; methodology, J.C. and M.C.; formal analysis, A.L.C.; investigation, K.L.V. and A.-P.S.; resources, R.M.C.; data curation, M.A.; writing—original draft preparation, K.L.V. and M.A.; writing—review and editing, K.L.V., R.M.C., N.C.O.M. and A.-P.S.; visualization, K.L.V., N.C.O.M. and M.A.; supervision, J.C.; project administration, A.L.C. and J.C. All authors have read and agreed to the published version of the manuscript.

Funding: This research received no external funding.

Institutional Review Board Statement: This study did not require ethical approval.

Informed Consent Statement: Not applicable.

Data Availability Statement: The original contributions presented in this study are included in the article. Further inquiries can be directed to the corresponding author.

Acknowledgments: We would like to thank Janet Lee for her work and guidance.

Conflicts of Interest: The authors declare no conflicts of interest.

References

1. National Comprehensive Cancer Network (NCCN). Practice Guidelines in Oncology: Breast Cancer. Version 5.2021. Available online: https://www.nccn.org/professionals/physician_gls/pdf/breast.pdf (accessed on 22 November 2024).
2. Kocher, R.; Emanuel, E.J.; DeParle, N.-A.M. The Affordable Care Act and the future of clinical medicine: The opportunities and challenges. *Ann. Intern. Med.* **2010**, *153*, 536–539. [CrossRef]
3. Lang, J.E.; Summers, D.E.; Cui, H.; Carey, J.N.; Viscusi, R.K.; Hurst, C.A.; Waer, A.L.; Ley, M.L.B.; Sener, S.F.; Vijayasekaran, A. Trends in post-mastectomy reconstruction: A SEER database analysis. *J. Surg. Oncol.* **2013**, *108*, 163–168. [CrossRef] [PubMed]
4. Duraes, E.F.R.; Durand, P.; Duraes, L.C.; Orra, S.; Moreira-Gonzalez, A.; de Sousa, J.B.; Djohan, R.S.; Zins, J.; Bernard, S.; Schwarz, G.S. Comparison of preoperative quality of life in breast reconstruction, breast aesthetic and non-breast plastic surgery patients: A cross-sectional study. *J. Plast. Reconstr. Aesthet. Surg.* **2016**, *69*, 1478–1485. [CrossRef]
5. Santosa, K.B.; Qi, J.; Kim, H.M.; Hamill, J.B.; Wilkins, E.G.; Pusic, A.L. Long-term Patient-Reported Outcomes in Postmastectomy Breast Reconstruction. *JAMA Surg.* **2018**, *153*, 891–899. [CrossRef] [PubMed]
6. Cortina, C.S.; Bergom, C.R.; Kijack, J.; Thorgerson, A.A.; Huang, C.-C.S.; Kong, A.L. Postmastectomy breast reconstruction in women aged 70 and older: An analysis of the National Cancer Database (NCDB). *Surgery* **2021**, *170*, 30–38. [CrossRef]
7. Retrouvey, H.; Solaja, O.; Gagliardi, A.R.; Webster, F.; Zhong, T. Barriers of Access to Breast Reconstruction: A Systematic Review. *Plast. Reconstr. Surg.* **2019**, *143*, 465e–476e. [CrossRef] [PubMed]
8. Chen, H.; Zhang, M.; Wang, M.; Zhang, P.; Bai, F.; Wu, K. Immediate Breast Reconstruction in De Novo Metastatic Breast Cancer: An Analysis of 563 Cases Based on the SEER Database. *Clin. Breast Cancer* **2019**, *19*, e135–e141. [CrossRef]
9. U.S. Congress. 105th Congress, 1st Session. (1997). Pub. L. 105-277, The Women's Health and Cancer Rights Act of 1997. Available online: https://babel.hathitrust.org/cgi/pt?id=pst.000043022663&seq=1 (accessed on 16 November 2022).
10. American College of Surgeons. *National Accreditation Program for Breast Centers Standards Manual*; American College of Surgeons: Chicago, IL, USA, 2018.
11. Brennan, M.E.; Spillane, A.J. Uptake and predictors of post-mastectomy reconstruction in women with breast malignancy–systematic review. *Eur. J. Surg. Oncol.* **2013**, *39*, 527–541. [CrossRef]
12. Morrow, M.; Li, Y.; Alderman, A.K.; Jagsi, R.; Hamilton, A.S.; Graff, J.J.; Hawley, S.T.; Katz, S.J. Access to Breast Reconstruction After Mastectomy and Patient Perspectives on Reconstruction Decision Making. *JAMA Surg.* **2014**, *149*, 1015–1021. [CrossRef]
13. Chattha, A. A Comparison of Outcomes and Resource Utilization Between Plastic Surgeons and General Surgeons in Implant-Based Breast Reconstruction—PubMed. Available online: https://pubmed.ncbi.nlm.nih.gov/31135507/ (accessed on 16 November 2022).
14. Longacre, C.F.; Marmor, S.; Altman, A.M.; Hui, J.Y.; Jensen, E.H.; Tuttle, T.M. Patterns of Treatment and Survival among American Indian and Alaska Native Women with Breast Cancer, 2000–2015. *J. Health Care Poor Underserved* **2020**, *31*, 1308–1322. [CrossRef]
15. Kuhlefelt, C.; Homsy, P.; Repo, J.P.; Jahkola, T.; Kauhanen, S. Health-Related Quality of Life After Breast Reconstruction: Comparing Outcomes Between Reconstruction Techniques Using the BREAST-Q. *World J. Surg.* **2022**, *46*, 2695–2705. [CrossRef] [PubMed]
16. Mishra, A. Coping in Post-Mastectomy Breast Cancer Survivors and Need for Intervention: Systematic Review. *Breast Cancer Basic Clin. Res.* **2023**, *17*, 11782234231209126. [CrossRef] [PubMed]
17. Kirkpatrick, D.R.; Markov, N.P.; Fox, J.P.; Tuttle, R.M. Initial Surgical Treatment for Breast Cancer and the Distance Traveled for Care. *Am. Surg.* **2021**, *87*, 1280–1286. [CrossRef] [PubMed]
18. Connors, S.K.; Leal, I.M.; Nitturi, V.; Iwundu, C.N.; Maza, V.; Reyes, S.; Acquati, C.; Reitzel, L.R. Empowered Choices: African-American Women's Breast Reconstruction Decisions. *Am. J. Health Behav.* **2021**, *45*, 352–370. [CrossRef]
19. Restrepo, D.J.; Boczar, D.; Huayllani, M.T.; Sisti, A.; Gabriel, E.; McLaughlin, S.A.; Bagaria, S.; Spaulding, A.C.; Rinker, B.D.; Forte, A.J. Influence of Race, Income, Insurance, and Education on the Rate of Breast Reconstruction. *Anticancer Res.* **2019**, *39*, 2969–2973. [CrossRef]
20. Sergesketter, A.R.; Thomas, S.M.; Lane, W.O.; Orr, J.P.; Shammas, R.L.; Fayanju, O.M.; Greenup, R.A.; Hollenbeck, S.T. Decline in Racial Disparities in Postmastectomy Breast Reconstruction: A Surveillance, Epidemiology, and End Results Analysis from 1998 to 2014. *Plast. Reconstr. Surg.* **2019**, *143*, 1560–1570. [CrossRef]
21. Albornoz, C.R.; Bach, P.B.; Pusic, A.L.; McCarthy, C.M.; Mehrara, B.J.; Disa, J.J.; Cordeiro, P.G.; Matros, E. The influence of sociodemographic factors and hospital characteristics on the method of breast reconstruction, including microsurgery: A U.S. population-based study. *Plast. Reconstr. Surg.* **2012**, *129*, 1071–1079. [CrossRef]
22. Anderson, S.R.; Sieffert, M.R.; Talarczyk, C.M.R.; Johnson, R.M.; Fox, M.J.P. Geographic Variation in Breast Reconstruction Modality Use Among Women Undergoing Mastectomy. *Ann. Plast. Surg.* **2019**, *82*, 382–385. [CrossRef]
23. Meade, A.E.; Cummins, S.M.; Farewell, J.T.; Duque, S.; Mulqueen, S.K.; Chuah, A.; Zhang, A.Y. Breaking Barriers to Breast Reconstruction among Socioeconomically Disadvantaged Patients at a Large Safety-net Hospital. *Plast. Reconstr. Surg. Glob. Open* **2022**, *10*, e4410. [CrossRef]
24. Connors, S.K.; Goodman, M.S.; Myckatyn, T.; Margenthaler, J.; Gehlert, S. Breast reconstruction after mastectomy at a comprehensive cancer center. *Springerplus* **2016**, *5*, 955. [CrossRef]

25. Bailey, C.M.; Selber, J.; Liu, J.; Lee, C.N.; Offodile, A.C. Current Practice and Perceptions Regarding Cost Communication in Breast Cancer Reconstruction: Survey Results of the American Society of Plastic Surgeons. *Ann. Surg. Oncol.* **2021**, *28*, 376–385. [CrossRef] [PubMed]
26. Boczar, D.; Restrepo, D.J.; Sisti, A.; Huayllani, M.T.; Spaulding, A.C.; Gabriel, E.; Bagaria, S.; McLaughlin, S.; Parker, A.S.; Forte, A.J. Influence of Facility Characteristics on Access to Breast Reconstruction: A 12-Year National Cancer Database Analysis. *Anticancer. Res.* **2019**, *39*, 6881–6885. [CrossRef] [PubMed]
27. Vangsness, K.L.; Juste, J.; Sam, A.-P.; Munabi, N.; Chu, M.; Agko, M.; Chang, J.; Carre, A.L. Post-Mastectomy Breast Reconstruction Disparities: A Systematic Review of Sociodemographic and Economic Barriers. *Medicina* **2024**, *60*, 1169. [CrossRef]
28. Hawley, S.T.; Griggs, J.J.; Hamilton, A.S.; Graff, J.J.; Janz, N.K.; Morrow, M.; Jagsi, R.; Salem, B.; Katz, S.J. Decision Involvement and Receipt of Mastectomy Among Racially and Ethnically Diverse Breast Cancer Patients. *J. Natl. Cancer Inst.* **2009**, *101*, 1337–1347. [CrossRef]
29. Yang, R.L.; Newman, A.S.; Reinke, C.E.; Lin, I.C.; Karakousis, G.C.; Czerniecki, B.J.; Wu, L.C.; Kelz, R.R. Racial disparities in immediate breast reconstruction after mastectomy: Impact of state and federal health policy changes. *Ann. Surg. Oncol.* **2013**, *20*, 399–406. [CrossRef] [PubMed]
30. Connors, S.K.; Goodman, M.S.; Myckatyn, T.; Margenthaler, J.; Gehlert, S. Racial Disparities in Breast Reconstruction at a Comprehensive Cancer Center. *J. Racial Ethn. Health Disparities* **2022**, *9*, 2323–2333. [CrossRef]
31. Alderman, A.K.; Hawley, S.T.; Janz, N.K.; Mujahid, M.S.; Morrow, M.; Hamilton, A.S.; Graff, J.J.; Katz, S.J. Racial and Ethnic Disparities in the Use of Postmastectomy Breast Reconstruction: Results From a Population-Based Study. *J. Clin. Oncol.* **2009**, *27*, 5325–5330. [CrossRef]
32. Doren, E.L.; Park, K.; Olson, J. Racial disparities in postmastectomy breast reconstruction following implementation of the affordable care act: A systematic review using a minority health and disparities research framework. *Am. J. Surg.* **2023**, *226*, 37–47. [CrossRef]
33. Soni, S.E.; Lee, M.C.; Gwede, C.K. Disparities in Use and Access to Postmastectomy Breast Reconstruction Among African American Women. *Cancer Control* **2017**, *24*, 1073274817729053. [CrossRef]
34. Schafer, R.E.; Ho, I.; Potoczak, P.S.; Misra-Hebert, A.; Nowacki, A.S.; Schwarz, G.S. Legislative Impact and Persistent Disparities: Postmastectomy Breast Reconstruction Rates in the United States among 224,506 Patients. *Plast. Reconstr. Surg.* **2025**, *155*, 854e–862e. [CrossRef]
35. Wirth, L.S.; Hinyard, L.; Keller, J.; Bucholz, E.; Schwartz, T. Geographic variations in racial disparities in postmastectomy breast reconstruction: A SEER database analysis. *Breast J.* **2019**, *25*, 112–116. [CrossRef] [PubMed]
36. Wareham, C.; Bertaux, B.; Chahine, E.; Homsy, C.; Perry, D.; Persing, S.; Nardello, S.; Chatterjee, A. Geographical Presence of Plastic Surgeons in Relation to Breast Surgeons in the United States for Breast Reconstruction. *J. Surg. Oncol.* **2025** *in press*. [CrossRef] [PubMed]
37. Stankowski, T.J.; Schumacher, J.R.; Hanlon, B.M.; Tucholka, J.L.; Venkatesh, M.; Yang, D.-Y.; Poore, S.O.; Neuman, H.B. Barriers to Breast Reconstruction for Socioeconomically Disadvantaged Women. *Breast Cancer Res. Treat.* **2022**, *195*, 413–419. [CrossRef] [PubMed]

cancers

MDPI

Article

Clinician Recommendation for Hereditary Genetic Testing in Participants at Increased Risk for Hereditary Cancer

Emerson Delacroix [1,2,*], Sarah Austin [2], John D. Rice [3], Elena Martinez Stoffel [2], Erika Koeppe [2], Jennifer J. Griggs [2,4] and Ken Resnicow [1,5,6]

1 Department of Health Behavior & Health Equity, University of Michigan, Ann Arbor, MI 48109, USA; kresnic@umich.edu
2 Department of Internal Medicine, Michigan Medicine, Ann Arbor, MI 48109, USA; austinse@med.umich.edu (S.A.); estoffel@med.umich.edu (E.M.S.); eskoeppe@med.umich.edu (E.K.); jengrigg@med.umich.edu (J.J.G.)
3 Department of Biostatistics, University of Michigan, Ann Arbor, MI 48109, USA; jdrice@umich.edu
4 Department of Health Management and Policy, University of Michigan, Ann Arbor, MI 48109, USA
5 Rogel Cancer Center, Michigan Medicine, Ann Arbor, MI 48109, USA
6 Division of Epidemiology & Community Health, University of Minnesota, Minneapolis, MN 55455, USA
* Correspondence: emmed@umich.edu

Simple Summary: Genetic testing (GT) is a valuable tool in managing hereditary cancer risk but remains underutilized. This study explores the role of clinician recommendations in GT uptake, focusing on demographic and cancer history variables. From 784 respondents, a subset with heightened hereditary cancer risk who had not completed GT was analyzed. The results revealed that only 14.0% received clinician recommendations for GT, and younger adults with fewer financial concerns and higher education levels were less likely to receive recommendations. These findings underscore the need for enhanced clinician education regarding GT indications and the integration of electronic medical record tools to better identify eligible patients. Addressing these barriers through clinician-focused education and decision-support systems can improve the standardization and uptake of GT recommendations, ultimately enhancing cancer management.

Abstract: Background: Despite clinical utility in managing hereditary cancers, genetic testing (GT) remains underutilized. While barriers include knowledge gaps and cost, clinician recommendation is a major driver of GT uptake, with rates varying by cancer type and family cancer history documentation. **Methods:** Adult participants ($\geq$18 years) were recruited through multiple sources to complete a cancer family history survey for a larger intervention trial. Participants with personal or family history indicating increased hereditary cancer risk who had not undergone GT (N = 3001) were invited to complete a baseline survey. Multivariable logistic regression was used to analyze associations between demographics and cancer history by receipt of a clinician recommendation for GT. **Results:** Among 784 respondents, most were White (84.6%), female (58.4%), and over age 51 (75.3%), with 58.2% reporting a diagnosis of cancer. Only 14.0% reported receiving a clinician recommendation for GT, with lower recommendation rates among younger adults (20.1%), those reporting no financial stress (10.7%), and those with higher education (12.0%). Multivariate analysis showed participants who did not report financial stress (p = 0.049) were less likely to receive a recommendation. **Discussion:** These findings highlight disparities in GT recommendation by clinicians. Increased clinician education about indications for GT, the implementation of electronic medical record tools to facilitate the identification of patients with guideline-concordant personal and/or biological-relative cancer history, and patient-facing interventions could standardize the dissemination of recommendations for GT. **Conclusions:** Future efforts that focus on increasing clinician

Cancers **2025**, *17*, 1994

https://doi.org/10.3390/cancers17121994

education and electronic decision support should identify individuals with personal and/or biological-relative cancer history meeting criteria for GT.

Keywords: adults; genetic testing; genetic risk; adherence; hereditary cancer

1. Introduction

As many as 1 in every 10 individuals diagnosed with advanced cancer has an underlying genetic susceptibility to cancer [1]; however, many patients do not undergo clinically indicated genetic testing (GT) for cancer susceptibility despite its utility in the detection, prevention, and treatment of hereditary cancers [2–6]. Groups with particularly low rates of GT include individuals who are of older age, are racial and ethnic minorities, and/or have a personal/family history of cancer other than breast cancer [4,7–10]. Barriers to the uptake of GT include knowledge gaps, cost concerns, and a lack of clinician recommendation [1,11,12].

Several studies have demonstrated that clinician recommendation drives GT uptake [2,4–6,8,13–20]. Few patients seek testing without a clinician referral [13,21]. Factors that influence clinician recommendation for GT include cancer type, having documentation of a comprehensive biological-relative history of cancer, and awareness of national and international guidelines for GT. Rates of recommendation for GT are higher among individuals with breast and/or gynecologic cancers associated with hereditary breast and ovarian cancer syndrome (HBOC) and Lynch syndrome, with biologic females tested at a higher rate than their male counterparts [8,9,13]. Rates of recommendation for GT are lower for individuals with prostate and colorectal cancers (CRC), and for those without a personal history of cancer but whose biological-relative history of cancer indicates a higher risk for hereditary cancer syndromes [13].

The purpose of this study was to examine the determinants and correlates of receiving a clinician recommendation for GT within a sample of patients meeting national guidelines for GT for cancer susceptibility. This study adds to our previous work by including individuals who had not undergone GT, and we account for the cancer type and family history present [13].

2. Materials and Methods

Study surveys used previously validated measures to assess perceived benefits and barriers to GT [13]. Respondents self-reported a recommendation for GT with a single item developed from prior studies: "Has a doctor or other health care provider ever recommended that you get cancer genetic testing?" (1) Yes, (2) No, (3) I don't remember [22]. Responses two and three were collapsed to simplify analysis. Participants reporting (1) Yes, were subsequently asked, "Who recommended the cancer genetic testing? (Choose all that apply)" Fill-in response options were recoded (Table 1).

Analyzed descriptive variables are detailed in Table 2 and included gender identification (trichotomized into female, male, non-binary/transgender), age (current) (trichotomized into years 18–50, 51–70, >70), education (dichotomized into vocational or less, bachelor's or higher), household financial stress (dichotomized into living comfortably, getting by or finding it (very) difficult), insurance status (dichotomized into public (Medicare, Medicaid, Tri-care, Veterans Affairs, Indian Health) or private (employer-funded; other)), race and ethnicity (choose all that apply), and employment status (trichotomized into employed, unemployed/student, and retired/disabled).

Table 1. Participant characteristics, N = 784. Descriptive statistics of baseline survey respondents including receipt of a recommendation for GT.

Demographic Variables	Level	Overall (n = 784)
Gender: *n* (%)	Female	458 (58.4%)
	Male	318 (40.6%)
	Non-binary, genderqueer, or transgender	7 (0.9%)
	Missing	1 (0.1%)
	Total gender	784 (100.0%)
Race and Ethnicity: *n* (%)	American Indian or Native American, Alaskan Native	8 (1.0%)
	Asian or Asian American	17 (2.2%)
	Black or African American	35 (4.5%)
	Hispanic/Latinx-only	29 (3.7%)
	Middle Eastern or North African	7 (0.9%)
	Other (includes multiracial)	13 (1.7%)
	White or European American, non-Hispanic	663 (84.6%)
	Missing	12 (1.5%)
	Total race and ethnicity	784 (100.0%)
Ashkenazi Jewish ancestry: *n* (%)	Yes	133 (17.0%)
	No	610 (77.8%)
	Missing	41 (5.2%)
	Total ancestry	784 (100.0%)
Age (in years): *n* (%)	18–50	194 (24.7%)
	51–70	375 (47.8%)
	71 or older	215 (27.4%)
	Total age	784 (100.0%)
Education: *n* (%)	Less than high school, HS diploma or GED, vocational certificate, or associate's	242 (30.9%)
	Bachelor's degree or higher	540 (68.9%)
	Missing	2 (0.3%)
	Total education	784 (100.0%)
Employment: *n* (%)	Currently employed (full or part time), or volunteer	348 (44.4%)
	Unemployed or student	32 (4.1%)
	Retired, homemaker, or disabled	404 (51.5%)
	Total employment	784 (100.0%)
Financial stress on present income: *n* (%)	Living comfortably	485 (61.9%)
	Getting by, finding it (very) difficult	286 (36.5%)
	Missing or prefer not to answer	13 (1.7%)
	Total financial stress	784 (100.0%)
Health insurance type: *n* (%)	Public/government	370 (47.2%)
	Private	414 (52.8%)
	Total insurance	784 (100.0%)

Table 1. *Cont.*

Demographic Variables	Level	Overall (n = 784)
Years since cancer diagnosis: *n* (%)	Less than 1 1 to 2 More than 2 Missing Total years since diagnosis	52 (6.6%) 85 (10.8%) 319 (40.7%) 328 (41.8%) 784 (100%)
Eligibility for MiGHT: *n* (%)	Level 1 Breast, CRC, endometrial, or prostate < 51 years; or ovarian or pancreatic any age	98 (12.5%)
	Level 2 Breast, CRC, endometrial, or prostate > 50-years; or other cancer types	400 (51.0%)
	Level 3 No personal history of cancer	286 (36.5%)
	Total eligible	784 (100%)
Received recommendation for cancer GT: *n* (%)	No or do not recall Yes Total recommended	674 (86.0%) 110 (14.0%) 784 (100.0%)

Table 2. Data on 110 participants for "Who recommended cancer GT? (Choose all that apply)". Of the 110 participating reporting receipt of GT referral, 17 participants reported that more than one clinician recommended GT, n = 13 reported two clinicians, and n = 4 participants reported that three clinicians recommended GT.

Who Recommended GT?	Level	Recommended GT
Generalist	Primary care provider, family physician	31 (23.7%)
	Physician assistant	5 (3.8%)
	Nurse	1 (0.8%)
	Total generalists	37 (28.2%)
Specialists	Dermatologist	1 (0.8%)
	Endocrinologist	4 (3.1%)
	Gastroenterologist	2 (1.5%)
	Genetic specialist (genetic counselor, clinical geneticist)	9 (6.9%)
	Neuromuscular specialist	1 (0.8%)
	Obstetrics/gynecologist	12 (9.2%)
	Oncologist	44 (33.6%)
	Surgeon	12 (9.2%)
	Urologist	2 (1.5%)
	Total specialists	87 (66.4%)
Others (i.e., fellow, do not recall)	Relative	2 (1.5%)
	Undefined healthcare professional	5 (3.8%)
	Total others	7 (5.3%)
Total	Recommendations for GT	131 (100%)

To test our hypothesis that participants with a personal diagnosis of a cancer type that is prominent in known hereditary cancer syndromes would be more likely to receive a clinician recommendation for GT, we trichotomized subjects' cancer histories into three levels (Figure 1) according to the National Comprehensive Cancer Network® (NCCN®) Clinical Practice Guidelines in Oncology (NCCN Guidelines®), which are widely used in the United States. Level 1 cancer history includes individuals with a personal diagnosis of early age-of-onset breast, colorectal, endometrial/uterine, or prostate cancers (diagnosed age < 50 years) or personal diagnosis of ovarian or pancreatic cancers (diagnosed at any age). Level 2 cancer history includes individuals with a personal history any other cancer diagnosis (including Level 1 cancer types diagnosed at age > 50 years) [22]. Level 3 cancer history includes individuals without a personal history of cancer (eligible for genetic testing based on their family cancer history only). The rationale for categorizing cancer histories like this is that the cancer diagnoses in Level 1 have been specifically highlighted in genetic testing guidelines for >10 years and rely on personal history only. In contrast, Level 2 cancer histories include additional cancer types and/or older ages of diagnosis plus family cancer history meeting criteria that have more recently been included in expanded guidelines for clinical GT such as the NCCN Guidelines® for pancreatic cancer at any age [23]. Furthermore, individuals with Level 3 cancer history are identified only by their family history of cancer, with no personal history of cancer.

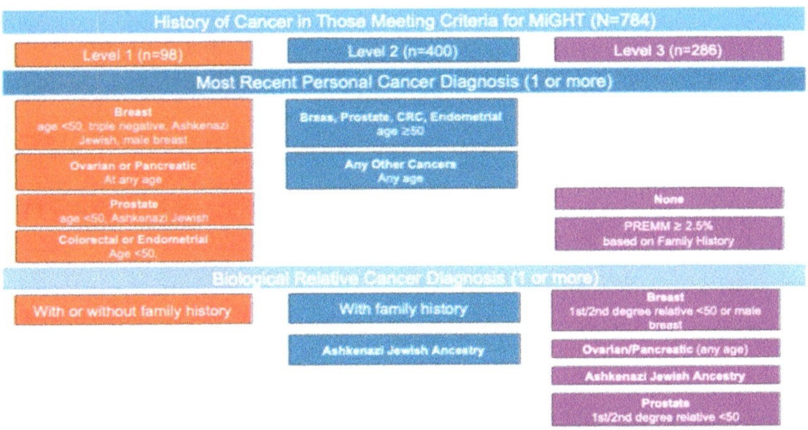

Figure 1. MiGHT subjects were categorized into one of three levels based on personal and biological-relative cancer histories.

As part of recruitment for a large trial evaluating interventions to promote the uptake of genetic testing for cancer susceptibility, adults were invited to complete a family health history survey eliciting a detailed family history of cancer diagnoses in first- and second-degree relatives (MiGHT Study clinical trials.gov (NCT05162846) [22]. Subjects were recruited from community oncology practices in the state of Michigan, cancer registries, oncology, gastroenterology, and primary care clinics at an academic medical center, community health fairs, and radio and newspaper advertisements. Regardless of sex assigned at birth, all participants were shown all cancer types (bladder, breast, cervical, colorectal, endometrial, lung, melanoma, ovarian, pancreatic, prostate, and ten others), and patients could report multiple primary cancers. The University of Michigan Medical School Institutional Review Board approved this research (HUM00180616, HUM00217689, HUM00231415). MiGHT is registered with clinicaltrials.gov (NCT05162846).

Individuals whose personal and/or family cancer histories met clinical guideline-based criteria for GT (N = 3001) received an email invitation from the study team with a unique link to complete a brief survey to assess eligibility for the clinical trial. Individuals were excluded if they had already completed GT (n = 932), had a GT appointment scheduled (n = 64), did not have access to a phone or internet connection (n = 155), were under age 18 (n = 1), did not communicate in English (n = 7), or were deceased (n = 15); 831 individuals provided informed consent for the trial.

Consenting subjects (n = 831) were asked to complete a baseline survey that included questions about hereditary GT knowledge, receipt of clinician recommendations about GT, and motivators and barriers to genetic testing uptake. Reminder emails to complete the baseline survey were sent 1 day, 3 days, 5 days, and 10 days after consent. Initially up-to eight, and later five, reminder phone calls were made one to three times each week for four weeks.

We examined factors associated with receipt of a clinician recommendation for cancer genetic testing (assessed by self-report) and used multivariable logistic regression to assess the association of demographic factors, cancer diagnoses, and receipt of clinician recommendation for cancer GT.

Data for these analyses are drawn from the baseline survey of a larger intervention clinical trial. Those who signed written consent were enrolled and offered USD 10.00 for survey completion. Reminders were sent 1 day, 3 days, 5 days, and 10 days after consent. Data were analyzed using R Foundation for Statistical Computing by R version 4.2.1 Core team (2024) Vienna, Austria and SPSS Statistics for Mac version 29 by IBM Corporation Armonk, New York (USA) (2024). The dataset supporting this study is available upon request from the corresponding author due to the timing of the published dataset and this article.

3. Results

3.1. Population Descriptions

Of the 831 consenting participants, 799 (96.1%) completed baseline surveys, and 784 received of a recommendation for GT (yes/no or I don't remember) and were included in this analysis. Demographic variables, cancer type, and receipt of a recommendation for GT are summarized by frequency in Table 1. Of the 784 respondents, the majority were female (58.4%), White (84.6%), and over the age of 51 years (75.3%). The majority reported low household financial stress (61.9%), private (employer-funded) health insurance (52.8%), and a bachelor's or advanced degree (68.9%).

Of the 2878 cancer diagnoses reported, the most common were breast (n = 640, 22.2%), followed by skin, (n = 546, 19.0%), (see Supplemental Table S1). A total of 498 (63.5%) participants reported a personal cancer diagnosis, with 98 (12.5%) reporting Level 1 cancer histories, 400 (51.0%) reporting Level 2 cancer histories, and 286 (36.5%) reporting no personal history of cancer (Level 3) and qualifying for GT based on their biological relatives' cancer history only.

Among the 286 (36.5%) participants with no personal history of cancer (Level 3) only 12.5% reported receipt of a recommendation for GT. Of the individuals in Level 3, 43.6% were over age 50.

Of those reporting receiving a recommendation for GT, Table 2, the majority (n = 87, 66.4%) received recommendation from a clinical specialist such as an oncologist, urologist, gastroenterologist, surgeon, obstetrician/gynecologist, or endocrinologist.

3.2. Univariate Analysis

Overall, 110 (14.0%) respondents reported receiving a clinician recommendation for GT, with individuals over 50 years old (75.3%), those with households feeling financially comfortable (51.8%), and those with higher education (12.0%) less likely to report receipt of a recommendation (Table 3). Females reported receiving a recommendation more frequently than males (17.0% vs. 9.4%, $p = 0.006$), Table 3.

Table 3. Univariate analysis of clinician recommendation for GT by demographics, N = 784. The *p*-values are from chi-square tests for within-group comparisons.

		Reported Recommendation for GT			
Variables	Level	Yes n	Total n	% of Variation	Statistical Significance
Gender	Female	78	458	17.0%	p = 0.006
	Male	30	318	9.4%	
	Non-binary or transgender	2	7	28.6%	
	Total	110	783	14.0%	
Age (in years)	18–50	39	194	20.1%	p = 0.003
	51–70	53	375	14.1%	
	71 and older	18	215	8.4%	
	Total	110	784	14.0%	
Education	≤Vocational	45	242	18.6%	p = 0.043
	Bachelor's degree or higher	65	540	12.0%	
	Total	110	784	14.0%	
Employment	Unemployed, volunteer, or student	5	32	15.6%	p = 0.201
	Working full or part time	57	348	16.4%	
	Retired or disabled	48	404	11.9%	
	Total	110	784	14.0%	
Financial stress	Getting by or finding it (very) difficult	57	286	19.9%	p < 0.001
	Living comfortably	52	485	10.7%	
	Total	109	771	14.1%	
Health insurance	Private	63	414	15.2%	p = 0.311
	Public	47	370	12.7%	
	Total	110	784	14.0%	
Years since cancer diagnosis	Less than 1	12	52	23.1%	p = 0.055
	1 to 2	17	85	20.0%	
	More than 2	40	319	12.5%	
	Total	69	456	15.1%	
Eligibility for MiGHT	Level 1	28	98	28.6%	p < 0.001
	Level 2	46	400	11.5%	
	Level 3	36	286	12.6%	
	Total	110	784	14.0%	

3.3. Multivariate Analysis

Patients exhibiting variables including low financial stress (p = 0.049), Level 2 cancer types (p = 0.007), and Level 3 (p = <0.001) cancer history were significantly less likely to report receiving a recommendation for testing, Table 4. Gender, age, and education level were significant in univariate analysis, though not in multivariate.

Table 4. Multivariate of clinician recommendation for GT by demographics, n = 768. Note 14 cases were excluded due to missing values.

Independent Variables	Levels	Odds Ratio (OR)	95% CI for OR	*p*-Value
Gender	Female	1.0		
	Male	0.64	0.396–1.042	$p = 0.073$
	Non-binary	1.80	0.308–10.548	$p = 0.514$
Age (in years)	18–50	1.0		
	51–70	0.82	0.474–1.403	$p = 0.461$
	71 or older	0.52	0.237–1.138	$p = 0.102$
Education	≤Vocational	1.0		
	Bachelor's degree or higher	0.71	0.449–1.108	$p = 0.130$
Employment	Unemployed, volunteer, or student	1.0		
	Working full or part time	1.21	0.422–3.485	$p = 0.720$
	Retired, homemaker, or disabled	1.00	0.340–2.966	$p = 2.996$
Financial stress	Getting by or finding it (very) difficult	1.0		
	Living comfortably	0.63	0.402–0.998	$p = 0.049$
Health insurance coverage	Private	1.0		
	Public vs. private	0.92	0.548–1.529	$p = 0.735$
Eligibility for MiGHT	Level 1	1.0		
	Level 2	0.44	0.247–0.798	$p = 0.007$
	Level 3	0.32	0.177–0.574	$p < 0.001$

4. Discussion

In this analysis of U.S. adults, we found several predictors of who is receiving a recommendation from their healthcare provider to undergo cancer GT. Our key findings were that despite every participant in this study meeting clinical guidelines for clinical GT, only 14.0% reported that their healthcare clinician recommended GT. This finding may not represent the true population rate, as this study included only individuals who did not undergo GT; however, it reinforces that a lack of clinician recommendation may be a driving factor in the underutilization of GT among eligible individuals. It is possible that recall bias is a factor in reporting receipt of a referral, noting that some studies report that participants may not recall receiving GT [24,25].

While in univariate analyses, males were significantly less likely to receive a recommendation than females, this effect was no longer significant in multivariate analysis, which adjusted for other sociodemographic and clinical factors, suggesting this was likely confounded by some factors, particularly cancer history and perceived financial stress. This contradicts previous findings, where gender was a significant predictor of uptake of GT, even when adjusting for other sociodemographic factors [13]. This could highlight a difference in sampling between our study and others, with ours including only individuals who have not undergone GT. Another difference between our study and previous reports in the literature is that our analysis included a relatively high proportion of males and individuals with a wide range of personal and/or family histories of cancer, as well as those without a personal history of cancer. Age and education were also significant in univariate analysis and not significant in multivariate. Age may affect patient access to care, treatment, and adherence, as it may correlate with health status or comorbidities. Age may interact with gender to dilute its observed effect in our multivariate model.

Participants reporting living comfortably at the present received fewer recommendations for testing. The previous study found no effect of financial stress on recommendation, though the difference could be due to the difference between perceived income and actual income. Why living comfortably is associated with a lower recommendation rate is unclear and merits further exploration. One possible explanation is that those that report higher incomes may have providers that are less likely to perceive they need a recommendation assuming these patients will advocate for themselves and ask for GT. Or it is possible those with lower financial stress may have already had GT, excluding them from this study, leading to sampling bias.

The type of cancer history was a strong predictor of clinician recommendation. Specifically, compared to those with a personal history of Level 1 cancers with a well-established recommendation for testing (pancreatic cancer or ovarian cancer at any age, personal history of either breast cancer > age 50, colon cancer > age 50, uterine cancer > age 50, prostate cancer > age 50), those with other, less striking personal cancer histories (Level 2) were significantly less likely in multivariate analyses to be recommended GT. Those with personal history of Level 1 cancers based on well-established clinical guidelines comprised only 12.5% of our sample—this is because many individuals with Level 1 cancers were not eligible for our study because they reported having already undergone GT. Our findings suggest that while clinicians are referring patients with Level 1 cancer histories for GT, there is still a need for continuing education to improve identification and referrals for patients with Level 2 cancer diagnoses and those without a personal cancer diagnosis (Level 3), whose family history of cancer informs eligibility for GT. Additionally, these findings may be in part due to selection bias in our sample, as only individuals who had not previously completed genetic testing were included. Individuals with higher motivation likely already completed genetic testing, leaving only the less-motivated individuals in these groups in our study cohort.

In our findings, the majority of "yes" recommendations tended to come from specialists (66.4%), particularly oncologists (33.6%), who are predominantly responsible for placing referrals for GT. This aligns with the existing literature, which suggests that specialists are more engaged in the GT referral process due to their specific roles and expertise.

Taken together, our findings indicate significant disparities in rates of recommendation for GT by financial stress, age, and cancer history and type. This points to a need to increase clinicians' familiarity with indications for GT and specifically a need to identify males and those who meet GT criteria due to family cancer history alone.

Although males are less likely to receive testing recommendations from clinicians, data suggest that they are just as likely as their female counterparts to follow through with GT if it is recommended [13]. Although clinician recommendation rates are particularly high for females with breast cancer, recommendation rates for females with other cancer types merit attention [8,13,18], as well as those for females with intersectional identities, such as those involving race, sexual orientation, gender identity, or gender presentation [6,18,26]. Clinicians could receive education on current American Medical Association guidelines for inclusive language when making clinical recommendations for those who do not identify as cisgender, heterosexual, or monogamous to ensure referrals are placed in visits with high clinician–patient rapport. Efforts to promote guideline-concordant recommendations for GT could include both clinician and patient-facing interventions. For clinicians, this may include post-graduate continuing medical education or maintenance of certification requirements in current GT guidelines, evidence-based approaches to encourage testing completion. Clinicians could also benefit from evidenced-based digital approaches to identify eligible patients and communicate the value of GT [3]. Additionally, best practice alerts in electronic records could include conversation starters for specific diagnoses in conjunction with quality improvement programs that decrease barriers to referrals for genetic counseling and testing, increase motivation to test, or improve the coordination of care efforts across specialties. For patients meeting GT guidelines, the alerts may include secured-portal or SMS messages with conversation starters to empower advocating for testing with their clinicians as well as links to patient-initiated testing options through clinical laboratories that include information about potential out-of-pocket costs. Independent clinical testing laboratories with relationships to specific clinicians or clinics could provide test results within the patient's electronic medical record with referral recommendations for genetic counseling services, cascade testing, or testing for other genes. Finally, electronic medical records are inconsistent in containing a complete family health history, limiting appropriate referral to germline testing. Increased adherence to updating family cancer history in EMRs could improve provider compliance with national and international genetic testing guidelines.

5. Conclusions

While recommendation rates remain strong for Level 1 cancer types and those reporting greater financial stress, patients who are older, have Level 2 cancer types, or have no personal history of cancer could benefit from healthcare clinicians' recognition of indications for genetic referrals for patients with less striking personal and/or family cancer histories (Levels 2 and 3). The impact of a clinician recommendation on testing uptake is substantial, and the impact is similar between sexes and cancer types, suggesting that focused efforts are needed to promote increasing clinician recommendations, particularly for males and those without a personal history.

Supplementary Materials: The following supporting information can be downloaded at: https://www.mdpi.com/article/10.3390/cancers17121994/s1, Supplemental Table S1. Reported Cancer.

Author Contributions: Conceptualization, E.D., S.A. and K.R.; Data curation, E.D., S.A., J.D.R. and E.K.; Formal analysis, E.D., S.A., J.D.R. and K.R.; Funding acquisition, E.M.S., J.J.G. and K.R.; Investigation, E.D., S.A., J.D.R., E.M.S., E.K. and K.R.; Methodology, E.D., S.A., J.D.R. and K.R.; Project administration, E.D., S.A. and E.K.; Resources, K.R.; Software, E.D., S.A. and J.D.R.; Supervision, E.M.S., J.J.G. and K.R.; Validation, E.D., S.A., J.D.R. and E.K.; Visualization, E.D., S.A., E.M.S., E.K. and K.R.; Writing—original draft, E.D., S.A., J.D.R., E.M.S., E.K., J.J.G. and K.R.; Writing—review & editing, E.D., S.A., J.D.R., E.M.S., E.K., J.J.G. and K.R. All authors have read and agreed to the published version of the manuscript.

Funding: This research was funded by National Institutes of Health, National Cancer Institute, grant number U01CA232827, mPIs Stoffel, Griggs, and Resnicow.

Institutional Review Board Statement: The University of Michigan Medical School Institutional Review Board (IRBMED) approved contacting patients who met the eligibility criteria with the applications (HUM00192898; protocol 2021.076, 4 January 2022), (HUM00217689, 9 August 2022), and (HUM00231415, 17 March 2023) for those who completed a family health history survey with the application (HUM00180616) and consented to future study invitations. All participants signed an electronic consent form prior to enrolling in the study, and the study is registered in ClinicalTrials.gov (NCT05162846).

Informed Consent Statement: Informed consent was obtained from all subjects involved in the study.

Data Availability Statement: The dataset supporting this study are available upon request from the corresponding author due to timing of the published dataset and this article. They will be available from the University of Michigan Library, Deep Blue Data at DOI: https://doi.org/10.7302/0tqr-dn38.

Acknowledgments: Research reported in this publication was supported by the National Cancer Institutes of Health under Award Number P30CA046592 for the use of the following Rogel Cancer Center Health Communications Shared Resource: Center for Health Communications Research, who designed the web-based portal for MiGHT Aim 2.

Conflicts of Interest: The authors declare no conflicts of interest.

References

1. Robinson, D.R.; Wu, Y.-M.; Lonigro, R.J.; Vats, P.; Cobain, E.; Everett, J.; Cao, X.; Rabban, E.; Kumar-Sinha, C.; Raymond, V.; et al. Integrative clinical genomics of metastatic cancer. *Nature* **2017**, *548*, 297–303. [CrossRef] [PubMed]
2. Haverfield, E.V.; Esplin, E.D.; Aguilar, S.J.; Hatchell, K.E.; Ormond, K.E.; Hanson-Kahn, A.; Atwal, P.S.; Macklin-Mantia, S.; Hines, S.; Sak, C.W.-M.; et al. Correction to: Physician-directed genetic screening to evaluate personal risk for medically actionable disorders: A large multi-center cohort study. *BMC Med.* **2021**, *19*, 288. [CrossRef]
3. Gornick, M.C.; Ryan, K.A.; Scherer, A.M.; Roberts, J.S.; De Vries, R.G.; Uhlmann, W.R. Interpretations of the Term "Actionable" when Discussing Genetic Test Results: What you Mean Is Not What I Heard. *J. Genet. Couns.* **2019**, *28*, 334–342. [CrossRef]
4. Hamilton, J.G.; Symecko, H.; Spielman, K.; Breen, K.; Mueller, R.; Catchings, A.; Trottier, M.; Salo-Mullen, E.E.; Shah, I.; Arutyunova, A.; et al. Uptake and acceptability of a mainstreaming model of hereditary cancer multigene panel testing among patients with ovarian, pancreatic, and prostate cancer. *Genet. Med.* **2021**, *23*, 2105–2113. [CrossRef]
5. Bednar, E.M.; Nitecki, R.; Krause, K.J.; Rauh-Hain, J.A. Interventions to improve delivery of cancer genetics services in the United States: A scoping review. *Genet. Med.* **2022**, *24*, 1176–1186. [CrossRef] [PubMed]
6. Cragun, D.; Bonner, D.; Kim, J.; Akbari, M.R.; Narod, S.A.; Gomez-Fuego, A.; Garcia, J.D.; Vadaparampil, S.T.; Pal, T. Factors associated with genetic counseling and BRCA testing in a population-based sample of young Black women with breast cancer. *Breast Cancer Res. Treat.* **2015**, *151*, 169–176. [CrossRef]
7. Shaw, J.; Bulsara, C.; Cohen, P.A.; Gryta, M.; Nichols, C.B.; Schofield, L.; O'sullivan, S.; Pachter, N.; Hardcastle, S.J. Investigating barriers to genetic counseling and germline mutation testing in women with suspected hereditary breast and ovarian cancer syndrome and Lynch syndrome. *Patient Educ. Couns.* **2018**, *101*, 938–944. [CrossRef] [PubMed]
8. Evaluation of Genomic Applications in Practice and Prevention (EGAPP) Working Group; Recommendations from the EGAPP Working Group. Genetic testing strategies in newly diagnosed individuals with colorectal cancer aimed at reducing morbidity and mortality from Lynch syndrome in relatives. *Genet. Med.* **2009**, *11*, 35–41. [CrossRef]
9. Sharaf, R.N.; Myer, P.; Stave, C.D.; Diamond, L.C.; Ladabaum, U. Uptake of genetic testing by relatives of lynch syndrome probands: A systematic review. *Clin. Gastroenterol. Hepatol.* **2013**, *11*, 1093–1100. [CrossRef]
10. Katapodi, M.C.; Northouse, L.; Pierce, P.; Milliron, K.J.; Liu, G.; Merajver, S.D. Differences between women who pursued genetic testing for hereditary breast and ovarian cancer and their at-risk relatives who did not. *Oncol. Nurs. Forum* **2011**, *38*, 572–581. [CrossRef]
11. Smith-Uffen, M.; Bartley, N.; Davies, G.; Best, M. Motivations and barriers to pursue cancer genomic testing: A systematic review. *Patient Educ. Couns.* **2021**, *104*, 1325–1334. [CrossRef] [PubMed]
12. Loeb, S.; Li, R.; Nolasco, T.S.; Ba, N.B.; Cheng, H.H.; Becker, D.; Leader, A.E.; Giri, V.N. Barriers and facilitators of germline genetic evaluation for prostate cancer. *Prostate* **2021**, *81*, 754–764. [CrossRef]
13. Delacroix, E.; Hanson, E.N.; Austin, S.; Carr, G.; Kidwell, K.M.; Griggs, J.J.; Stoffel, E.M.; Gerido, L.H.; Hawley, S.T.; Bacon, E.; et al. Effects of cancer type and sex on genetic testing for clinician recommendation and uptake. *J. Men's Health* **2023**, *19*, 23–30.
14. Greve, V.; Odom, K.; Pudner, S.; Lamb, N.E.; Cooper, S.J.; East, K. Characteristics and experiences of patients from a community-based and consumer-directed hereditary cancer population screening initiative. *HGG Adv.* **2022**, *3*, 100055. [CrossRef] [PubMed]
15. Mallen, A.R.; Conley, C.C.; Fuzzell, L.; Ketcher, D.; Augusto, B.M.; McIntyre, M.; Barton, L.V.; Townsend, M.K.; Fridley, B.L.; Tworoger, S.S.; et al. I think that a brief conversation from their provider can go a very long way": Patient and provider perspectives on barriers and facilitators of genetic testing after ovarian cancer. *Support. Care Cancer* **2021**, *29*, 2663–2677. [CrossRef] [PubMed]
16. Vaimberg, E.; Demers, L.; Ford, E.; Sabatello, M.; Stevens, B.; Dasgupta, S. Project Inclusive Genetics: Exploring the impact of patient-centered counseling training on physical disability bias in the prenatal setting. *PLoS ONE* **2021**, *16*, e0255722. [CrossRef]
17. Scott, D.; Friedman, S.; Telli, M.L.; Kurian, A.W. Decision Making About Genetic Testing Among Women With a Personal and Family History of Breast Cancer. *JCO Oncol. Pract.* **2020**, *16*, e37–e55. [CrossRef]
18. Muller, C.; Lee, S.M.; Barge, W.; Siddique, S.M.; Berera, S.; Wideroff, G.; Tondon, R.; Chang, J.; Peterson, M.; Stoll, J.; et al. Low Referral Rate for Genetic Testing in Racially and Ethnically Diverse Patients Despite Universal Colorectal Cancer Screening. *Clin. Gastroenterol. Hepatol.* **2018**, *16*, 1911–1918.e2. [CrossRef]

19. Vysotskaia, V.; Kaseniit, K.E.; Bucheit, L.; Ready, K.; Price, K.; Johansen Taber, K. Clinical utility of hereditary cancer panel testing: Impact of PALB2, ATM, CHEK2, NBN, BRIP1, RAD51C, and RAD51D results on patient management and adherence to provider recommendations. *Cancer* **2020**, *126*, 549–558. [CrossRef]
20. Halverson, C.M.E.; Wessinger, B.C.; Clayton, E.W.; Wiesner, G.L. Patients' willingness to reconsider cancer genetic testing after initially declining: Mention it again. *J. Genet. Couns.* **2020**, *29*, 18–24. [CrossRef]
21. Krakow, M.; Ratcliff, C.L.; Hesse, B.W.; Greenberg-Worisek, A.J. Assessing Genetic Literacy Awareness and Knowledge Gaps in the US Population: Results from the Health Information National Trends Survey. *Public Health Genom.* **2017**, *20*, 343–348. [CrossRef] [PubMed]
22. Gerido, L.H.; Griggs, J.J.; Resnicow, K.; Kidwell, K.M.; Delacroix, E.; Austin, S.; Hanson, E.N.; Bacon, E.; Koeppe, E.; Goodall, S.; et al. The Michigan Genetic Hereditary Testing (MiGHT) study's innovative approaches to promote uptake of clinical genetic testing among cancer patients: A study protocol for a 3-arm randomized controlled trial. *Trials* **2023**, *24*, 105. [CrossRef] [PubMed]
23. NCCN®. *NCCN Referencing Guidance*; NCCN: Plymouth Meeting, PA, USA, 2024; pp. 1–2. Available online: https://www.nccn.org/docs/default-source/business-policy/nccn-referencing-guidance.pdf?sfvrsn=ad8525f_2 (accessed on 28 May 2025).
24. Wing, S.E.; Hu, H.; Lopez, L.; Solomon, I.; Shen, J.; Raquel, C.; Sur, M.; Chao, J.; Cristea, M.; Fakih, M.; et al. Recall of Genomic Testing Results Among Patients with Cancer. *Oncologist* **2021**, *26*, e2302–e2305. [CrossRef] [PubMed]
25. Jacobs, C.; Dancyger, C.; Smith, J.A.; Michie, S. Accuracy of recall of information about a cancer-predisposing BRCA1/2 gene mutation among patients and relatives. *Eur. J. Hum. Genet.* **2015**, *23*, 147–151. [CrossRef]
26. For the PROMISE study team; Hann, K.E.J.; Freeman, M.; Fraser, L.; Waller, J.; Sanderson, S.C.; Rahman, B.; Side, L.; Gessler, S.; Lanceley, A. Awareness, knowledge, perceptions, and attitudes towards genetic testing for cancer risk among ethnic minority groups: A systematic review. *BMC Public Health* **2017**, *17*, 503. [CrossRef]

cancers

MDPI

Article

Relationship Among Body Mass Index, Survival, Cancer Treatment and Health-Related Quality of Life Among Older Patients with Bladder Cancer

Mitesh Rajpurohit [1,†], Mojgan Golzy [1,*,†], Nai-Wei Chen [1], Katie S. Murray [2] and Geoffrey Rosen [3,4]

[1] Department of Biomedical Informatics, Biostatistics and Medical Epidemiology, University of Missouri at Columbia, Columbia, MO 65201, USA; mrrf9t@health.missouri.edu (M.R.); naiwei.chen@health.missouri.edu (N.-W.C.)

[2] Department of Urology, NYU-Langone Health, New York, NY 10016, USA; katie.murray@nyulangone.org

[3] Department of Urology, Oregon Health & Science University, Portland, OR 97201, USA; geoff.rosen@gmail.com

[4] Division of Urology, Department of Surgery, VA Portland Health Care, Portland, OR 97239, USA

* Correspondence: golzym@health.missouri.edu; Tel.: +1-573-8842348

† These authors contributed equally to this work.

Simple Summary: This study explored how body weight (measured by BMI) affects survival, quality of life, and daily activities in older adults with bladder cancer. We analyzed data from over 8000 patients aged 65 and older and found that people with higher BMI (overweight or obese) tended to live longer after bladder cancer diagnosis than those with a normal or underweight BMI. Overweight patients also reported the best overall physical and mental well-being. However, severe obesity came with downsides—these individuals had the most difficulty performing daily tasks like bathing and dressing. Meanwhile, underweight patients also struggled with daily activities. The findings suggest that while extra weight may improve survival and, to some extent, quality of life, extreme obesity can reduce a person's ability to stay independent. This study highlights the complex relationship between body weight, survival, and well-being in older adults with bladder cancer.

Abstract: Background: The relationship between body composition and bladder cancer outcomes is complex. While a higher body mass index (BMI) has been associated with an increased risk of bladder cancer development, its impact on survival outcomes is less clear. This study aimed to explore the association between BMI, survival, health-related quality of life, and the performance of ADLs in a cohort of older patients with bladder cancer. Methods: Data were obtained from the Surveillance, Epidemiology, and End Results-Medicare Health Outcomes Survey, including patients diagnosed with bladder cancer who had recorded BMI values. Analysis of variance was used to assess the association between BMI categories and patient demographics as well as cancer/treatment characteristics. Generalized linear models examined the impact of BMI on health-related quality of life, as measured by the physical and mental component summary scores when controlling for confounding variables. Kaplan–Meier survival curves across BMI categories were compared using log-rank tests. Results: The final cohort consisted of 8013 patients (age ≥ 65) with a mean age of 77.7 ± 7.1 years, the majority of whom were White (85.6%) and male (74.8%). We observed no significant association between BMI and cancer/treatment characteristics. The severely obese subgroup had the highest rate of disability in performing ADLs (18.3%) followed by the underweight subgroup (10.3%). Overweight patients exhibited the highest physical and mental component summary scores, indicating better health-related quality of life. BMI was a significant predictor of overall

https://doi.org/10.3390/cancers17071200

survival, with overweight, obese, and severely obese patients demonstrating improved survival compared to those with healthy or underweight BMI. These findings remained statistically significant in multivariable analysis. Conclusions: Our findings suggest a dual role of BMI in older patients with bladder cancer: higher BMI provides a survival advantage and, to an extent, a QoL advantage. At the same time, severe obesity did lead to the lowest QoL despite improved survival outcomes. These results underscore the complex interplay between BMI, survival, and QoL in this bladder cancer population.

Keywords: health-related quality of life; activity of daily living; bladder cancer; body mass index; physical and component summary scores

1. Background

Bladder cancer (BC) is a disease found mostly in the population aged 55 and above with an average age at diagnosis of 73 [1]. In 2024 alone, it was estimated to have affected 83,190 individuals in the United States and led to 16,840 deaths [2]. Following a BC diagnosis, patients often experience a significant decline in functional status and overall health compared to their pre-diagnosis state [3]. Poor general health and impaired ability to perform activities of daily living (ADLs) are among the strongest risk factors for depression in older BC patients [4]. The association between BC outcomes and body mass index (BMI) is widely researched. A 2023 umbrella review showed that being overweight and underweight were positively and negatively associated with increased incidences of BC, respectively [5,6].

Various studies have reported the effect of BC on activities of daily living (ADLs). A 2017 systematic review showed that almost half of those who are treated with radical cystectomy are frail or prefrail [7]. These individuals more frequently develop postoperative adverse events such as major complications and early mortality. Another study by Monfardini et al. found that more than 55% of patients with bladder and renal cancer had at least one Cumulative Illness Rating Scale grade three (severe) or four (extremely severe) comorbidity [8]. Persons affected by BC often have smoking exposure, high BMI, and are insufficiently active [9]. Our previous study demonstrated that patient clusters based on mental and physical functioning exhibit significantly different survival outcomes, independent of BC disease severity or treatment type [10]. Additionally, within two years of diagnosis, a quarter of BC patients experience substantial changes in quality of life [11]. The association between body mass index (BMI) and BC survival is not clear, with some studies showing better outcomes and others showing worse outcomes [12]. Some studies have found that patients with higher BMI had better survival within the first five years after radical cystectomy. Other studies have found that patients with higher BMI had better outcomes [13–15].

There is also considerable interest in the relationship between BMI and Health-Related Quality of Life (HRQoL) in BC survivors across settings [16–19]. Generally, a higher BMI is consistently linked to lower HRQoL, highlighting the negative impact of obesity on survivors' well-being [20]. However, the studies also reveal variability in the magnitude of these effects, pointing to the influence of demographic, clinical, and treatment-related variables.

This study aims to clarify the relationship between BMI, HRQoL, and survival in BC patients aged 65 and older. Herein, we will (1) evaluate the impact of BMI on health-related quality of life (HRQoL) in patients with BC and (2) assess the association between BMI and survival in these patients.

2. Methods

Study Design: This is a population-based retrospective cross-sectional cohort study conducted using the Surveillance, Epidemiology, and End Results-Medicare Health Outcomes Survey (SEER-MHOS).

Study Population: This study utilized data from the SEER-MHOS database spanning 1999 to 2021 [21,22]. SEER-MHOS offers a unique opportunity for cancer research by integrating cancer-specific data with health-related quality of life (HRQOL) information for Medicare Advantage enrollees. This large, longitudinal dataset enables the investigation of long-term cancer impacts on HRQOL, encompassing physical, emotional, and social well-being, as well as the reverse relationship.

Our study focused on older patients with bladder cancer (BC). We included individuals aged $\geq$ 65 years who had a documented BC diagnosis and a recorded body mass index (BMI), our primary variable of interest. To ensure a more homogeneous study population, we excluded patients with a survival duration of less than six months, minimizing potential confounding from individuals experiencing rapid mortality.

For patients with multiple records, we selected the most recent survey as the baseline to ensure consistency in follow-up calculations for survival analysis. Given that some patients had recurrent BC diagnoses, older survey records—some dating back as far as a decade—might not accurately represent their current health status. Therefore, we prioritized the most recent survey to capture the latest clinical information, enhancing the relevance and reliability of our analysis.

Data Quality: The SEER-MHOS dataset maintains high data quality through rigorous auditing and validation processes. These measures ensure that the resource remains a reliable and valuable tool for cancer research. SEER-MHOS spans over two decades (1999–2021), providing a large sample for analyzing long-term trends. Additionally, SEER captures approximately 28% of the U.S. population, offering comprehensive cancer surveillance data with demographic diversity [23]. SEER-MHOS maintains high data quality through rigorous data collection protocols, periodic audits, and standardized validation processes. SEER follows strict case ascertainment procedures, while MHOS ensures self-reported HRQOL measures are collected consistently across survey cycles [22]. The linkage between SEER and MHOS allows researchers to study cancer patients' health outcomes with high reliability.

Outcome Measures: Outcome variables of interest included (1) HRQoL measured by the physical component summary (PCS), and mental component summary (MCS), (2) overall ability to perform ADLs (ADLs), and (3) survival.

The physical component summary (PCS) is a comprehensive measure of physical health, derived from responses across multiple domains, including physical functioning, role limitations due to physical health, bodily pain, and general health perceptions. It is a summary score ranging from 0 to 100, with a higher score indicating better physical health. The mental component summary (MCS) is a comprehensive measure of mental health, derived from responses across multiple domains, including general mental health, role limitations due to emotional problems, social functioning, and vitality. Like the PCS, it is a summary score ranging from 0 to 100, with a higher score indicating better mental health [24]. ADLs consist of bathing, dressing, eating, sitting on/standing up from a chair, walking, and using the toilet. The overall ADL ability was classified into three categories: "No difficulty in any ADL", "Difficulty in at least one ADL", and "Disability in at least one ADL".

Independent Variable: The primary independent variable was BMI (kg/m^2), with the following classifications: BMI < 18.5 as "Underweight"; 18.5 $\leq$ BMI < 25 as "Normal weight"; 25 ≤ BMI < 30 as "Overweight"; 30 ≤ BMI < 40 as "Obesity"; and 40 ≤ BMI as "Severe obesity".

Covariates: Additional baseline characteristics (including age, gender, race, marital status, home ownership, education level, income, and smoking status); cancer characteristics (including surgery, chemotherapy, and stage of cancer); comorbidities (including muscular disease, depressive symptoms for more than two weeks of the last year, pre-existing comorbid health conditions [computed as a summed disease burden of self-reported physician diagnosed hypertension, cardio-vascular disease, chronic pulmonary obstruction disease, diabetes mellitus, gastrointestinal disease, stroke, and other cancer]); and time from the first cancer diagnosis to the survey.

Statistical Analysis: Patient characteristics at the baseline were summarized with descriptive statistics and presented as frequencies (percentages) for categorical variables and means (standard deviations) for continuous variables in the text and table. Bivariate analyses were stratified by the level of BMI categories. The chi-square test of independence was used to assess the association of the categorical outcome (e.g., ADL) and BMI categories. Analysis of variance (ANOVA) was used to assess the association of numeric outcomes (e.g., HR-QoL, PCS, and MCS) and BMI categories. All assumptions were inspected, and a non-parametric test such as Kruskal–Wallis was used when the normality assumption was violated [25].

To further evaluate the effect of BMI categories on HR-QoL (e.g., PCS and MCS), a generalized linear model (GLM) was used, adjusting for covariates [26]. Covariates in the GLM model included age, gender, race, income, home ownership, education, smoking status, surgery type, chemotherapy, cancer stage, pre-existing depression symptoms, muscular disease, pre-existing comorbid health conditions, and time from the first cancer diagnosis to the survey. Residual analysis was applied to check assumptions in linear regression. To account for the skewness in the MCS, the Box–Cox transformation ($MCS_{cox} = [MCS^{\lambda} - 1]/\lambda$) was used with optimal lambda (λ) = 2.25 [27]. The effect of BMI categories was evaluated on the transformed the MCS in a multivariable GLM. Additionally, a log-rank test corresponding to Kaplan–Meier survival analysis was used to assess whether there was any significant difference in survival probability across BMI categories [28,29]. All tests of statistical significance were two-sided with a significance level of 0.05. Analyses were performed with SAS version 9.4 (SAS Institute, Inc., Cary, NC, USA) [30].

3. Results

We included 33,145 SEER-MHOS records of 18,827 patients with BC (Figure 1). We excluded 14,259 records prior to BC diagnosis, 565 records prior to age 65, and 539 records with less than 6 months of post-survey survival. We excluded 5001 records without BMI data. This left us with 12,781 surveys related to 8013 patients. We only included the last survey from each patient, leaving us with 8013 surveys from an equal number of patients.

The mean age at the time of survey of the sample set was 77.68 years with a standard deviation of 7.08 years. Most of the participants were male (74.8%) and White (85.6%). The majority were married (58.7%), homeowners (74.5%), high school graduates or less educated (54.7%), earning an annual income of USD 20,000 to 49,000 (37.9%), non-smokers (85.7%), and in the overweight BMI category (40.7%) (Table 1).

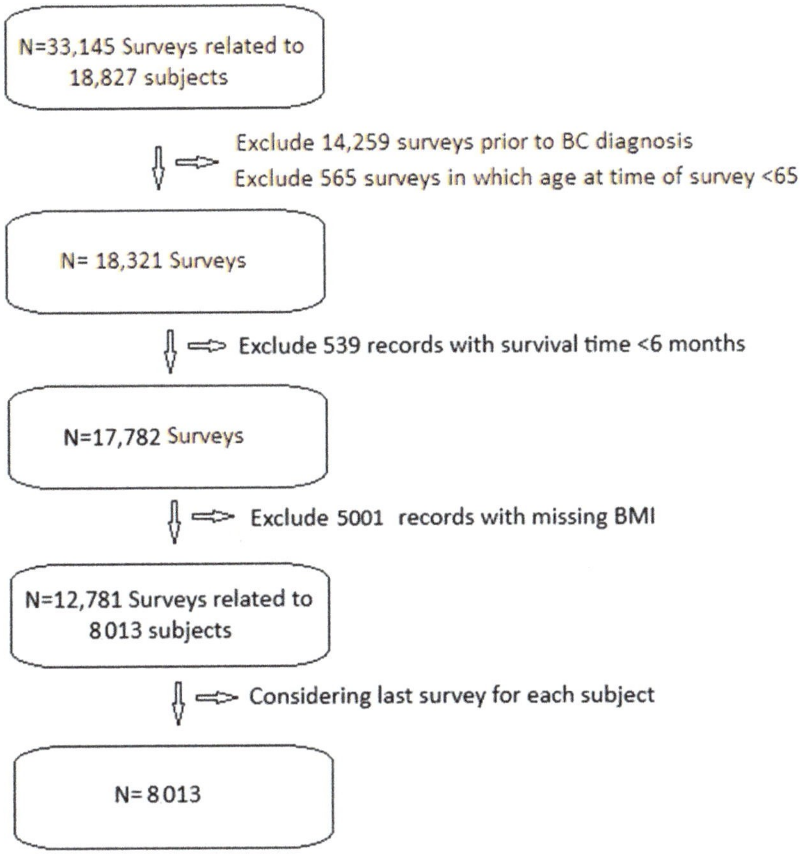

Figure 1. Study flow diagram.

Table 1. Summary statistics of demographic and socioeconomic variables.

Variables	Level	Overall (N = 8013)
Age at survey Mean (SD)		77.68 (7.08)
Gender: *n* (%)	Female	2017 (25.2%)
	Male	5996 (74.8%)
Marital status: *n* (%)	Married	4706 (58.7%)
	Other	3237 (40.4%)
	Unknown	70 (0.9%)
Home Ownership: *n* (%)	Owner	5966 (74.5%)
	Other	1803 (22.5%)
	Unknown	244 (3.0%)
Race: *n* (%)	White	6860 (85.6%)
	Hispanic	463 (5.8%)
	Black or African American	345 (4.3%)
	Asian or Pacific Islander	309 (3.9%)
	American Indian or Alaskan native	25 (0.3%)
	Another race or multi-race	11 (0.1%)

Table 1. *Cont.*

Variables	Level	Overall (N = 8013)
Education: *n* (%)	2–4 years	2640 (33.0%)
	Above 4 years	861 (10.7%)
	High school or less	4380 (54.7%)
	Unknown	132 (1.6%)
Income: *n* (%)	Less than USD 20,000	2026 (25.3%)
	USD 20,000—49,999	3036 (37.9%)
	USD 50,000 or more	1490 (18.6%)
	Unknown	1461 (18.2%)
Smoking status: *n* (%)	Yes	1025 (12.8%)
	Not at all	6865 (85.7%)
	Don't know or missing	123 (1.5%)
Body mass index group, kg/m^2: *n* (%)	Underweight (BMI < 18.5)	181 (2.3%)
	Healthy range (18.5 ≤ BMI < 25)	2638 (32.9%)
	Overweight (25 ≤ BMI < 30)	3258 (40.7%)
	Obesity (30 ≤ BMI < 40)	1756 (21.9%)
	Severe Obesity (40 ≤ BMI)	180 (2.2%)

3.1. Cancer Charateristics and BMI Association

The time from diagnosis to survey completion was correlated with time since cancer diagnosis, with the shortest interval for those with severe obesity and the longest for underweight individuals ($p < 0.001$, Table 2). Survival was also correlated with BMI ($p < 0.001$), with shortest survival for severe obese and underweight patients and longest survival for overweight patients.

Table 2. Mean and standard deviation of time in months since first cancer diagnosis to survey and survival time in months since time of survey.

	Overall	Underweight	Healthy	Overweight	Obesity	Severe Obesity
Months since first cancer diagnosis to survey ($p < 0.001$)	102 ± 84	118 ± 94	107 ± 88	101 ± 83	96 ± 79	87± 70
Survival time since survey ($p < 0.001$)	57 ± 37	41 ± 29	53 ± 37	60 ± 38	59 ± 38	53 ± 33

Months since first cancer diagnosis to survey reports the time elapsed from the initial diagnosis to study inclusion, regardless of potential disease-free intervals.

The cancer stage at diagnosis was not correlated with BMI at survey completion ($p = 0.17$, Table 3). Similarly, there was no statistically significant correlation between BMI and the type of surgical treatment ($p = 0.24$) or receipt of chemotherapy ($p = 0.57$).

Table 3. Distribution of cancer characteristics overall and by BMI categories.

Variables	Overall	Underweight	Healthy	Overweight	Obesity	Severe Obesity
Stage ($p = 0.17$)						
Non-muscle invasive	6519 (81%)	149 (82%)	2128 (81%)	2632 (81%)	1461 (83%)	149 (83%)
Muscle invasive	1196 (15%)	21 (12%)	405 (15%)	509 (16%)	234 (13%)	*
Metastatic	298 (3.7%)	*	105 (4.0%)	117 (3.6%)	61 (3.5%)	*

Table 3. *Cont.*

Variables	Overall	Underweight	Healthy	Overweight	Obesity	Severe Obesity
Surgery ($p = 0.24$)						
Cystectomy	980 (12%)	20 (11%)	343 (13%)	413 (13%)	187 (11%)	17 (9%)
Transurethral	3722 (46%)	86 (48%)	1230 (47%)	1526 (47%)	802 (46%)	88 (49%)
None/unknown	3311 (41%)	75 (41%)	1065 (40%)	1329 (41%)	767 (44%)	75 (42%)
Chemotherapy ($p = 0.57$)						
Yes	969 (12%)	17 (9%)	310 (12%)	414 (13%)	208 (12%)	20 (11%)
None/unknown	7044 (88%)	164 (91%)	2328 (88%)	2844 (87%)	1548 (88%)	160 (89%)

* Numbers are masked per CMS policy.

3.2. Physical and Mental Component Summary Scores and BMI Association

The overall mean PCS score in the sample population was 37.3 ± 12.1, with the highest score in the overweight category (38.5) and the lowest in the severe obesity category (30.7). The overall mean MCS score was 51.6 ± 11.4, with the highest mean observed in the overweight category (52.3) and the lowest in the severe obesity category (46.5) (Figure 2).

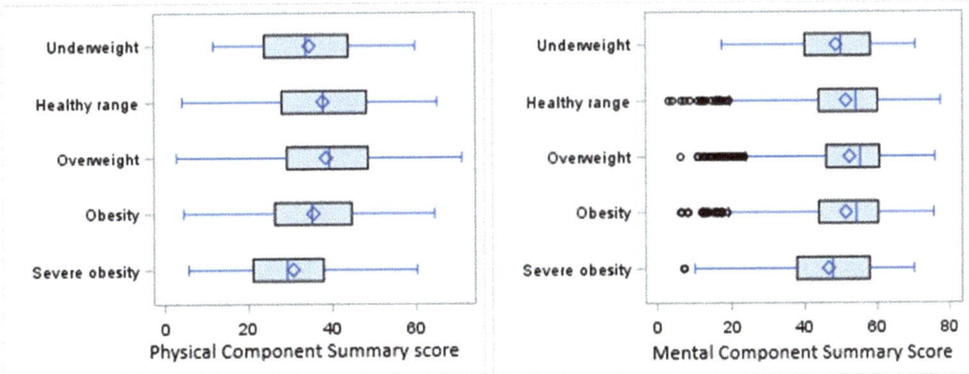

Figure 2. Box plots for PCS and MCS scores by BMI categories.

The results of ANOVA showed a significant difference in PCS scores among the BMI categories ($F_{(4,7495)} = 32.66$, $p < 0.0001$). The distribution of the MCS scores was right-skewed, and so the nonparametric Kruskal–Wallis (KW) test was performed for univariate analysis of the MCS scores, indicating a significant difference in distribution of the MCS among the BMI categories (KW *p*-value < 0.0001).

When looking at the PCS and MCS scores over time from 2007 to 2019, we observed a trend towards higher scores ($p < 0.0001$, Figure 3) for the MCS, signifying improved mental health over time. No significant overall change in the PCS scores was observed ($p = 0.9$). From 2007 to 2019, we observed a stable PCS score for the healthy-range, overweight, and obesity subgroups over time, a trend towards higher scores for the underweight subgroup, and a trend towards lower scores for sever obese subjects over time.

ADLs and BMI Association: There was a significant difference in ADL ability correlated with BMI ($p < 0.0001$, Table 4). Severely obese individuals had the highest percentage of individuals with at least one ADL difficulty (57.8%) and the highest for disabilities (18.5%), while underweight and obese patients had similar levels of overall disability (45.4% having difficulty with one ADL and no disability for both). Healthy-range and overweight individuals had fewer ADL difficulties and disabilities, with a majority having no difficulties.

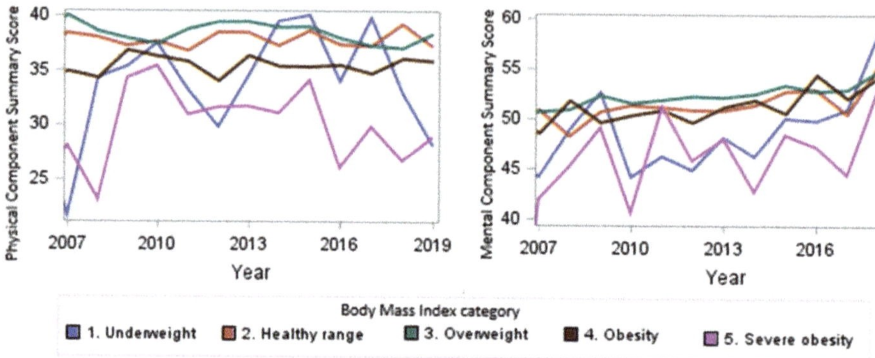

Figure 3. PCS and MCS score trends by year.

Table 4. Frequency and column percentages of overall ADL ability by BMI categories.

Ability to Perform ADLs * ($p < 0.0001$)	Underweight	Healthy Range	Overweight	Obesity	Severe Obesity
No difficulty in any ADLs	77 (44.3%)	1525 (59.3%)	1926 (60.8%)	838 (48.5%)	41 (23.7%)
Difficulty in at least one ADL	79 (45.4%)	867 (33.7%)	1103 (34.8%)	784 (45.4%)	100 (57.8%)
Disability in at least one ADL	18 (10.3%)	180 (7%)	141 (4.4%)	106 (6.1%)	32 (18.5%)

* Frequency missing = 196.

3.3. Survival Analysis by BMI

Kaplan–Meier survival analysis demonstrated that the median survival time after survey completion was 81.8 months. Our findings highlight a significant variability in survival outcomes among different BMI categories, with underweight and normal-weight individuals experiencing the worst survival (log-rank test $p < 0.0001$, Figure 4).

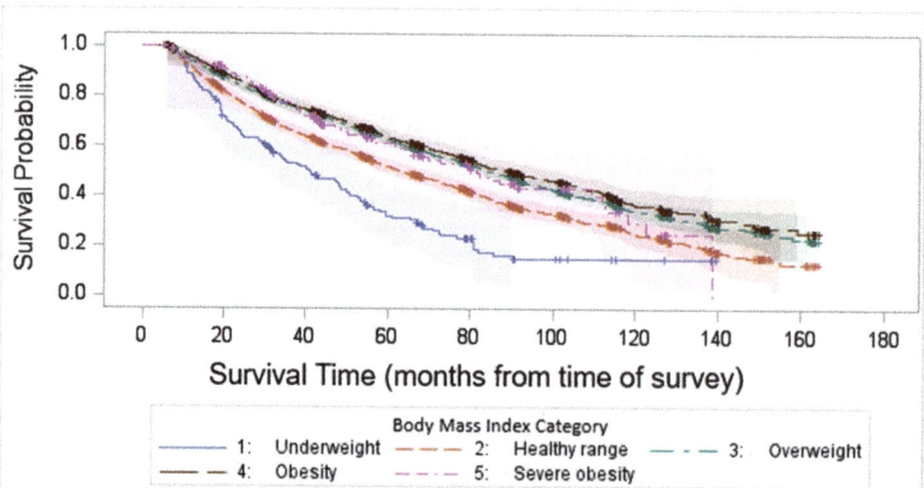

Figure 4. Kaplan–Meier survival time after survey completion by BMI categories.

We compared the KM survival curves among BMI groups with first BC diagnosis as the baseline, and we observed a similar result which shows the consistency of the result. Figure 5, rather than capturing uninterrupted disease duration, reports the time elapsed from the initial diagnosis to study inclusion, regardless of potential disease-free intervals.

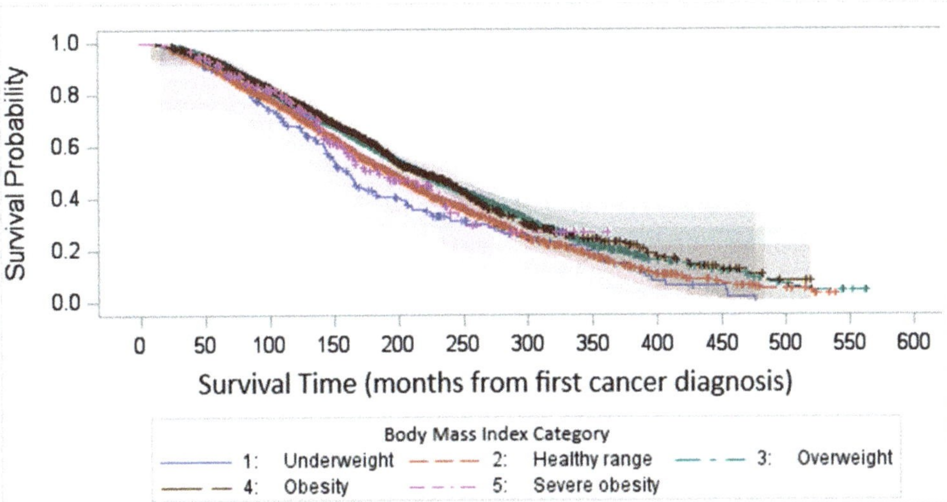

Figure 5. Kaplan–Meier survival time after first cancer diagnosis by BMI categories.

3.4. Multivariable Regression Analysis of PCS and MCS Outcomes

In multivariate analysis, with the normal range BMI as the reference, underweight, and severe obesity had significantly lower PCS and MCS scores (Table 5). Obese patients had significantly lower PCS scores, and overweight patients had significantly better mental health than the normal range BMI. Modeling results also revealed that age is negatively associated with both the PCS and MCS results, indicating that older age results in lower scores. Race and gender were not associated with the PCS, but females and White participants had a significantly better MCS outcome. Variables such as depression symptoms, non-house ownership, low income, and the number of comorbidities were linked to significantly lower PCS and MCS scores. Smoking, muscular diseases, and undergoing cystectomy are also linked to significantly lower PCS scores. The bladder cancer stage, surgical intervention, receipt of intravenous chemotherapy, and time from the first cancer diagnosis to the survey were not significantly associated with the MCS outcome. The time from the first cancer diagnosis to the survey has no significant effect on either the PCS (p = 0.4066) or MCS scores (p = 0.9082).

Table 5. Estimates of effect of patient characteristics on PCS and transformed MCS outcomes in multivariable GLMs.

	PCS Outcome			Transformed MCS Outcome		
Variables	Estimate	SE	p Value	Estimate	SE	p Value
	BMI Group (reference: Healthy range)					
Underweight	−1.74	0.89	0.05	−199.88	104.24	0.0552
Overweight	0.34	0.30	0.2541	76.69	35.50	0.0308
Obesity	−2.15	0.36	<0.0001	27.40	42.66	0.5208
Severe obesity	−5.72	0.91	<0.0001	−321.00	106.35	0.0026
Age	−0.30	0.02	<0.0001	−5.68	2.29	0.0131

Table 5. *Cont.*

Variables	PCS Outcome Estimate	SE	*p* Value	Transformed MCS Outcome Estimate	SE	*p* Value
Time from first cancer diagnosis	0.00	0.00	0.4066	0.02	0.18	0.9082
Gender (reference: Male)						
Female	−0.36	0.30	0.2335	78.99	35.25	0.0251
Race (reference: White)						
Black or American African	0.56	0.64	0.3853	−256.98	75.43	0.0007
Other	−0.03	0.44	0.9536	−335.63	51.21	<0.0001
Depression (reference: No)						
Yes	−2.46	0.37	<0.0001	−1351.7	43.28	<0.0001
Muscular disease (reference: No)						
Yes	−0.51	0.33	0.1245	79.14	39.28	0.044
Surgery (reference: None/Unknown)						
Cystectomy	−1.07	0.48	0.0257	−25.02	56.47	0.6578
Transurethral	−0.31	0.29	0.2723	−30.89	33.47	0.356
Chemotherapy (reference: No)						
Yes	−0.43	0.41	0.2985	27.04	48.59	0.5779
Stage (reference: Non-muscle invasive)						
Metastatic	−0.18	0.70	0.7995	−55.37	81.70	0.498
Muscle invasive	0.19	0.41	0.6396	−39.42	48.29	0.4144
Income (reference: USD 20,000-49,999)						
≥USD 50,000	1.11	0.37	0.0028	137.17	43.73	0.0017
<USD 20,000/Unknown	−0.84	0.29	0.0044	−126.47	34.56	0.0003
Home Ownership (reference: Owner)						
Other	-0.98	0.31	0.0015	−205.11	36.09	<0.0001
Education (reference: High school or less)						
2–4 years	0.72	0.29	0.0128	104.81	33.76	0.0019
>4 years	2.07	0.45	<0.0001	125.71	52.75	0.0172
Smoker (reference: None/unknown)						
Yes	−2.08	0.39	<0.0001	−43.75	45.97	0.3413
Number of comorbidities (reference: 2 or fewer)						
≥5	−5.23	0.34	<0.0001	−153.73	39.57	0.0001
3 or 4	−11.07	0.42	<0.0001	−513.70	49.60	<0.0001

4. Discussion

Our final cohort data are in line with prior studies both in terms of age [1]. sex [31], and race [32]. Our study highlights the complex interplay between BMI, demographic factors, and patient-reported HRQoL outcomes in older patients with BC. The significant association between obesity and lower physical component summary (PCS) scores aligns with the previous literature, suggesting that excess body weight may contribute to physical limitations and reduced mobility, ultimately impacting overall physical well-being [20]. Our study indicates low PCS scores for underweight individuals as well. Interestingly, overweight individuals demonstrated significantly better mental component summary (MCS) scores compared to those with normal-range BMI, which may indicate potential psychological resilience or benefits associated with a slightly higher body weight [33].

Age was a determinant of both physical and mental health, with increasing age negatively associated with PCS and MCS scores. This finding is expected, as aging is often accompanied by a decline in physical function, increased comorbidities, and potential psychosocial challenges, such as reduced social engagement and loss of independence.

While race and gender did not significantly impact PCS scores, females and White individuals had significantly higher MCS scores. This may reflect differences in social support, healthcare access, coping mechanisms, or cultural perceptions of mental health, warranting further exploration into underlying psychosocial or systemic factors.

Socioeconomic and health-related variables played a significant role in both PCS and MCS outcomes. Depression symptoms, lower income, lack of home ownership, and a higher number of comorbidities were strongly linked to poorer HRQoL across both dimensions. These results underscore the importance of addressing social determinants of health in improving patient well-being. Additionally, smoking, muscular diseases, and undergoing cystectomy were associated with lower PCS scores, suggesting that these conditions contribute to significant physical health burdens.

The time from the first cancer diagnosis to the survey has no significant effect on either the PCS or MCS scores.

Notably, cancer-related variables such as cancer stage, surgery type, chemotherapy, and time from the first cancer diagnosis to the survey did not significantly impact MCS outcomes. This finding suggests that while cancer treatment can impose physical stress, mental health outcomes may be more influenced by pre-existing conditions, coping mechanisms, and social support rather than the specific cancer treatment characteristics.

Our findings also highlight a significant variability in survival outcomes among different BMI categories, with underweight and normal-weight individuals experiencing the worst survival. This aligns with prior research suggesting that low BMI may be associated with higher frailty, reduced physiological reserves, and increased vulnerability to disease-related complications [34]. The poor survival in the underweight group may reflect underlying malnutrition, muscle wasting (sarcopenia), or more advanced disease states at original diagnosis.

Interestingly, overweight and obese individuals demonstrated better survival outcomes [15]. Several other studies also reported that higher BMI is associated with better survival in bladder cancer patients [35,36]. While obesity is typically associated with higher risks of chronic diseases, higher BMI in bladder cancer patients may provide protective benefits. These may include greater metabolic reserves during periods of severe illness, better tolerance to treatment-related stress, and differences in inflammatory responses. However, it remains unclear whether these benefits are directly due to excess body weight or other underlying factors such as muscle mass, nutritional status, or differences in treatment received.

We compared Kaplan–Meier (KM) survival curves among BMI groups using two different baseline time points: the time of the survey (Figure 4) and the first cancer diagnosis (Figure 5). This analysis aimed to identify any inconsistencies between the approaches. Our findings demonstrated a consistent pattern across both methods. In this dataset, the average time from the first bladder cancer (BC) diagnosis to the most recent survey (i.e., inclusion in the study) was 8.5 years (102 months). However, it is important to acknowledge that BC can recur following initial treatment. For patients with recurrent BC, there may have been periods of disease-free survival between episodes of recurrence.

4.1. Limitations

This study has several limitations that should be considered when interpreting the findings. In terms of sample selection, our analysis was based on data obtained from the SEER–MHOS database, which comprises survey information on bladder cancer patients enrolled in the Medicare Advantage Program from participating registries. As a result, the study population may not fully represent the diverse demographics of the broader U.S. population, nor can the findings be generalized to other countries. Nonetheless, our data are in line with prior studies both in terms of age [1], sex [31], and race [32].

As BMI was the main variable of interest, we excluded individuals with missing BMI, which may introduce the potential for selection bias if the missingness is not random, as these individuals may differ systematically from those included in the analysis. This study occurred over a long timeframe over which the management of bladder cancer significantly changed, and it continues to do so.

Regarding study design, the cross-sectional nature of this study limits its ability to establish causality and exploration of temporal relationships between BMI, physical and mental component summary (PCS and MCS) scores, and activities of daily living (ADLs) disabilities. Consequently, causal inferences or longitudinal insights into these associations cannot be drawn from the current findings.

4.2. Strengths of the Study

The SEER-MHOS data resource is one of the most comprehensive resources available for analyzing cancer patients. It provides a unique opportunity for cancer research by combining cancer-specific data with health-related quality of life (HRQOL) information for Medicare Advantage enrollees. This is a unique and large dataset that gives researchers the opportunity to study the long-term impact of cancer on health-related quality of life, including physical, emotional, and social well-being. Additionally, it can be used to compare cancer survival among different populations.

5. Conclusions

Our study underscores the multifaceted relationship between BMI, demographic and socioeconomic factors, and HRQoL outcomes, as well as survival disparities among BMI categories for older patients with bladder cancer. Future research should aim to further explore the mechanisms driving these associations and investigate targeted interventions to improve HRQoL and survival outcomes, particularly for high-risk groups such as underweight individuals and those with socioeconomic disadvantages. Integrating personalized treatment strategies that consider both physical and mental health factors could lead to better overall patient outcomes and quality of life.

Author Contributions: K.S.M. and M.G. purchased the bladder cancer data from SEER-MHOS for the WU ICTS grant. G.R. and M.G. conceptualized the initial idea. M.G. and M.R. analyzed the data, interpreted the results, and drafted the manuscript. N.-W.C. contributed to substantially revising the manuscript. All authors reviewed the manuscript. All authors have read and agreed to the published version of the manuscript.

Funding: This research received no external funding.

Institutional Review Board Statement: Approved by University of Missouri IRB via waiver as no patient identifiers included.

Informed Consent Statement: For SEER-MHOS data, investigators are not required to obtain individual patient consent because the data are considered a limited dataset, exempt from additional HIPAA requirements. However, the investigators have agreed to the SEER-MHOS Data Use Agreement (DUA) and adhered to specific data handling and security protocols.

Data Availability Statement: Data for this study were obtained from the SEER-MHOS link data resource. The SEER-MHOS database is available to outside investigators for research purposes (please see https://healthcaredelivery.cancer.gov/seer-mhos/obtain/overview.html) (accessed on 31 March 2025).

Conflicts of Interest: The authors declare that they have no competing interests.

List of Abbreviations

BC	Bladder cancer
BMI	Body mass index.
SEER-MHOS	Surveillance: Epidemiology, and End Results-Medicare Health Outcomes Survey
PCS	Physical component summary
MCS	Mental component summary
ADL	ADL
HR-QoL	Health-related quality of life
ANOVA	Analysis of variance.
GLM	Generalized linear model
KW	Kruskal–Wallis

References

1. Siegel, R.L.; Giaquinto, A.N.; Jemal, A. Cancer statistics, 2024. *CA Cancer J. Clin.* **2024**, *74*, 12–49. [CrossRef]
2. American Cancer Society. Key Statistics for Bladder Cancer. Available online: https://www.cancer.org/cancer/types/bladder-cancer/about/key-statistics.html (accessed on 16 April 2024).
3. Ungerer, G.; Anwar, T.; Golzy, M.; Murray, K.S. Living with Bladder Cancer: Self-reported Changes in Patients' Functional and Overall Health Status Following Diagnosis. *Eur. Urol. Open Sci.* **2020**, *20*, 14–19. [CrossRef] [PubMed] [PubMed Central]
4. Oserowsky, A.; Anwar, T.; Lough, C.; Golzy, M.; Murray, K.S. The Significant Role of Depression in Elderly Patients with Bladder Cancer. *Eur. Urol. Open Sci.* **2021**, *33*, 11–18. [CrossRef] [PubMed] [PubMed Central]
5. Zhao, L.; Tian, X.; Duan, X.; Ye, Y.; Sun, M.; Huang, J. Association of body mass index with bladder cancer risk: A dose-response meta-analysis of prospective cohort studies. *Oncotarget* **2017**, *8*, 33990–34000. [CrossRef] [PubMed] [PubMed Central]
6. Chen, J.; Ke, K.; Liu, Z.; Yang, L.; Wang, L.; Zhou, J.; Dong, Q. Body Mass Index and Cancer Risk: An Umbrella Review of Meta-Analyses of Observational Studies. *Nutr. Cancer* **2023**, *75*, 1051–1064. [CrossRef] [PubMed]
7. Ethun, C.G.; Bilen, M.A.; Jani, A.B.; Maithel, S.K.; Ogan, K.; Master, V.A. Frailty and cancer: Implications for oncology surgery, medical oncology, and radiation oncology. *CA Cancer J. Clin.* **2017**, *67*, 362–377. [CrossRef] [PubMed]
8. Monfardini, S.; Morlino, S.; Valdagni, R.; Catanzaro, M.; Tafa, A.; Bortolato, B.; Petralia, G.; Bonetto, E.; Villa, E.; Picozzi, S.; et al. Follow-up of elderly patients with urogenital cancers: Evaluation of geriatric care needs and related actions. *J. Geriatr. Oncol.* **2017**, *8*, 289–295. [CrossRef]
9. Catto, J.W.F.; Rogers, Z.; Downing, A.; Mason, S.J.; Jubber, I.; Bottomley, S.; Conner, M.; Absolom, K.; Glaser, A. Lifestyle Variables in Patients with Bladder Cancer: A Contemporary Picture of Tobacco Smoking, Electronic Cigarette Use, BMI, and Levels of Physical Activity. *Eur. Urol. Focus* **2023**, *9*, 974–982. [CrossRef] [PubMed]
10. Golzy, M.; Beheshti, M.; Henslee, B.; Rosen, G.H.; Murray, K.S. Transition in Quality Of Life Among Older Patients With Bladder Cancer and Its Association With Treatment: A Clustering Approach. *JU Open Plus* **2024**, *2*, e00090. [CrossRef]
11. Golzy, M.; Rosen, G.H.; Kruse, R.L.; Hooshmand, K.; Mehr, D.R.; Murray, K.S. Holistic Assessment of Quality of Life Predicts Survival in Older Patients with Bladder Cancer. *Urology* **2023**, *174*, 141–149. [CrossRef] [PubMed]
12. Arthuso, F.Z.; Fairey, A.S.; Boulé, N.G.; Courneya, K.S. Associations between body mass index and bladder cancer survival: Is the obesity paradox short-lived? *Can. Urol. Assoc. J.* **2022**, *16*, E261–E267. [CrossRef] [PubMed] [PubMed Central]
13. Chromecki, T.F.; Cha, E.K.; Fajkovic, H.; Rink, M.; Ehdaie, B.; Svatek, R.S.; Karakiewicz, P.I.; Lotan, Y.; Tilki, D.; Bastian, P.J.; et al. Obesity is associated with worse oncological outcomes in patients treated with radical cystectomy. *BJU Int.* **2013**, *111*, 249–255. [CrossRef] [PubMed]
14. Dabi, Y.; Rouscoff, Y.; Anract, J.; Delongchamps, N.B.; Sibony, M.; Saighi, D.; Zerbib, M.; Peyraumore, M.; Xylinas, E. Impact of body mass index on the oncological outcomes of patients treated with radical cystectomy for muscle-invasive bladder cancer. *World J. Urol.* **2017**, *35*, 229–235. [CrossRef]
15. Giert, M.; Zeman, F.; Denzinger, S.; Vetterlein, M.W.; Fisch, M.; Bastian, P.J.; Syring, I.; Ellinger, J.; Müller, S.C.; Herrmann, E.; et al. Influence of body mass index on clinical outcome parameters, complication rate and survival after radical cystectomy: Evidence from a prospective, European, multicenter study. *Urol. Int.* **2018**, *101*, 16–24. [CrossRef]
16. Revicki, D.A.; Kleinman, L.; Cella, D. A history of health-related quality of life outcomes in psychiatry. *Dialogues Clin. Neurosci.* **2014**, *16*, 127–135. [CrossRef]
17. Yin, S.; Njai, R.; Barker, L.; Siegel, P.Z.; Liao, Y. Summarizing health-related quality of life (HRQOL): Development and testing of a one-factor model. *Popul. Health Metr.* **2016**, *14*, 22. [CrossRef] [PubMed]
18. Carmona-Torres, J.M.; Rodriguez-Borrego, M.A.; Laredo-Aguilera, J.A.; Lopez-Soto, P.J.; Santacruz-Salas, E.; Cobo-Cuenca, A.I. Disability for basic and instrumental ADL in older individuals. *PLoS ONE* **2019**, *14*, e0220157. [CrossRef]

19. Katz, S. Assessing self-maintenance: ADL, mobility, and instrumental ADL. *J. Am. Geriatr. Soc.* **1983**, *31*, 721–727. [CrossRef]
20. Chung, J.; Kulkarni, G.S.; Bender, J.; Breau, R.H.; Guttman, D.; Maganti, M.; Matthew, A.; Morash, R.; Papadakos, J.; Jones, J.M. Modifiable lifestyle behaviours impact the health-related quality of life of bladder cancer survivors. *BJU Int.* **2020**, *125*, 836–842. [CrossRef] [PubMed] [PubMed Central]
21. SEER-Medicare Health Outcomes Survey (SEER-MHOS) Linked Data Resource-National Cancer Institute. Available online: https://healthcaredelivery.cancer.gov/seer-mhos/ (accessed on 26 March 2025).
22. Ambs, A.; Warren, J.L.; Bellizzi, K.M.; Topor, M.; Haffer, S.C.; Clauser, S.B. Overview of the SEER--Medicare Health Outcomes Survey linked dataset. *Health Care Financ. Rev.* **2008**, *29*, 5–21. [PubMed] [PubMed Central]
23. SEER-MHOS: Data Documentation and Methods. National Cancer Institute (NCI). USA. 2023. Available online: https://healthcaredelivery.cancer.gov/seer-mhos/aboutdata/documentation.html (accessed on 26 March 2025).
24. Ware, J.E.; Sherbourne, C.D. The MOS 36-Item Short-Form Health Survey (SF-36): I. Conceptual Framework and Item Selection. *Med. Care* **1992**, *30*, 473–483. Available online: https://www.jstor.org/stable/3765916 (accessed on 25 March 2025).
25. Kruskal, W.H.; Wallis, W.A. Use of ranks in one-criterion variance analysis. *J. Am. Stat. Assoc.* **1952**, *47*, 583–621. [CrossRef]
26. Nelder, J.A.; Wedderburn, R.W. Generalized Linear Models. *J. R. Stat. Soc. Ser. A (Gen.)* **1972**, *135*, 370–384. [CrossRef]
27. Box, G.E.P.; Cox, D.R. An analysis of transformations. *J. Roy. Statist. Soc. B* **1964**, *26*, 211–252.
28. Kaplan, E.L.; Meier, P. Nonparametric estimation from incomplete observations. *J. Amer. Statist. Assoc.* **1958**, *53*, 457–481. [CrossRef]
29. Mantel, N. Evaluation of survival data and two new rank order statistics arising in its consideration. *Cancer Chemother. Rep.* **1966**, *50*, 163–170. [PubMed]
30. *SAS 9.4 Help Documentation*; SAS Institute Inc: Cary, NC, USA, 2023.
31. Bladder Cancer Statistics from MOFFIT Cancer Center. Available online: https://www.moffitt.org/cancers/bladder-cancer/faqs/bladder-cancer-statistics/ (accessed on 19 March 2025).
32. Fang, W.; Yang, Z.; Chen, T.; Shen, X.; Zhang, C. Ethnicity and survival in bladder cancer: A population-based study based on the SEER database. *J. Transl. Med.* **2020**, *18*, 145. [CrossRef] [PubMed]
33. Zheng, N.; Zhuang, M.; Zhu, Y.; Wang, Y.; Ye, M.; Zhang, Y.; Zhan, Y. Association between psychological resilience and body mass index in a community-based population: A cross-sectional study. *Obes. Sci. Pract.* **2024**, *10*, e761. [CrossRef] [PubMed] [PubMed Central]
34. Clegg, A.; Young, J.; Iliffe, S.; Rikkert, M.O.; Rockwood, K. Frailty in elderly people. *Lancet* **2013**, *381*, 752–762. [CrossRef] [PubMed] [PubMed Central]
35. Bi, H.; Huang, Y.; Wang, G.; Ma, L.; Lu, M. Impact of body mass index and pretreatment hemoglobin level on prognosis following radical cystectomy for bladder cancer in males and females. *Urol. Int.* **2020**, *104*, 28–35. [CrossRef]
36. Psutka, S.P.; Boorjian, S.A.; Moynagh, M.R.; Schmit, G.D.; Frank, I.; Carrasco, A.; Stewart, S.B.; Tarrell, R.; Thapa, P.; Tollefson, M.K. Mortality after radical cystectomy: Impact of obesity vs. adiposity after adjusting for skeletal muscle wasting. *J. Urol.* **2015**, *193*, 1507–1513. [CrossRef]

cancers

MDPI

Article

The Impact of Homelessness on Lung Cancer Survival and Healthcare Utilization in the Hungarian Universal Healthcare System

Daniel Heilig [1], Ákos Szabó [2], Petra Fadgyas-Freyler [3] and Judit Simon [1,3,*]

1 Department of Health Economics, Center for Public Health, Medical University of Vienna, 1090 Vienna, Austria; daniel.heilig@meduniwien.ac.at
2 Department of Financial Accounting, Corvinus University of Budapest, 1093 Budapest, Hungary
3 Department of Health Policy, Corvinus University of Budapest, 1093 Budapest, Hungary
* Correspondence: judit.simon@meduniwien.ac.at

Simple Summary: This study looks at the health effects of homelessness in subjects diagnosed with lung cancer in a nationwide dataset in Hungary. Healthcare costs and survival analysis showed worse outcomes, with the length of experienced homelessness playing a key role.

Abstract: Differences in the lifestyle and health-service-seeking behavior of persons experiencing homelessness (PEH) are well known. However, a comprehensive estimation of the resulting healthcare utilization differences and health outcome impacts are so far under-researched, especially at the national level. We aim to close this gap of evidence for lung cancer within the Hungarian universal healthcare system. We analyzed lung cancer-related information for the PEH population in the Hungarian national central health insurance register dataset and a matched control population between 2015 and 2021. In this period, 11,857 people were registered as homeless for the majority of at least one year. To capture the effect of homelessness, we created a categorical "homelessness length index" (HLI) according to the proportion of time an individual experienced homelessness during the investigation period (HLI 0: 0; HLI 1: >0–1/3; HLI 2: >1/3–2/3; HLI 3: >2/3). PEH individuals were matched 1:5 with a non-PEH control sample adjusted for age, sex and region. We conducted Kaplan–Meier survival analysis and Cox proportional hazards (CPH) regression adjusted for age, sex, HLI and average lung cancer-related healthcare costs. Our final analysis sample consisted of 641 patients (233 PEH, 408 control) who were newly diagnosed with lung cancer during the observation period. The lung cancer prevalence in the PEH group was 1.97% as opposed to 0.69% in the control group. The Kaplan–Meier curve showed lower average survival times for the PEH group, compared to the control group. Lung cancer associated costs between diagnosis and death/censoring were substantially different with average per patient cumulative costs of EUR 3668 in the PEH group compared to EUR 6827 in the control group (2018 prices). This translated to an average 47% lower annual lung cancer-related healthcare cost per PEH patient. CPH analysis showed that after disease severity, the degree of time spent in homelessness had the most significant effect on mortality, with a HR of 1.47 associated with both HLI 2 and 3 (95% CI: 1.08–2.00 and 1.01–2.14, respectively). We find that in Hungary, homelessness is associated with a much higher lung cancer burden linked to a three-times-higher prevalence, lower overall survival and almost 50% lower annualized disease-specific healthcare costs. Worse outcomes are mainly driven by long-term homelessness. Results could not be further refined according to lifestyle-related factors due to data availability limitations.

Keywords: homelessness; lung cancer; survival analysis; healthcare costs; public health

1. Introduction

Many studies have noted the detrimental health effects of homelessness. A recent review and meta-analysis covering related studies found worse outcomes for people experiencing homelessness (PEH) in virtually all disease fields and all-cause mortality [1]. The definitions for homelessness can include different types but most broadly, a PEH is defined as a person lacking a fixed, adequate nighttime residence [2]. Nationwide studies on the health effects of homelessness, however, are virtually nonexistent due to homelessness being an issue that is rarely found in national databases with widespread coverage, due to PEH having no official insurance status or claim. This generally does not mean PEH receive no health care, but rather that examining healthcare utilization is not feasible. This study is based on Hungarian health insurance data with the unique opportunity to quantify the effects of homelessness on disease outcomes and healthcare utilization due to universal health coverage at the national level including PEH.

Lung cancer is the most common cancer-related cause of death worldwide, according to the World Health Organization (WHO) [3]. It has similar high mortality rates for both sexes but shows differences in outcomes across the socioeconomic spectrum [4]. It is also the most common cancer in the homeless population of a previous study [5]. These factors make it a suitable disease to compare survival outcomes between PEH and a control population. If a difference in survival is observed, it is also important to investigate the likely causes of this difference as far as possible in the given data.

Hungary has a single-payer universal healthcare system, where the National Health Insurance Fund (NHIF) provides high (around 95%) population coverage to roughly 9.7 million inhabitants [6]. This Bismarckian social insurance system requires an entitlement reason (and preferably a contribution payment) for insurance coverage such as employment, retirement status, student status, etc. One of these entitlement reasons can be homelessness. In order to gain this homeless status, providers specializing in care for PEH have the right to register their service users in the NHIF database, thus ensuring them full insurance coverage for the next six months [7]. All insured individuals have a unique patient identifier received at birth or by entering the national health insurance system at a later time point (e.g., foreign citizens employed in Hungary). This identifier does not change during an individual's lifetime and is linked to their place of residence and, if applicable, the death date from the central registries. This system provides the possibility to track all registered PEH in Hungary at a national level over an extended period of time and observe the time spent in homelessness, as well as all health services received in the Hungarian health insurance system.

To see what impact homelessness has on lung cancer care costs and overall survival outcomes in a universal healthcare system such as Hungary, we conducted a retrospective cohort study with administrative healthcare data provided by the Hungarian NHIF.

2. Materials and Methods

2.1. Data Source

The central NHIF dataset contains records for all publicly reimbursed health services used by insured individuals, including primary care, specialist outpatient care, inpatient care, accident and emergency care, transport, pharmaceuticals, medical imaging, etc. Due to the type of reimbursement, fee-for-service (FFS) in the form of a so-called German point system mixed with Diagnosis-Related Groups (DRGs) for acute inpatient care, the NHIF database contains ICD-10 (International Statistical Classification of Diseases and

Related Health Problems 10. Revision) diagnostic codes, admission-related DRGs and ATC (Anatomical Therapeutic Chemical Classification) pharmaceutical codes at an individual patient-level. Through linkage with the death registry, the recorded date of death of each individual who died in the observed period is also available. Due to death registry data being mostly available without cause-of-death information, all survival analyses in this study reflect all-cause mortality.

2.2. Study Sample

For our study sample, we selected all individuals from the NHIF database, whose typical entitlement (>6 months) reason was homelessness in any given year between 2015 and 2021 (PEH sample). We then created a matched control group of the same sex and age from the same region of residence with a one-to-five case-to-control ratio (control sample). Our study thus draws lung cancer cases from the resulting total (Figure 1). We then compared these two samples for newly diagnosed lung cancer outcomes and costs. Consequently, data from all persons out of the homeless and matched populations who had a diagnosis of lung cancer between 2010 and 2021 were extracted for analysis. Diagnoses of lung cancer were defined as any healthcare services received for a main diagnosis of C34 according to the ICD-10 classification system [8]. Cases of lung cancer between 2010 and 2014 were only used to filter for newly diagnosed cases from 2015 onwards, without a previous record of a C34 diagnosis. They were not used in the main analysis since we wanted to capture the entire disease progression as far as possible including survival times and received healthcare services from first diagnosis to death alongside the time spent in homelessness. Furthermore, some lung cancer cases newly diagnosed after 2015 had to be excluded because their lung cancer diagnoses were dated after their registered death dates (Figure 1). This is most likely due to the cancer having been found during autopsy, since Hungary has one of the highest autopsy rates in Europe [9].

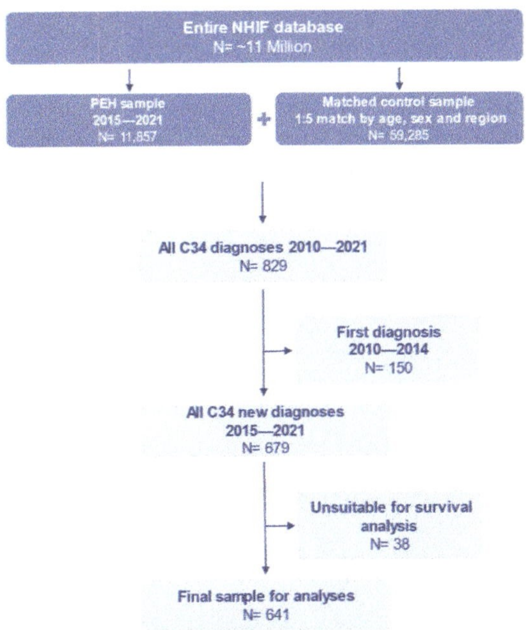

Figure 1. Study sample.

We stratified the sample according to the share of time spent in homeless status between 2015 and 2021. For this, a categorical variable called the homelessness length index (HLI), was created where Category 0 stands for no time spent as homeless, i.e., the control cohort. Categories 1, 2 and 3 of the HLI were defined as up to 1/3, >1/3 up to 2/3 and >2/3 of the total observation time spent as homeless, respectively. The decision for thirds was made after sensitivity testing different groupings of the share of time. Overall, stratification by thirds showed the most homogenous groups with the most stable differences between groups. This stratification also proved to have the best model fit. To judge the model fit in comparison, we used the concordance index as proposed by Harrel et al. [10,11]. This final three-stage categorization also aligns with the three-group typology for homelessness by Kuhn and Culhane [12] representing transitional, episodic and chronic homelessness.

For health service utilization costs, all costs that were registered in the database linked with the diagnosis code for lung cancer (C34) were summed up on an individual patient level annually in 2018 prices. The discounting of later years was performed according to the rates given by the UNECE Statistical Database [12]. All cost data used in this analysis were given in Hungarian Forint (HUF), so there was no need to approximate them via assigned DRG points as would be the norm in many other healthcare insurance datasets. Furthermore, to compare these costs to other healthcare systems, we converted them into Euros and purchase power parity-adjusted Euros (PPPEUR) by using the appropriate exchange rates and PPP conversion factors given by the UNECE and Eurostat [13,14]. In the NHIF dataset, costs are split into five categories: inpatient, pharmaceuticals, outpatient, radio-diagnostics and "other". "Other costs" contains item-based medicine and item-based devices, implants and procedures. These assets are expensive and, therefore, in the case of some products (e.g., medicaments without Health Technology Assessment (HTA) approval) require special approval (compassionate use). Some chemotherapy products are also included in this category.

2.3. Statistical Analyses

For survival outcomes, we compared median survival times and five-year survival and graphically plotted survival curves using the Kaplan–Meier approach [15]. Survival times were calculated from the date of the index lung cancer diagnosis until the recorded date of death, if available, or the date of censoring otherwise. All individuals still at risk at the end of 2021 were right censored. Furthermore, we restricted the maximum observation period to 5 years for all individuals since that was the longest period with sufficient data in both groups for stratification.

To take into account the effects of other parameters on survival such as age, sex and healthcare cost differences, we calculated the Cox proportional hazards (CPH) regression [16]. This multivariate regression approach is the most widely used method to infer the effect of different variables on survival outcomes in medical research [17]. The average yearly healthcare cost was also used as a control variable to explore the extent of mortality hazard differences that could be associated with differential healthcare resource use between the PEH and control groups. We conducted the CPH analyses in a stepwise approach by adding more variables one by one into different models and rerunning the analysis. Better-performing variables that described the same characteristics were chosen. Since no staging information was available, we used metastatic cancer codes as a proxy for more severe stages of lung cancer. To identify these, we flagged all patients where C77–C79 codes were registered in addition to the initial lung cancer diagnosis. The confidence interval was set to 95% and a p value of <0.05 was considered statistically significant. All analyses were conducted using R statistical software version 4.1.1. This study was based on the official data provision process of the National Health Insurance Fund of Hungary [18] (approval number: I043-46-2023, date of approval: 5 April 2023). Since data were handled directly on the NHIF servers and only aggregated secondary data were published here, the study was exempt from additional ethics approval.

3. Results

3.1. Sample Descriptives

For the period 2015–2021, there were 11,857 individuals who were classified as having homeless status (PEH sample) and 59,285 individuals in the matched control cohort. In the PEH sample, 23% (n = 2762) were females. Lung cancer was the most common cancer observed, with a prevalence of approximately 20% (Appendix A, Table A1).

Of the total 71,142 individuals in the analysis sample, 641 were newly diagnosed with lung cancer during the observation period (Figure 1). There were 233 PEH cases (PEH group) compared to 408 control cases (control group) corresponding to prevalence rates of 1.97% and 0.69%, respectively (Table 1).

Table 1. Sample characteristics.

	All PEH Sample	Control Sample	New Lung Cancer Cases	
			PEH Group	Control Group
Total (N/%)	11,857 (17%)	59,285 (83%)	233 (36%)	408 (64%)
Males (N/%)	9095 (77%)	45,475 (77%)	196 (82%)	372 (85%)
Females (N/%)	2762 (23%)	13,810 (23%)	43 (18%)	68 (15%)
Age in 2015 (mean ± SD)	43 (±12)	43 (±12)	53 (±7)	55 (±7)
Males	44 (±12)	44 (±12)	53 (±7)	56 (±7)
Females	41 (±12)	41 (±12)	53 (±6)	53 (±6)
Age at C34 diagnosis (mean ± SD)	-	-	56 (±7)	58 (±7)
Males	-	-	56 (±7)	58 (±7)
Females	-	-	56 (±6)	56 (±6)
Number of years registered as homeless (mean ± SD)	2.1 (±1.5)	-	1.9 (±1.3)	-
Percentage of time registered as homeless (mean ± SD)	33% (±25)	-	40% (±29)	-
Homelessness Length Index (HLI, N/%):				
HLI 1	8095 (68% †)	-	138 (59% ‡)	-
HLI 2	2292 (19% †)	-	52 (22% ‡)	-
HLI 3	1470 (12% †)	-	43 (19% ‡)	-

† % refers to the entire PEH sample (N = 11,857). Percentages are rounded to the nearest full number and do not add up to 100%. ‡ % refers to a PEH sample with a lung cancer diagnosis (N = 233).

Considering homelessness, lung cancer cases were overrepresented in the higher HLI groups with a prevalence of 3.06% in the HLI 3 group, 2.31% in the HLI 2 group and 1.58% in the HLI 1 group (Table 1).

3.2. Healthcare Costs

We summed up all healthcare costs associated with a C34 diagnosis between the index diagnosis and death or censoring. This amounted to an average of HUF 1,136,568 per lung cancer case in the PEH group and HUF 2,115,777 per lung cancer case in the control group, translating into a 46% lower average total lung cancer treatment cost per PEH patient. These costs corresponded to EUR 3564 and EUR 6635 (2018 prices) and to PPP EUR 12,052 and PPP EUR 22,436 (2018 prices), respectively [13]. The difference in annualized cost per patient was similarly 47% less in the PEH group (Table 2). The inpatient costs were the most similar: only 20% lower per patient in the PEH group. In contrast, pharmaceutical costs were the most different, over 80% lower per PEH patient, although these costs were only a minor fraction of the total costs for both groups (3% for PEH vs. 8% for control). A considerable part of lung cancer costs was recorded in the "other costs" category (49% for PEH vs. 59% for control) (Table 2).

Table 2. Lung cancer associated healthcare costs (in 2018 prices, HUF and PPP EUR).

	HUF		EUR		PPP EUR		Difference PEH vs. Control	Percentage of Total Costs	
	PEH	Control	PEH	Control	PEH	Control		PEH	Control
Average C34 associated **total** healthcare costs per patient	1,136,568	2,115,777	3564	6635	12,052	22,436	−46%	100%	100%
Average C34 associated **total** healthcare costs **per patient year**	675,562	1,276,978	2119	4004	7163	13,541	−47%	100%	100%
Average C34 associated **inpatient** costs **per patient year**	295,223	366,925	926	1151	3131	3890	−20%	44%	29%
Average C34 associated **pharmaceuticals** costs **per patient year**	19,119	100,084	60	314	203	1,061	−81%	3%	8%
Average C34 associated **outpatient** costs **per patient year**	15,008	26,245	47	82	159	278	−43%	2%	2%
Average C34 associated **radio-diagnostics** costs **per patient year**	15,410	29,328	48	92	163	311	−47%	2%	2%
Average C34 associated **other** costs **per patient year**	330,802	754,397	1037	2366	3508	8000	−56%	49%	59%

Source: NHIF data, exchange rates from Eurostat [14] PPP EUR rates from OECD [19].

3.3. Survival

Figure 2 shows the Kaplan–Meier survival curves stratified by group. After an initial big drop in survival representing the high mortality rates of certain lung cancers in the first year, the Kaplan–Meier survival curves of the two groups converged before further clear separation after two years (Figure 2). The median survival times were 292 days (95% CI: 200–419) for the PEH group and 330 (95% CI: 419–447) for the control group. The difference when only looking at a single homelessness category, however, was not statistically significant ($p = 0.3$). Kaplan–Meier survival analysis by HLI category was only possible for the first year due to sample size issues. This showed a clear separation of HLI 2 and 3 from HLI 0 and 1, meaning that persons experiencing long-term, chronic homelessness showed a significantly lower initial average survival time when compared to no or episodic homelessness (Appendix A, Figure A1). To test this observed difference and measure its magnitude, we used CPH regression analysis.

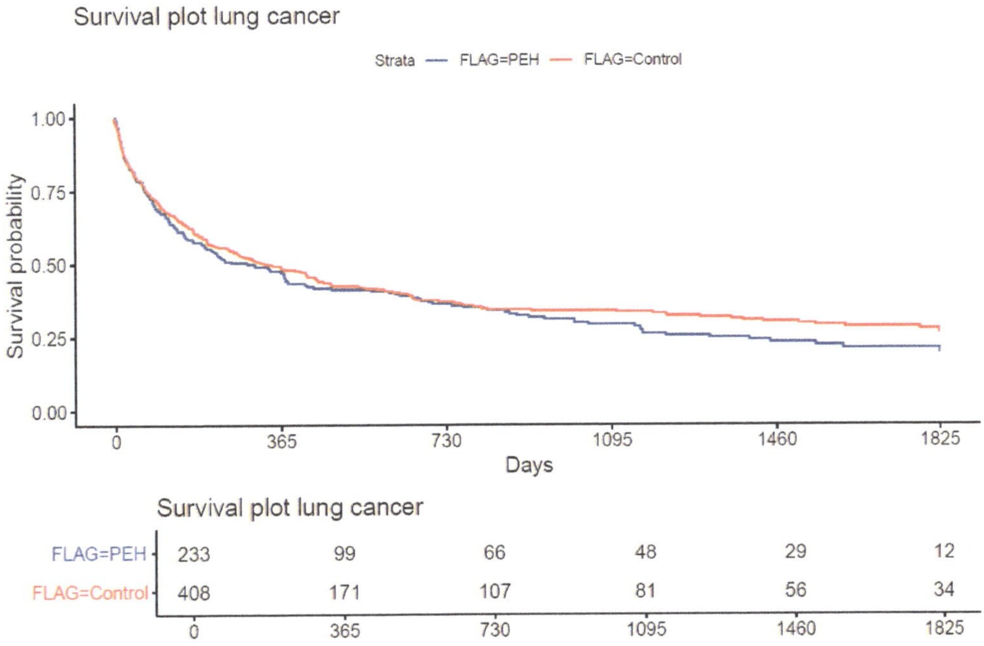

Figure 2. Kaplan–Meier survival plot (p = 0.3).

All-cause mortality hazard ratios (HRs) were tested for significance for different CPH models, including different homelessness stratification approaches and control variables. We found significant interactions between all-cause mortality and age, HLI, lung cancer-specific healthcare costs and metastatic cancer stages. As shown by the rising concordance index, the model performance improved with each variable addition after settling on the most fitting way to stratify the sample by the level of homelessness.

First, we controlled for age and sex in all six models shown in the table. Although female sex showed a reduced HR, this did not reach statistical significance in our study. Nevertheless, based on previous evidence about sex-based differences in lung cancer survival and the potential magnitude of female sex impact in our data, sex remained included as a standard control variable in all models [20,21]. Age showed a significant association with all-cause mortality (HR = 1.04, 95% CI 1.02–1.05) that was robust across all models. Being one year older increased the hazard of dying in the given period by 4%, keeping all other factors constant (Models 4–6) (Table 3).

Models 2 and 3, which included homelessness as a dummy or continuous variable, did not deliver significant results as opposed to Model 4 where homelessness experience was stratified based on the aforementioned sensitivity analysis and literature [12]. While compared to the control cohort, short-term homelessness (HLI 1: 59% of the PHE group) showed no significant difference, mortality hazard increased significantly by more than 50% for episodic or long-term homelessness represented in our sample by HLI 2 and 3 (HR = 1.59, 95% CI: 1.18–2.16; and HR = 1.66, 95% CI: 1.15–2.41, respectively). Between HLI 2 and 3, the HRs only differed slightly when controlled for other factors (Models 5 and 6) (Table 3).

Table 3. Cox proportional hazards (CPH) regression results.

CPH	HR (95% CI)					
	Model 1	Model 2	Model 3	Model 4	Model 5	Model 6
Age at diagnosis	**1.03 (1.01–1.05) ***	**1.03 (1.01–1.05) ***	**1.03 (1.01–1.05) ***	**1.03 (1.02–1.05) ***	**1.04 (1.02–1.05) ***	**1.03 (1.02–1.05) ***
Female sex	0.83 (0.63–1.02)	0.83 (0.63–1.02)	0.83 (0.63–1.01)	0.88 (0.67–1.16)	0.89 (0.67–1.18)	0.92 (0.69–1.21)
Homelessness yes/no	-	1.02 (0.99–1.47)	-	-	-	-
Homelessness in years	-	-	0.99 (0.91–1.07)	-	-	-
HLI						
1	-	-	-	0.96 (0.75–1.24)	0.98 (0.76–1.26)	1.03 (0.80–1.32)
2	-	-	-	**1.59 (1.18–2.16) ***	**1.51 (1.11–2.05) ***	**1.47 (1.08–2.00) ***
3	-	-	-	**1.66 (1.15–2.41) ***	**1.50 (1.03–2.18) ***	**1.47 (1.01–2.14) ***
Total annualized lung cancer associated healthcare costs (per HUF 100,000)	-	-	-	-	**0.97 (0.96–0.98) ***	**0.97 (0.96–0.98) ***
Metastatic cancer	-	-	-	-	-	**2.37 (1.92–2.93) ***
Concordance index	0.563	0.565	0.563	0.584	0.675	0.690

HR: hazard ratio. **Bold** * = significant variables at $p < 0.05$.

To control for costs in the model, we included annualized lung cancer-associated healthcare costs on an individual level. Higher costs were associated with a significantly lower mortality hazard (−0.03 per additional HUF 100,000). However, the overall magnitude of this association was only marginal when compared to the associations with longer-term homelessness or disease severity (Models 5 and 6).

Metastatic cancer had by far the strongest association with mortality differences. With an HR of 2.37 (95% CI: 1.92–2.93), patients with metastatic cancer diagnoses were more than twice as likely to die at any point during the observation period than those without. Furthermore, the differential results between Models 4 to 6 indicate that in total about 25–40% of the excess mortality hazard for HLI 2 and 3 was explainable by lower lung cancer-specific healthcare costs and a higher prevalence of metastatic cancer cases in these groups (Table 3).

4. Discussion

Generally, the Hungarian population of PEH we covered in this study is similar to those in other studies; for example, the percentage of females in our study's PEH population (23%) is in line with the average sex distribution in homeless populations according to a recent systematic review [22].

Our study shows that homelessness is not only associated with an increase in lung cancer prevalence for the Hungarian PEH population, but this increase is linked to the magnitude of time spent in homelessness. The high general prevalence and it being the most common cancer in the PEH population is in line with a previous study [5].

This higher prevalence is likely to be due to multiple factors. First, there is usually a much higher smoking rate amongst PEH populations [23]. Consequently, a previous study found excess rates of many smoking attributable cancer types in the homeless population of Boston [24]. A second factor that has been proposed to influence lung cancer prevalence is pulmonary tuberculosis infections, being up to five times as prevalent among PEH as in the non-homeless population [25,26]. Since our study was based on administrative data, we could not control for any of these factors.

Our cost estimates of EUR 3668 and EUR 6827 for PEH and controls (EUR 5519 between both groups) are along the lines of the EUR 4157 average treatment costs for lung cancer in Hungary from Inotai et al. based on earlier data from 2000 to 2012 [27]. Our average treatment cost results of PPP EUR 18,661 also compare to the respective treatment costs of EUR 25,063, EUR 17,777 and EUR 32,500 from France, England and Germany, as described by McGuire et al. in 2015 [28].

We found only a limited positive impact of higher healthcare costs on lowering mortality hazard, which may be reflective of the high fatality rate and standardized treatment patterns for lung cancer. These results may also simply reflect the increased treatment costs associated with a longer survival time. Overall, we found only limited evidence that survival differences between PEH and controls with lung cancer are caused by significantly different healthcare utilization. Our differential survival results are rather indicative of more metastatic cancer cases within the PEH group, most likely due to later diagnosis and lower general ability to battle lung cancer, especially in the case of episodic and long-term homelessness (HLI 2 and 3).

A previous study in the USA found that a deficit in quality of life, as experienced by PEH, lowered overall survival [29] and that from a survival perspective, the main focus should lie on preventing people from experiencing long-term homelessness [30]. Although we were not able to reflect on quality of life, our findings are in line with this conclusion, showing that transitional or short-term homelessness (HLI 1) had no significant impact on survival, while longer-term homelessness increased the mortality hazard by around 50%. These findings also support the hypothesis that a large proportion of socio-economic differences in survival, which have been observed in other studies summarized by Redondo-Sánchez et al. [4], are the result of differences in lifestyle and general resilience rather than experienced differences in treatment.

It has to be noted though that these findings may only be generalizable to universal healthcare systems similar to those in Hungary where PEH can have full access to public healthcare services. In less equitable healthcare systems, it is likely that a similar analysis, if feasible, would yield different results. From a public health perspective, however, Hungary's policy of providing PEH with full access to public healthcare services seems to influence survival to some degree with the median survival time of 292 days among PEH with lung cancer when compared to a study from Seattle, where the PEH lung cancer patient median survival time was 211 days [31].

Further research may expand this study by looking at different cancer types and other chronic diseases in the context of homelessness and outcomes. It would also be important to assess whether previously experienced homelessness retains its legacy effect on disease outcome and survival even if a certain time spent out of homelessness has passed.

Our study is based on administrative health insurance data, which brings some general data limitations with it. Firstly, no data on privately funded healthcare service use are available in the NHIF database. For the current study, it is very unlikely that homeless people would have used private services and paid out-of-pocket, but this may not be true for the control group, which can lead to some downward bias in the magnitude of health service utilization differences. On the other hand, since the majority of lung cancer treatment is conducted in inpatient or outpatient specialist care settings, relevant services would be covered in the dataset as standard. A second general limitation is due to known up-coding activities as a consequence of FFS reimbursement [32,33]. However, these biases would appear in both groups (PEH and control) equally and, therefore, would not affect the comparative results of the analyses. The third important administrative limitation of our dataset is the potential selection bias of homeless cases. Since PEH status is registered when accessing some type of health or care service provision, not all homeless individuals in Hungary are registered by the NHIF. Those who appear in the NHIF dataset are likely to be in a more fragile health status requiring acute care. Yet again, in the case of lung cancer, this bias may not be of particular importance in comparison to some chronic diseases. Lastly, due to the ICD code format, we were not able to reflect on cancer staging information and the potentially differential impacts of small- and non-small-cell lung cancers on survival, healthcare utilization and cost differences that may also drive some of the group differences [34]. However, we tried to catch some of these differences by controlling for metastatic cancer codes which coincided with lung cancer diagnoses.

5. Conclusions

The results of this study imply that equitable healthcare provision for diagnosed lung cancer cases may only influence negative survival outcome differences faced by homeless people to a certain degree. The evidence on prevalence, metastatic stages and survival differences indicates that the lung cancer disease burden is considerably higher in the PEH group, which on average should lead to higher yearly costs with no difference in access. The lower average costs for the PEH group, as seen in this case study for lung cancer from Hungary, however, show that mere access does not necessarily lead to higher utilization. Additional emphasis on screening, early detection and tackling issues that lead to long-term homelessness is also needed to improve outcomes for this vulnerable group. Earlier detection and treatment could not only improve survival and quality of life but also limit the downstream costs of more severe lung cancer cases. Overall, our findings support the need for broader, more complex policies to improve healthcare utilization among PEH with lung cancer.

Author Contributions: D.H. and J.S. conceptualized the study and developed the methods. P.F.-F. contributed to the data acquisition. Á.S., D.H. and P.F.-F. contributed to data cleaning. D.H. analyzed the data supported by P.F.-F. under J.S.'s supervision. All authors contributed to the interpretation of results. D.H. prepared the first draft of the manuscript which was revised by P.F.-F. and J.S. All authors have read and agreed to the published version of the manuscript.

Funding: This study received no external funding and no author has any financial interest in the results of this study.

Institutional Review Board Statement: This study was based on the official data provision process of the National Health Insurance Fund of Hungary [17] (approval number: I043-46-2023, date of approval: 5 April 2023). Since data were handled directly on the NHIF servers and only aggregated secondary data were exported, this study was exempt from additional ethics approval. This study does not reflect the NHIF's official opinion; it is solely the work of the authors listed.

Informed Consent Statement: Patient consent was waived due to no subjects being identifiable in the present study.

Data Availability Statement: Due to the sensible nature of the NHIF individual health data, the underlying data can only be described in aggregate form and are not available to the general public. Requests to access the data should be directed to the NHIF.

Conflicts of Interest: The authors declare no conflicts of interest.

Appendix A

Table A1. Ten most common cancers by case percentage in the PEH population.

Cancer ICD 10 Code	Percentage of All Cancer Cases
C34	19.8%
C79	6.4%
C32	6.0%

Table A1. *Cont.*

Cancer ICD 10 Code	Percentage of All Cancer Cases
C78	5.9%
C77	4.6%
C10	3.4%
C53	3.1%
C13	2.9%
C18	2.5%
C67	2.5%

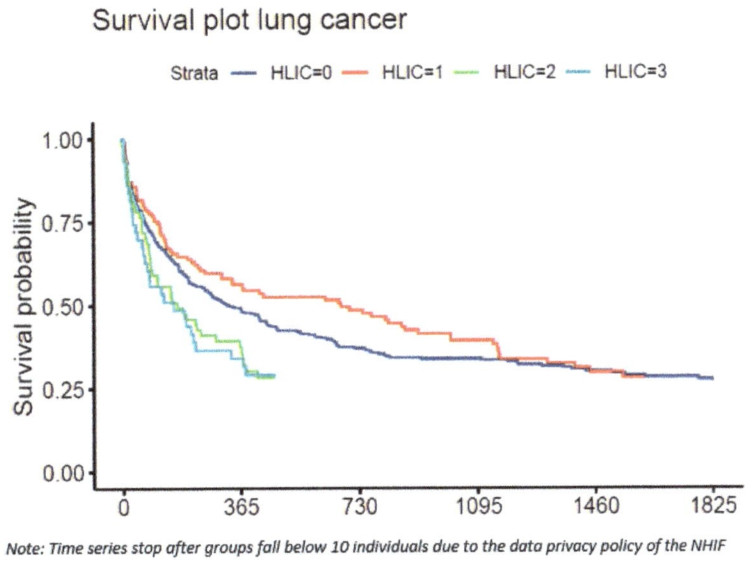

Figure A1. KM survival plot by HLI category ($p = 0.004$).

References

1. Fornaro, M.; Dragioti, E.; De Prisco, M.; Billeci, M.; Mondin, A.M.; Calati, R.; Smith, L.; Hatcher, S.; Kaluzienski, M.; Fiedorowicz, J.G.; et al. Homelessness and health-related outcomes: An umbrella review of observational studies and randomized controlled trials. *BMC Med.* **2021**, *20*, 224. [CrossRef]
2. Tipple, G.; Speak, S. Definitions of homelessness in developing countries. *Habitat Int.* **2005**, *29*, 337–352. [CrossRef]
3. Lung cancer n.d. Available online: https://www.who.int/news-room/fact-sheets/detail/lung-cancer (accessed on 29 August 2024).
4. Redondo-Sánchez, D.; Petrova, D.; Rodríguez-Barranco, M.; Fernández-Navarro, P.; Jiménez-Moleón, J.J.; Sánchez, M.-J. Socio-Economic Inequalities in Lung Cancer Outcomes: An Overview of Systematic Reviews. *Cancers* **2022**, *14*, 398. [CrossRef] [PubMed]
5. Holowatyj, A.N.; I Heath, E.; Pappas, L.M.; Ruterbusch, J.J.; Gorski, D.H.; A Triest, J.; Park, H.K.; Beebe-Dimmer, J.L.; Schwartz, A.G.; Cote, M.L.; et al. The Epidemiology of Cancer Among Homeless Adults in Metropolitan Detroit. *JNCI Cancer Spectr.* **2019**, *3*, pkz006. [CrossRef]
6. OECD Data Explorer Healthcare coverage n.d. Available online: https://data-explorer.oecd.org/vis?fs[0]=Topic,1%7CHealth#HEA#%7CHealthcare%20coverage#HEA_COV#&pg=0&fc=Topic&bp=true&snb=1&vw=tl&df[ds]=dsDisseminateFinalDMZ&df[id]=DSD_HEALTH_PROT@DF_HEALTH_PROT&df[ag]=OECD.ELS.HD&df[vs]=1.0&pd=2010,&dq=HUN.A..PT_POP.&ly[cl]=TIME_PERIOD&to[TIME_PERIOD]=false (accessed on 12 June 2024).
7. Tasks of the National Health Insurance Fund of Hungary (Hungarian acronym: NEAK)—NEAK n.d. Available online: https://www.neak.gov.hu/oldalak/nyelvi-oldalak/english (accessed on 7 March 2025).

8. World Health Organization. International Statistical Classification of Diseases and Related Health Problems (10th ed.) 2019. Available online: https://icd.who.int/browse10/2019/en (accessed on 24 March 2025).
9. Menyhárt, O.; Fekete, J.T.; Győrffy, B. Demographic shift disproportionately increases cancer burden in an aging nation: Current and expected incidence and mortality in Hungary up to 2030. *Clin. Epidemiol.* **2018**, *10*, 1093–1108. [CrossRef]
10. Harrell, F.E.; Lee, K.L.; Mark, D.B. Prognostic/Clinical Prediction Models: Multivariable Prognostic Models: Issues in Developing Models, Evaluating Assumptions and Adequacy, and Measuring and Reducing Errors. Tutorials in Biostatistics. *Stat. Methods Clin. Stud.* **2005**, *1*, 223–249. [CrossRef]
11. Hartman, N.; Kim, S.; He, K.; Kalbfleisch, J.D. Pitfalls of the concordance index for survival outcomes. *Stat. Med.* **2023**, *42*, 2179–2190. [CrossRef]
12. Kuhn, R.; Culhane, D.P. Applying Cluster Analysis to Test a Typology of Homelessness by Pattern of Shelter Utilization: Results from the Analysis of Administrative Data. *Am. J. Community Psychol.* **1998**, *26*, 207–232. [CrossRef]
13. Exchange Rates and PPPs by Indicator, Country and Year. UNECE Statistical Database n.d. Available online: https://w3.unece.org/PXWeb2015/pxweb/en/STAT/STAT__20-ME__6-MEER/30_en_MECCExchPPPsNEWY_r.px/ (accessed on 1 September 2024).
14. Statistics—Eurostat n.d. Available online: https://ec.europa.eu/eurostat/databrowser/view/ERT_BIL_EUR_A/default/table?lang=en (accessed on 24 February 2025).
15. Kaplan, E.L.; Meier, P. Nonparametric Estimation from Incomplete Observations. *J. Am. Stat. Assoc.* **1958**, *53*, 457–481. [CrossRef]
16. Cox, D.R. Regression Models and Life-Tables. *J. R. Stat. Soc. Ser. B* **1972**, *34*, 187–202. [CrossRef]
17. Kumar, M.; Sonker, P.K.; Saroj, A.; Jain, A.; Bhattacharjee, A.; Saroj, R.K. Parametric survival analysis using R: Illustration with lung cancer data. *Cancer Rep.* **2020**, *3*, e1210. [CrossRef]
18. Tájékoztató a Közadatok Újrahasznosításáról—NEAK n.d. Available online: http://www.neak.gov.hu/felso_menu/rolunk/kozerdeku_adatok/kozadatok_igenylese/kozadat_ujrahasznositas (accessed on 20 February 2025).
19. OECD Data Explorer—Annual Purchasing Power Parities and exchange rates n.d. Available online: https://data-explorer.oecd.org/vis?tm=purchasing%20power&pg=0&snb=44&vw=tb&df[ds]=dsDisseminateFinalDMZ&df[id]=DSD_NAMAIN10@DF_TABLE4&df[ag]=OECD.SDD.NAD&df[vs]=2.0&dq=A.EU27_2020+EA20+HUN...PPP_B1GQ.......&lom=LASTNPERIODS&lo=10&to[TIME_PERIOD]=false (accessed on 24 February 2025).
20. May, L.; Shows, K.; Nana-Sinkam, P.; Li, H.; Landry, J.W. Sex Differences in Lung Cancer. *Cancers* **2023**, *15*, 3111. [CrossRef] [PubMed]
21. Yu, X.Q.; Yap, M.L.; Cheng, E.S.; Ngo, P.J.; Vaneckova, P.; Karikios, D.; Canfell, K.; Weber, M.F. Evaluating Prognostic Factors for Sex Differences in Lung Cancer Survival: Findings from a Large Australian Cohort. *J. Thorac. Oncol.* **2022**, *17*, 688–699. [CrossRef]
22. Barry, R.; Anderson, J.; Tran, L.; Bahji, A.; Dimitropoulos, G.; Ghosh, S.M.; Kirkham, J.; Messier, G.; Patten, S.B.; Rittenbach, K.; et al. Prevalence of Mental Health Disorders Among Individuals Experiencing Homelessness: A Systematic Review and Meta-Analysis. *JAMA Psychiatry* **2024**, *81*, 691–699. [CrossRef]
23. Soar, K.; Dawkins, L.; Robson, D.; Cox, S. Smoking amongst adults experiencing homelessness: A systematic review of prevalence rates, interventions and the barriers and facilitators to quitting and staying quit. *J. Smok. Cessat.* **2020**, *15*, 94–108. [CrossRef]
24. Baggett, T.P.; Chang, Y.; Porneala, B.C.; Bharel, M.; Singer, D.E.; Rigotti, N.A. Disparities in Cancer Incidence, Stage, and Mortality at Boston Health Care for the Homeless Program. *Am. J. Prev. Med.* **2015**, *49*, 694–702. [CrossRef] [PubMed]
25. Preda, M.; Tănase, B.C.; Zob, D.L.; Gheorghe, A.S.; Lungulescu, C.V.; Dumitrescu, E.A.; Stănculeanu, D.L.; Manolescu, L.S.C.; Popescu, O.; Ibraim, E.; et al. The Bidirectional Relationship between Pulmonary Tuberculosis and Lung Cancer. *Int. J. Environ. Res. Public Health* **2023**, *20*, 1282. [CrossRef]
26. Dias, M.; Gaio, R.; Sousa, P.; Abranches, M.; Gomes, M.; Oliveira, O.; Correia-Neves, M.; Ferreira, E.; Duarte, R. Tuberculosis among the homeless: Should we change the strategy? *Int. J. Tuberc. Lung Dis.* **2017**, *21*, 327–332. [CrossRef]
27. Inotai, A.; Abonyi-Tóth, Z.; Rokszin, G.; Vokó, Z. Prognosis, Cost, and Occurrence of Colorectal, Lung, Breast, and Prostate Cancer in Hungary. *Value Heal. Reg. Issues* **2015**, *7*, 1–8. [CrossRef]
28. McGuire, A.; Martin, M.; Lenz, C.; Sollano, J.A. Treatment cost of non-small cell lung cancer in three European countries: Comparisons across France, Germany, and England using administrative databases. *J. Med. Econ.* **2015**, *18*, 525–532. [CrossRef]
29. Sloan, J.A.; Zhao, X.; Novotny, P.J.; Wampfler, J.; Garces, Y.; Clark, M.M.; Yang, P. Relationship Between Deficits in Overall Quality of Life and Non-Small-Cell Lung Cancer Survival. *J. Clin. Oncol.* **2012**, *30*, 1498–1504. [CrossRef] [PubMed]
30. Flike, K.; Aronowitz, T. Factors That Influence Quality of Life in People Experiencing Homelessness: A Systematic Mixed Studies Review. *J. Am. Psychiatr. Nurses Assoc.* **2022**, *28*, 128–153. [CrossRef] [PubMed]
31. Concannon, K.F.; Thayer, J.H.; Wu, Q.V.; Jenkins, I.C.; Baik, C.S.; Linden, H.M. Outcomes Among Homeless Patients with Non–Small-Cell Lung Cancer: A County Hospital Experience. *JCO Oncol. Pr.* **2020**, *16*, e1004–e1014. [CrossRef]
32. Joiner, K.A.; Lin, J.; Pantano, J. Upcoding in medicare: Where does it matter most? *Health Econ. Rev.* **2024**, *14*, 1. [CrossRef]

33. Bowblis, J.R.; Brunt, C.S. Medicare Skilled Nursing Facility Reimbursement and Upcoding. *Health Econ.* **2014**, *23*, 821–840. [CrossRef]
34. Travis, W.D.; Rush, W.; Flieder, D.B.; Falk, R.; Fleming, M.V.; Gal, A.A.; Koss, M.N. Survival Analysis of 200 Pulmonary Neuroendocrine Tumors with Clarification of Criteria for Atypical Carcinoid and Its Separation from Typical Carcinoid. *Am. J. Surg. Pathol.* **1998**, *22*, 934–944. [CrossRef]

cancers

MDPI

Article

A Retrospective Analysis of Breast Cancer Mortality among Jewish and Muslim Arab Women in Israel: The Role of Sociodemographic Factors

Ronit Pinchas-Mizrachi [1,*] and Dan Bouhnik [2]

[1] Faculty of Nursing, Jerusalem College of Technology, Jerusalem 91160, Israel
[2] Department of Computer Science, Jerusalem College of Technology, Jerusalem 91160, Israel; bouhnik@jct.ac.il
* Correspondence: pinchasm@g.jct.ac.il

Simple Summary: Breast cancer is a major health concern worldwide, with mortality rates varying between ethnic groups. In Israel, Jewish and Muslim Arab women have different socioeconomic backgrounds and lifestyle factors that may influence breast cancer outcomes. This study investigates disparities in breast cancer mortality between these two groups and examines how factors such as number of children, socioeconomic status, and place of residence affect mortality rates. By analyzing data from over 800,000 Israeli women over a 30-year period, the researchers aim to understand the complex interplay among ethnicity, sociodemographic factors, and breast cancer mortality. The findings of this study could help identify key risk factors and protective elements specific to each ethnic group. This information is crucial for developing targeted intervention programs to reduce disparities and improve breast cancer outcomes for both Jewish and Muslim Arab women in Israel.

Abstract: Breast cancer mortality rates vary across ethnic groups in Israel, where protective factors such as high fertility and breastfeeding rates may be moderated by socioeconomic factors and mammography rates. We aim to investigate disparities in breast cancer mortality between Jewish and Muslim Arab women in Israel and examine how sociodemographic variables and number of children are associated with mortality. Our retrospective follow-up study uses data from the Israeli Central Bureau of Statistics and multivariable Cox regression models, adjusting for age, number of children, country of origin, locality size, and socioeconomic status. Compared to Jewish women, Muslim Arab women exhibited lower breast cancer mortality rates. However, after adjusting for multiple sociodemographic variables, no significant differences persisted between Jewish and Muslim Arab women. Having more than three children was associated with lower mortality among Muslim Arab women but not among Jewish women. European/American origin, larger localities, and medium socioeconomic status were associated with higher mortality. Sociodemographic factors may therefore explain the disparities in breast cancer mortality between Jewish and Muslim Arab women in Israel. Targeted intervention programs that consider the unique characteristics and risk factors of different ethnic groups are needed to reduce disparities and improve outcomes.

Keywords: breast cancer mortality; ethnic disparities; socioeconomic status; reproductive factors; Israeli women; health inequalities

1. Introduction

Breast cancer is the second leading cause of death worldwide and the cancer with the second-highest incidence rate [1]. According to the World Health Organization, in 2020, 2.3 million females were diagnosed with breast cancer worldwide. The incidence and related mortality from breast cancer continue to grow despite remarkable advances in early detection and treatment [2,3]. In Israel, the survival rate for breast cancer is relatively high, with an estimated five-year survival rate of around 88% [4].

Breast cancer morbidity and mortality is associated with various sociodemographic risk factors. The risk of breast cancer morbidity increases with age [5]. Previous studies have found higher breast cancer mortality rates among Black women as compared to White women [6]. Among Jewish women of Ashkenazi descent, genetic characteristics have been found that are associated with breast cancer morbidity [7]. In a previous study we conducted, lower breast cancer mortality rates were found among women living in non-urban areas as compared to women living in urban areas [8].

Various other factors affect breast cancer incidence. Women of lower socioeconomic status tend to develop breast cancer less frequently than women of higher socioeconomic status [9,10], but they face a higher risk of breast cancer mortality [2] and worse survival outcomes [11,12]. They also tend to undergo mammography screening less frequently [13,14] and are at a higher risk of late-stage diagnosis [15,16]. Reproductive factors such as young maternal age at first birth [17,18], hormonal treatments [19,20], pregnancy and childbirth [21,22], and breastfeeding [21,23,24] influence breast cancer incidence. Breastfeeding and a long duration of breastfeeding have been found to be protective factors against breast cancer morbidity [23,24]. Breastfeeding can help reduce the short-term increase in breast cancer risk following pregnancy and provides additional protective benefits over time [21]. Women of lower socioeconomic status tend to breastfeed less [25].

As of 2022, Arab citizens of Israel constitute approximately 21.1% of the total population [26]. They tend to live in small- and medium-sized localities rather than large ones [27]. Compared to Jewish women, they are, on average, younger at first birth [28], less likely to use hormonal medications [29], undergo mammography [30], or enter the labor market [31] but are more likely to breastfeed for longer [32,33]. Historically, Israel's Arab Muslim population has been characterized by particularly high fertility rates, but these have decreased over the years [34]. Previous studies have found that Arab women have lower breast cancer incidence and mortality than do Jewish women, though these gaps have recently been narrowing [29,35]. In summary, the Arab community is characterized by factors that can offer protection against breast cancer but also by factors that may negatively impact survival rates. Additionally, all-cause mortality rates are higher among Arabs as compared to Jewish women.

In this study, we aim to investigate breast cancer mortality disparities between Jewish and Muslim Arab women in Israel. Our study examines how sociodemographic factors (age, socioeconomic status, locality size, education) and number of children are associated with breast cancer mortality in each ethnic group. Elucidating the interplay of ethnicity, sociodemographic factors, reproductive history, and breast cancer mortality in Israel offers insight toward reducing disparities and improving outcomes.

2. Materials and Methods

We conducted a retrospective follow-up study on breast cancer mortality among Israeli women over a 30-year period, from 1 January 1990, to 31 December 2020. The data for this study were collected by the Israeli Central Bureau of Statistics from the Population Registry, Education Registry, and Ministry of Health. The study group included 817,445 Israeli women born between 1940 and 1960, of whom 743,090 were Jewish (90.9%) and 74,355 were Muslim Arab (9.1%).

Data on birth year, ethnicity (Jewish/Arab), religion, country of origin, number of children, and locality size were collected from the Population Registry. The number of children was dichotomized into "3 children or less" and "more than 3 children". The "country of origin" variable was defined by the woman's father's birth country in one of three categories: 1. Israel, 2. Asia/Africa, or 3. Europe/America/Australia. Locality size was dichotomized into small (up to 20,000 inhabitants) and large (more than 20,000 inhabitants).

The socioeconomic status variable was constructed by combining two variables: education (obtained from the Central Bureau of Statistics' Education Registry, which is based on educational data from various sources such as educational institutions, administrative files, surveys, censuses, administrative data, and more) and the socioeconomic status of residential areas (for the 20% of the population whose education data were missing). The categorization was based on the distribution of these variables in Israeli society. High socioeconomic status was determined by 15 or more years of education or a residential area socioeconomic score of 8–10. Medium status was determined by 11–14 years of education or a residential area score of 6–7. Low status was determined by up to 10 years of education or a residential area score of 1–5.

The outcome variable was breast cancer mortality, and death year was obtained from the Ministry of Health. For all variables except education, missing data were below one percent.

First, we examined the distributions for age, number of children, country of origin, locality size, and socioeconomic status, and analyzed differences between the groups relative to these variables. The statistical significance of differences was calculated using the Chi-square test for categorical variables and the *t*-test for age (Table 1).

Table 1. Distribution of research variables among Jewish and Muslim Arab women.

		Jewish (n = 743,090)	Muslim Arab (n = 74,355)	p
Age		39.08 (5.66)	37.99 (5.90)	<0.001
Number of children		2.45 (1.95)	4.87 (3.54)	<0.001
Country of origin	Asia/Africa	33.4%	4.0%	<0.001
	Europe/America	44.0%	1.4%	
	Israel	22.6%	94.6%	
Locality size	Small	84.6%	55.3%	<0.001
	Large	15.4%	44.7%	
Socioeconomic status	Low	23.7%	84.7%	<0.001
	Medium	43.2%	11.8%	
	High	33.1%	3.6%	

Next, we examined mortality rates per 10,000 women by ethnicity, number of children, country of origin, locality size, and socioeconomic status. In assessing the disparities' effect size between groups and their statistical significance, the Adjusted Hazard Ratio (AHR) for breast cancer mortality was calculated after adjusting for age (Table 2).

Table 2. Breast cancer mortality rate by research variables among study population (n = 817,455).

		Breast Cancer Mortality per 10,000 Women	AHR (Age-Adjusted Hazard Ratio), 99% CI	p
Ethnicity	Jewish	105.40	1.00	
	Muslim Arab	84.33	0.866 (0.778–0.964)	<0.001
Number of children	0–3	106.54	1.00	
	>3	95.19	0.902 (0.845–0.962)	<0.001
Country of origin	Asia/Africa	96.47	1.00	
	Israel	105.06	1.068 (0.997–1.143)	0.013
	Europe/America	107.59	1.109 (1.031–1.192)	<0.001
Locality size	Small	84.30	1.00	
	Large	107.70	1.229 (1.136–1.330)	<0.001
Socioeconomic status	Low	99.96	1.00	
	Medium	111.94	1.179 (1.101–1.262)	<0.001
	High	97.27	1.019 (0.945–1.098)	0.526

Then, via regression and adjusted Kaplan–Meier curves, we created multivariable models to evaluate the relationship between ethnicity and breast cancer mortality. The first model included age, ethnicity, number of children, and country of origin. The second model included those four variables and locality size. The third model included all the variables of the second model, as well as socioeconomic status (Table 3).

Table 3. Multivariate Cox models for breast cancer mortality prediction among study population (n = 817,445).

		Model 1	Model 2	Model 3
		HR (99% CI)	HR (99% CI)	HR (99% CI)
Ethnicity	Jewish	1.00	1.00	1.00
	Muslim Arab	0.815 (0.722–0.920)	0.849 (0.752–0.960)	0.904 (0.793–1.031)
Number of children	0–3	1.00	1.00	1.00
	>3	0.925 (0.963–0.992)	0.938 (0.875–1.007)	0.924 (0.861–0.992)
Country of origin	Asia/Africa	1.00	1.00	1.00
	Israel	1.044 (0.972–1.120)	1.046 (0.974–1.123)	1.060 (0.985–1.140)
	Europe/America	1.166 (1.078–1.260)	1.181 (1.092–1.277)	1.173 (1.083–1.270)
Locality size	Small		1.00	1.00
	Large		1.219 (1.124–1.322)	1.189 (1.095–1.291)
Socioeconomic status	Low			1.00
	Medium			1.140 (1.060–1.227)
	High			0.970 (0.893–1.364)

We found significant interactions ($p < 0.001$) among ethnicity, socioeconomic status, and number of children and breast cancer mortality. We found significant interactions between ethnicity and socioeconomic status, as well as between ethnicity and number of children and the prediction of breast cancer mortality. Therefore, we decided to separately examine the role of each of the following in predicting breast cancer mortality among Jewish and Muslim Arab women: number of children, country of origin, locality size, and socioeconomic status (Table 4).

Table 4. Breast cancer mortality rate by research variables among Jewish (n = 743,090) and Muslim Arab women (n = 74,355).

		Model A: Jewish (n = 743,090)	**Model B: Muslim Arab (n = 74,355)**
		Age adjusted HR (99% CI)	Age adjusted HR (99% CI)
Number of children	0–3	1.00	1.00
	>3	0.960 (0.896–1.028)	0.751 (0.609–0.927)
Country of origin	Asia/Africa	1.00	1.00
	Israel	1.08 (1.001–1.146)	0.651 (0.159–4.466)
	Europe/America	1.185 (1.096–1.282)	0.703 (0.373–1.326)
Locality size	Small	1.00	1.00
	Large	1.217 (1.115–1.329)	1.177 (0.954–1.451)
Socioeconomic status	Low	1.00	1.00
	Medium	1.146 (1.064–1.235)	1.309 (1.015–1.796)
	High	0.988 (0.912–1.071)	1.591 (1.052–2.613)

It is important to note that for individuals who immigrated from Israel during the follow-up period and did not return by the end of the follow-up, and for whom information on their death was not obtained, survival data were calculated up to the year in which they immigrated from Israel. In other words, such individuals contributed survival years until the year they left Israel.

3. Results

Significant differences were found between Jewish and Muslim Arab women concerning age, number of children, country of origin, locality size, and socioeconomic status ($p < 0.001$).

Higher all-cause mortality rates were found among Muslim Arab women as compared to Jewish women (AHR = 1.658, 99% CI (1.612, 1.704)) but lower breast cancer mortality rates were found among Muslim Arab women (AHR = 0.866, 99% CI (0.778, 0.964)) (Figure 1). After adjusting for age, lower breast cancer mortality rates were found among women with more than three children (AHR = 0.902; 99% CI (0.845–0.962)), those of Asian/African origin as compared to European/American origin (AHR = 1.109, 99% CI (1.031–1.192)) and Israeli origin (AHR = 1.068, 99% CI (0.997–1.143), $p = 0.013$), those living in smaller localities (AHR = 1.229, 99% CI (1.136, 1.330)), and those with low socioeconomic status as compared to medium socioeconomic status (AHR = 1.179, 99% CI = 1.101, 1.252). No significant difference was found between high and low socioeconomic status (AHR = 1.019, 99% CI = 0.945, 1.098) (Table 2, Figure 1).

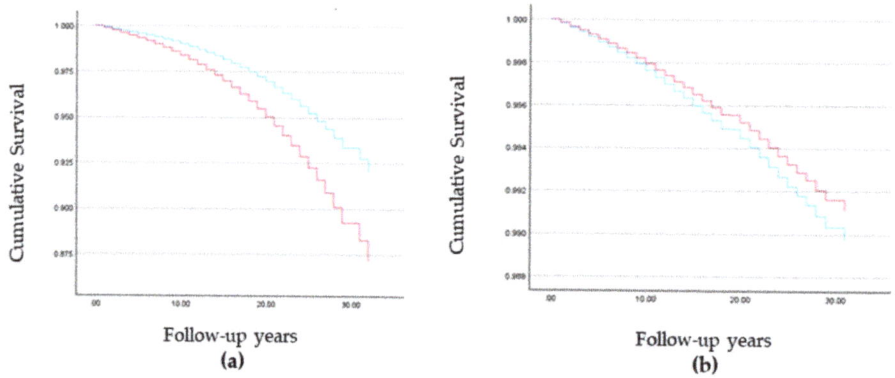

Figure 1. Kaplan–Meier survivor curves among the study population: Jewish women (blue line) and Muslim Arab women (red line): (**a**) All-cause mortality rates and (**b**) breast cancer mortality rates.

As displayed in Table 3, Model 1 accounted for age, ethnicity, number of children, and country of origin. It found lower breast cancer mortality rates among Muslim Arab women (HR = 0.815; 99% CI (0.722, 0.920)), those with more than three children (AHR = 0.925; 99% CI (0.963, 0.992)), and those of Asian/African origin as compared to European/American origin (AHR = 1.166, 99% CI (1.078–1.260)). No significant differences were found between Israeli and Asian/African origin. Model 2 accounted for the same variables, along with locality size. Likewise, it found lower breast cancer mortality rates among Muslim Arab women (HR = 0.849; 99% CI (0.752, 0.960)), those with more than three children (AHR = 0.938; 99% CI (0.875, 1.007), $p = 0.019$), those of Asian/African origin as compared to European/American origin (AHR = 1.181, 99% CI (1.092, 1.277)), and those living in smaller localities (AHR = 1.219, 99% CI (1.124, 1.322)). Similarly, no significant differences were found between Israeli and Asian/African origin. Model 3 accounted for the same variables as Model 2, along with socioeconomic status. It found no significant difference between Muslim Arab and Jewish women. Lower breast cancer mortality rates were found among those with more than three children (AHR = 0.924; 99% CI (0.861, 0.992)), those of Asian/African origin as compared to European/American origin (AHR = 1.173, 99% CI (1.083, 1.270)) and Israeli origin (AHR = 1.060, 99% CI (0.985, 1.140), $p = 0.004$), those living in smaller localities (AHR = 1.189, 99% CI (1.095, 1.291)), and those with low socioeconomic status as compared to medium socioeconomic status (AHR = 1.140, 99% CI (1.060, 1.227)). No significant difference was found between high and low socioeconomic status (AHR = 0.970, 99% CI (0.893, 1.364)).

We found significant interactions between ethnicity and both socioeconomic status and number of children and the prediction of breast cancer mortality. Accordingly, the study population was divided into two groups, Muslim Arab women and Jewish women, by Cox regression and adjusted Kaplan–Meier. The models were built for each group with the following variables being entered separately with age: number of children, country of origin, locality size and socioeconomic status.

Among Muslim Arab women, lower breast cancer mortality rates were found among those with more than three children (AHR = 0.751; 99% CI (0.609, 0.927)) and higher rates among those with high (AHR = 1.591, 99% CI (1.052, 2.631)) and medium socioeconomic status (AHR = 1.309, 99% CI (1.015, 1.796)) as compared to low. Country of origin and locality size were not significant predictors (Table 4, Figure 2).

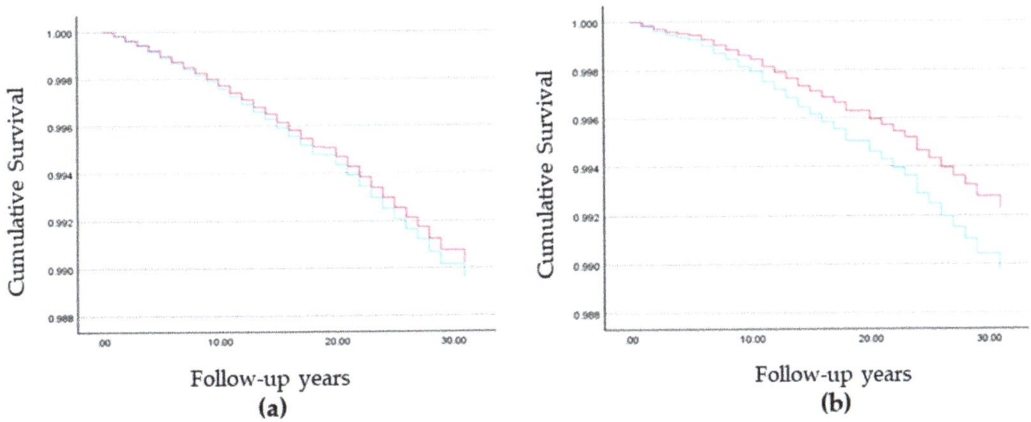

Figure 2. Kaplan–Meier survivor curves among the study population: 0–3 children (blue line) and >3 children (red line): (**a**) Breast cancer mortality among Jewish women and (**b**) Muslim Arab women.

Among Jewish women, number of children was not a significant predictor. Higher breast cancer mortality rates were found among those of European/American (AHR = 1.185, 99% CI (1.096, 1.282)) and Israeli origin (AHR = 1.080, 99% CI (1.001, 1.146)) as compared to those of Asian/African origin, those living in larger localities (AHR = 1.217, 99% CI (1.115, 1.329)), and those with medium socioeconomic status (AHR = 1.146, 99% CI (1.064, 1.235)) as compared to low socioeconomic status. No significant difference was found between high and low socioeconomic status (AHR = 0.988, 99% CI (0.912, 1.071)) (Table 4, Figures 2 and 3).

Overall, Muslim Arab women had lower breast cancer mortality rates as compared to Jewish women. Having more than three children was associated with lower rates in the overall population and among Muslim Arab women but not among Jewish women. Women of European/American origin had higher rates as compared to those of Asian/African origin, consistently among Jewish women but not among Muslim Arab women. Living in larger localities was associated with higher rates, consistently among Jewish women but not among Muslim Arab women. Medium socioeconomic status was associated with higher rates as compared to low status. Among Muslim Arab women, both high and medium status were associated with higher rates, while among Jewish women, only medium status was associated with higher rates as compared to low rate.

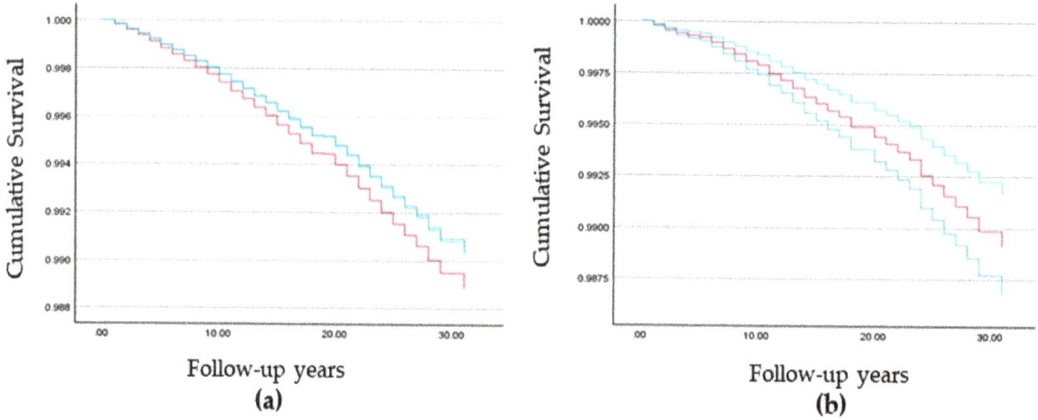

Figure 3. Kaplan–Meier survivor curves among the study population: low (blue line), medium (red line), and high socioeconomic status (green line): (**a**) Breast cancer mortality among Jewish women and (**b**) Muslim Arab women.

4. Discussion

This study investigated differences in breast cancer mortality between two groups and examined how factors such as number of children, socioeconomic status, and place of residence affect mortality rates. By analyzing data from over 800,000 Israeli women over a 30-year period, the researchers' goal was to understand the complex interrelationships among ethnicity, sociodemographic factors and breast cancer mortality.

Similar to previous studies among Muslim Arab women, we also found higher fertility rates [34], lower socioeconomic status [26], and higher tendency to live in smaller localities [27] as compared to Jewish women. Previous studies have also found genetic factors associated with breast cancer morbidity and mortality, with specific genetic characteristics identified among Jewish women of Ashkenazi descent [6,7]. In this study, lower breast cancer mortality was found among Jewish women whose countries of origin were Asia/Africa as compared to those originating from America/Europe. However, this finding was not observed among Muslim Arab women, possibly due to this community's homogeneity regarding country of origin.

Furthermore, this study found higher all-cause mortality rates among Arab women as compared to Jewish women, while breast cancer mortality was higher in Jewish women [29,35]. However, these disparities were not significant after adjusting for variables such as number of children, country of origin, locality size, and socioeconomic status. This may indicate that the differences in mortality between groups can be explained by those variables.

Previous studies have found that women of lower socioeconomic status (SES) have higher breast cancer mortality rates as compared to women of higher SES [2,11]. This disparity has been attributed to lower rates of mammography screening [13,14] later-stage diagnosis [15,16], and worse survival outcomes among women of lower SES [11]. However, a meta-analysis by Taheri et al. [12] suggests that the association between SES and breast cancer mortality rates may not be as strong as previously thought. In contrast to these findings, our study found higher breast cancer mortality rates among women of medium SES as compared to low SES, both among Jewish and Muslim Arab women. This can be explained by Israel's National Health Insurance Law, which allows all women to undergo mammography, significantly reducing the barrier to screening. Furthermore, the law provides women of low SES with access to treatment, potentially leading to higher survival rates.

Coinciding with our previous study [8], we found lower breast cancer mortality rates among Jewish women residing in non-urban areas as compared to those living in urban areas. This finding was not observed among Muslim Arab women, possibly due to differences in quality of life and air pollution exposure between Jewish and Arab communities [35].

Furthuremore, our study found intriguing results regarding breast cancer mortality rates among women of high socioeconomic status as compared to women of low socioeconomic status. In Jewish women, no significant differences in breast cancer mortality were found between high and low socioeconomic status groups. Conversely, in Arab Muslim women, a gradient of increasing breast cancer mortality risk was observed with higher socioeconomic status as compared to women of low socioeconomic status. This finding could be explained by the fact that Jewish women of high socioeconomic status have greater access to resources for extending survival from the disease, while Arab women of similar socioeconomic status have less access. It can be hypothesized that Arab women of high socioeconomic status are more likely to enter the labor market, which is still less common in Arab society [31]. This entry into the workforce may be associated with relatively lower breastfeeding rates. [33]. Furthermore, it can be speculated that Arab women of high socioeconomic status are less likely to breastfeed and less likely to marry and have their first child at a young age, which may increase the risk of morbidity. Previous studies have shown that breastfeeding is associated with a reduced risk of breast cancer [23], and thus, lower breastfeeding rates among Arab women of high socioeconomic status may partially explain the higher breast cancer mortality rates in this group.

Full-term pregnancy and childbirth have been found in previous studies to be protective factors against breast cancer morbidity in the long term [21,22]. However, regarding predictors of breast cancer mortality, we found a high number of children was protective in the general population and among Muslim Arab women but not among Jewish women. This phenomenon can be explained by several factors. Compared to Arab women in Israel, Jewish women tend to have lower breastfeeding rates, older age at breastfeeding, and older maternal age at first birth [28,33]. Arab women are more likely to breastfeed and report fewer difficulties and barriers to breastfeeding [32,33]. Arab women are less likely to enter the labor market [31] and less likely to use hormonal medications [29]. These factors, along with the tendency of Arab women to have a lower maternal age at first birth and to breastfeed more, may contribute to the lack of protective effect of a high number of children against breast cancer mortality in Jewish women as compared to Arab women in Israel.

This study has several limitations. First, it is based on administrative data. Cause of death was determined based on information collected from death certificates by the Ministry of Health. Another limitation was the lack of data on breast cancer incidence and prevalence rates among the studied groups. Such data would have provided a more comprehensive picture and enabled the evaluation of mortality disparities in relation to morbidity and survival disparities.

An additional limitation of our study is the use of parity as a dichotomous variable, with a single threshold of three or more children. While this threshold aligns with the average Israeli fertility rates, exploring different parity levels could provide more nuanced insights. Future research should consider a more granular analysis of parity to better understand how varying fertility rates in different populations might influence breast cancer outcomes.

The absence of education data for a relatively large portion of the population led the authors to use a composite variable of socioeconomic status instead.

5. Conclusions

This study's findings underscore the complex interplay of ethnicity, socioeconomic status, and reproductive factors in breast cancer mortality among Israeli women. The differential impact of risk factors between Jewish and Muslim Arab populations emphasizes the need for culturally sensitive, group-specific interventions. The paradoxical relationship between socioeconomic status and breast cancer mortality in the Israeli context, particularly among Muslim Arab women, warrants further investigation. Moreover, the varying protective effect of parity between ethnic groups suggests intricate interactions with factors such as breastfeeding practices and age at first birth. These results highlight the importance of developing nuanced research approaches and tailored prevention strategies that account for the specific risk profiles of different ethnic and socioeconomic groups. Future studies should aim to elucidate these complex relationships to inform more effective, targeted public health interventions and policies, ultimately reducing breast cancer mortality disparities in Israel's diverse population.

Author Contributions: Conceptualization, R.P.-M. and D.B.; methodology, R.P.-M.; software, D.B. and R.P.-M.; validation, R.P.-M.; formal analysis, R.P.-M.; investigation, R.P.-M.; resources, R.P.-M. and D.B.; data curation, R.P.-M.; writing—original draft preparation, R.P.-M.; writing—review and editing, D.B.; visualization, D.B.; supervision, D.B.; project administration, D.B.; funding acquisition, D.B. All authors have read and agreed to the published version of the manuscript.

Funding: This work was supported by Israel Academic College [Grant Number 112019] and Jerusalem College of Technology [Grant Number 012022RP].

Institutional Review Board Statement: This study was approved by the Ethics Committee of the CBS and the Population Registry Ethics Committee of Ramat Gan Academic College (No 1324).

Informed Consent Statement: Patient consent was waived due to the nature of the study as a retrospective mortality follow-up research using existing, anonymized data from national databases. The study design precludes individual consent and was approved by the institutional ethics committee.

Data Availability Statement: Data are available upon reasonable request.

Conflicts of Interest: The author declares that there are no known competing financial interests or personal relationships that could have appeared to influence the work reported in this paper.

References

1. Bray, F.; Ferlay, J.; Soerjomataram, I.; Siegel, R.L.; Torre, L.A.; Jemal, A. Global cancer statistics 2018: GLOBOCAN estimates of incidence and mortality worldwide for 36 cancers in 185 countries. *CA Cancer J. Clin.* **2018**, *68*, 394–424. [CrossRef] [PubMed]
2. Evelina, A.; Harvey, N.M. *Breast Cancer*; Exon Publications: Brisbane, Australia, 2022; Chapter 1.
3. Ferlay, J.; Colombet, M.; Soerjomataram, I.; Parkin, D.M.; Piñeros, M.; Znaor, A.; Bray, F. Cancer statistics for the year 2020: An overview. *Int. J. Cancer* **2021**, *149*, 778–789. [CrossRef] [PubMed]
4. Ben-Lessen, M.; Silverman, B.; Keinan-Boker, L. Breast Cancer in Israel: An update on morbidity and mortality data. In *Israel Center for Disease Control*; Ministry of Health: Singapore, 2022. Available online: https://www.health.gov.il/PublicationsFiles/breast_cancer_october2022.pdf (accessed on 1 May 2024).
5. Nasrazadani, A.; Marti, J.L.G.; Kip, K.E.; Marroquin, O.C.; Lemon, L.; Shapiro, S.D.; Brufsky, A.M. Breast cancer mortality as a function of age. *Aging* **2022**, *14*, 1186–1199. [CrossRef]
6. Giaquinto, A.N.; Miller, K.D.; Tossas, K.Y.; Winn, R.A.; Jemal, A.; Siegel, R.L. Cancer statistics for African American/Black People 2022. *CA Cancer J. Clin.* **2022**, *72*, 202–229. [CrossRef] [PubMed]
7. Díaz-Velásquez, C.E.; Gitler, R.; Antoniano, A.; Sefchovich, R.K.; De La Cruz-Montoya, A.H.; Martínez-Gregorio, H.; Rojas-Jiménez, E.A.; Penha, R.C.C.; Terrazas, L.I.; Wegman-Ostrosky, T.; et al. Evaluation of genetic alterations in hereditary cancer susceptibility genes in the Ashkenazi Jewish women community of Mexico. *Front. Genet.* **2023**, *14*, 1094260. [CrossRef] [PubMed]
8. Pinchas-Mizrachi, R.; Liptz, J.J.; Zalcman, B.G.; Romem, A. Disparities in Breast Cancer Mortality Rates in Israel among Urban and Rural Women. *Int. J. Environ. Res. Public Health* **2022**, *19*, 15785. [CrossRef]
9. DeSantis, C.E.; Ma, J.; Gaudet, M.M.; Newman, L.A.; Miller, K.D.; Goding Sauer, A.; Jemal, A.; Siegel, R.L. Breast cancer statistics, 2019. *CA Cancer J. Clin.* **2019**, *69*, 438–451. [CrossRef]
10. Tresilian, G.; Morgan, J.; Wyld, L.; Reed, M.; Martin, C.; Chater, T.; Pemberton, K.; Leung, K.C.; Audisio, R.; Thompson, A.; et al. A prospective cohort study to analyse the effect of socioeconomic deprivation on breast cancer stage at diagnosis, treatment allocation and outcomes in older women in the United Kingdom. *Eur. J. Surg. Oncol. (EJSO)* **2022**, *48*, e87. [CrossRef]
11. Ji, P.; Gong, Y.; Jiang, C.; Hu, X.; Di, G.; Shao, Z. Association between socioeconomic factors at diagnosis and survival in breast cancer: A population-based study. *Cancer Med.* **2020**, *9*, 1922–1936. [CrossRef]
12. Taheri, M.; Tavakol, M.; Akbari, M.E.; Almasi-Hashiani, A.; Abbasi, M. Relationship of Socio Economic Status, Income, and Education with the Survival Rate of Breast Cancer: A Meta-Analysis. *Iran. J. Public Health* **2020**, *48*, 1428–1438. [CrossRef]
13. Christiansen, S.R.; Autier, P.; Støvring, H. Change in effectiveness of mammography screening with decreasing breast cancer mortality: A population-based study. *Eur. J. Public Health* **2022**, *32*, 630–635. [CrossRef] [PubMed]
14. Luu, X.Q.; Lee, K.; Jun, J.K.; Suh, M.; Jung, K.-W.; Choi, K.S. Effect of mammography screening on the long-term survival of breast cancer patients: Results from the National Cancer Screening Program in Korea. *Epidemiol. Health* **2022**, *44*, e2022094. [CrossRef] [PubMed]

15. Orsini, M.; Trétarre, B.; Daurès, J.-P.; Bessaoud, F. Individual socioeconomic status and breast cancer diagnostic stages: A French case–control study. *Eur. J. Public Health* **2016**, *26*, 445–450. [CrossRef] [PubMed]
16. Bradley, C.J.; Given, C.W.; Roberts, C. Disparities in cancer diagnosis and survival. *Cancer* **2001**, *91*, 178–188. [CrossRef] [PubMed]
17. Evans, D.G.; Harkness, E.F.; Howel, S.; Woodward, E.R.; Howell, A.; Lalloo, F. Young age at first pregnancy does protect against early onset breast cancer in BRCA1 and BRCA2 mutation carriers. *Breast Cancer Res. Treat.* **2018**, *167*, 779–785. [CrossRef] [PubMed]
18. Haricharan, S.; Dong, J.; Hein, S.; Reddy, J.P.; Du, Z.; Toneff, M.; Holloway, K.; Hilsenbeck, S.G.; Huang, S.; Atkinson, R.; et al. Mechanism and preclinical prevention of increased breast cancer risk caused by pregnancy. *eLife* **2013**, *2*, e00996. [CrossRef] [PubMed]
19. Naghizadeh, S.; Faroughi, F.; Mirghafourvand, M. Investigating the relationship between breast and gynecological cancers and infertility and its treatments: A case-control study. *Eur. J. Cancer Prev.* **2023**, *32*, 600–607. [CrossRef]
20. Pompei, L.d.M.; Fernandes, C.E. Hormone Therapy, Breast Cancer Risk and the Collaborative Group on Hormonal Factors in Breast Cancer Article. *Rev. Bras. Ginecol. Obs.* **2020**, *42*, 233–234. [CrossRef]
21. Terry, M.B.; Liao, Y.; Kast, K.; Antoniou, A.C.; A McDonald, J.; Mooij, T.M.; Engel, C.; Nogues, C.; Buecher, B.; Mari, V.; et al. The Influence of Number and Timing of Pregnancies on Breast Cancer Risk for Women with BRCA1 or BRCA2 Mutations. *JNCI Cancer Spectr.* **2018**, *2*, pky078. [CrossRef]
22. Lund, E.; Nakamura, A.; Snapkov, I.; Thalabard, J.-C.; Olsen, K.S.; Holden, L.; Holden, M. Each pregnancy linearly changes immune gene expression in the blood of healthy women compared with breast cancer patients. *Clin. Epidemiol.* **2018**, *10*, 931–940. [CrossRef]
23. Islami, F.; Liu, Y.; Jemal, A.; Zhou, J.; Weiderpass, E.; Colditz, G.; Boffetta, P.; Weiss, M. Breastfeeding and breast cancer risk by receptor status—A systematic review and meta-analysis. *Ann. Oncol.* **2015**, *26*, 2398–2407. [CrossRef] [PubMed]
24. AlEdeilah, R.D.; Alanazi, O.H.A.; AlHarby, B.S.F.; Al Al Issa, M.S.; Al-Dhahry, S.A.S.; AlAnazi, A.N.K.; AlAnazi, H.O.H.; Alanazi, S.N.S. Breastfeeding as a Protective Factor against Breast Cancer: A Systematic Review. *Clin. Cancer Investig. J.* **2022**, *11*, 36–41. [CrossRef]
25. Foster, S.F.; Vazquez, C.; Cubbin, C.; Nichols, A.R.; Rickman, R.R.; Widen, E.M. Breastfeeding, socioeconomic status, and long-term postpartum weight retention. *Int. Breastfeed. J.* **2023**, *18*, 1–9. [CrossRef] [PubMed]
26. Alvakilli, N.; Publică, R.M.A.d.A.; Sirota, Y.; Valley, I.C.M.S.Y. DEMOGRAPHIC, ECONOMIC AND SOCIAL CHARACTERISTICS OF ISRAEL MINORITIES. *Adm. Publica* **2022**, 79–87. [CrossRef]
27. Haddad Haj-Yahya, N.; Khalaily, M.; Rudnitzky, A. *Statistical Report on Arab Society in Israel 2021*; Israel Democracy Institute: Jerusalem, Israel, 2022. Available online: https://en.idi.org.il/media/18218/statistical-report-on-arab-society-in-israel-2021.pdf (accessed on 1 May 2024).
28. Blickstein, I.; Baor, L. Trends in multiple births in Israel. *Harefuah* **2004**, *143*, 794–798, 839. [PubMed]
29. Tsanani, S.E.; Abu Ahmad, N.; Agbaria, M. Breast Cancer in Arab and Jewish Women in Northern Israel: A Retrospective Database Study. *Isr. Med. Assoc. J.* **2023**, *25*, 495–499.
30. Pinchas-Mizrachi, R.; Solnica, A.; Daoud, N. Religiosity Level and Mammography Performance among Arab and Jewish Women in Israel. *J. Relig. Health* **2020**, *60*, 1877–1894. [CrossRef] [PubMed]
31. Schein, A. Female labor force participation in Israel, 1955–2017. *Isr. Aff.* **2020**, *26*, 635–649. [CrossRef]
32. Keinan-Boker, L.; Shohat, T.; Wienstein, R.; Goldsmith, R.; Shimony, T.; Ophir, E.; Altman, H.; Amram, O.; Fisher, N.; Frost, D.; et al. *National Health and Nutrition Survey*; Ministry of Health: Singapore, 2014. Available online: https://www.gov.il/blobFolder/reports/mabat-infant/he/files_publications_units_ICDC_mabat-infant.pdf.pdf (accessed on 15 April 2024).
33. Zimmerman, D.R.; Kaplan, M.; Shoob, H.; Freisthler, M.; Toledano, M.; Stein-Zamir, C. Breastfeeding challenges and support in a high initiation population. *Isr. J. Health Policy Res.* **2022**, *11*, 1–10. [CrossRef]
34. Staetsky, L.D. Stalling fertility decline of Israeli Muslims and the demographic transition theory. *Popul. Stud.* **2019**, *73*, 317–333. [CrossRef]
35. Keinan-Boker, L.; Baron-Epel, O.; Fishler, Y.; Liphshitz, I.; Barchana, M.; Dichtiar, R.; Goodman, M. Breast cancer trends in Israeli Jewish and Arab Women, 1996–2007. *Eur. J. Cancer Prev.* **2013**, *22*, 112–120. [CrossRef] [PubMed]

cancers

MDPI

Article

Predictors of Clavien–Dindo Grade III–IV or Grade V Complications after Metastatic Spinal Tumor Surgery: An Analysis of Sociodemographic, Socioeconomic, Clinical, Oncologic, and Operative Parameters

Rafael De la Garza Ramos [1,2,*], Jessica Ryvlin [1], Ali Haider Bangash [1], Mousa K. Hamad [1,2], Mitchell S. Fourman [1,3], John H. Shin [4], Yaroslav Gelfand [1,2], Saikiran Murthy [1,2] and Reza Yassari [1,2]

1 Spine Research Group, Montefiore Medical Center, Albert Einstein College of Medicine, Bronx, NY 10467, USA; jessica.ryvlin@einsteinmed.org (J.R.); alihaider2022-010@stmu.edu.pk (A.H.B.); hamadmousa@gmail.com (M.K.H.); mfourman@montefiore.org (M.S.F.); ygelfand@montefiore.org (Y.G.); samurthy@montefiore.org (S.M.); ryassari@montefiore.org (R.Y.)

2 Department of Neurological Surgery, Montefiore Medical Center, Albert Einstein College of Medicine, Bronx, NY 10467, USA

3 Department of Orthopedic Surgery, Montefiore Medical Center, Albert Einstein College of Medicine, Bronx, NY 10467, USA

4 Department of Neurological Surgery, Massachusetts General Hospital, Harvard Medical School, Boston, MA 02115, USA; shin.john@mgh.harvard.edu

* Correspondence: rdelag@montefiore.org

Simple Summary: This research aims to understand the influence of sociodemographic, socioeconomic, clinical, oncologic, and operative parameters on a patient's risk of major complications or death within 30 days after surgery for spinal tumors that have spread from other parts of the body. The researchers looked at data from 165 patients who had this surgery at a major cancer center between 2012–2023. The findings suggest that a patient's background factors do not impact their short-term surgical outcomes. Instead, factors like the patient's overall health, spinal cord compression severity, and nutritional status seem more important. The research community may find these findings helpful in optimizing outcomes for patients undergoing complex spinal tumor surgeries.

Abstract: The rate of major complications and 30-day mortality after surgery for metastatic spinal tumors is relatively high. While most studies have focused on baseline comorbid conditions and operative parameters as risk factors, there is limited data on the influence of other parameters such as sociodemographic or socioeconomic data on outcomes. We retrospectively analyzed data from 165 patients who underwent surgery for spinal metastases between 2012–2023. The primary outcome was development of major complications (i.e., Clavien–Dindo Grade III–IV complications), and the secondary outcome was 30-day mortality (i.e., Clavien–Dindo Grade V complications). An exploratory data analysis that included sociodemographic, socioeconomic, clinical, oncologic, and operative parameters was performed. Following multivariable analysis, independent predictors of Clavien–Dindo Grade III–IV complications were Frankel Grade A–C, lower modified Bauer score, and lower Prognostic Nutritional Index. Independent predictors of Clavien–Dindo Grade V complications) were lung primary cancer, lower modified Bauer score, lower Prognostic Nutritional Index, and use of internal fixation. No sociodemographic or socioeconomic factor was associated with either outcome. Sociodemographic and socioeconomic factors did not impact short-term surgical outcomes for metastatic spinal tumor patients in this study. Optimization of modifiable factors like nutritional status may be more important in improving outcomes in this complex patient population.

Keywords: metastatic spinal tumors; outcomes; sociodemographic; socioeconomic; complications; mortality; Clavien–Dindo; vulnerability; modified Bauer score; health disparities

1. Introduction

Complication rates after oncologic surgery for metastatic spine disease are high [1–7]. Major adverse events such as unplanned return to the operating room or complications requiring management in an intensive care unit can all have a detrimental impact on a patient's postoperative course, potentially delaying chemotherapy or radiation treatment. Major complications, including perioperative mortality, are currently estimated to affect up to 35% of patients undergoing surgery, and the rate can be influenced by several risk factors [1–3,8,9].

Factors reported in the literature include older age, multilevel metastases, baseline performance status, frailty, malnutrition, and others [1,8–11]. Some studies have also found that race and insurance status affect the overall complication and non-routine discharge rate after spinal tumor surgery [12,13], but the association between multiple sociodemographic and socioeconomic factors with major complication rates or 30-day mortality has been understudied. In fact, most studies currently omit important covariates such as social vulnerability or primary language, which may play a role in the short-term morbidity and mortality of these patients and procedures.

Thus, the purpose of our study was to perform an exploratory data analysis into the association, if any, of sociodemographic, socioeconomic, clinical, oncologic, and operative parameters with the occurrence of Clavien–Dindo Grade III–IV or Grade V complications.

2. Materials and Methods

2.1. Study Design and Setting

This research investigation, which was carried out at an urban teaching hospital in a large metropolitan region, was retrospective and single-center. The hospital is affiliated to a cancer center that has been recognized by the National Cancer Institute. In July 2023, a query was made to our neurosurgical spine operative database to identify our potential research group.

2.2. Patients

We surgically managed 168 patients suffering from spinal metastases, spinal cord compression, pathologic vertebral compression fractures, and/or spinal mechanical instability between April 2012 and February 2023. Patients who met the following criteria were included: they had to be tracked until death or for at least 30 days after surgery, and they had to have comprehensive sociodemographic, socioeconomic, clinical, oncologic, operative, and follow-up data. These criteria resulted in the exclusion of 1% (2) patients for incomplete data and <1% (1) patient for loss prior to the minimum study follow-up time, leaving 98% (165 of 168) of the patients for final analysis. Among our analytic sample, surgical indications included metastatic spinal cord compression in 86% (142) of patients, pathologic vertebral compression fractures in 50% (83) of patients, 29% (48) of patients had unstable lesions, and 64% (106) of patients had potentially unstable lesions as identified by the Spinal Instability Neoplastic Score (SINS). Surgical decompression was performed for patients with myelopathy, motor weakness, or inability to ambulate if they presented within 48 h of impairment; internal fixation was performed in patients who were at risk for iatrogenic instability from surgical decompression or patients with a SINS indicative of potential instability or instability.

2.3. Variables

Collected sociodemographic and socioeconomic data included age, sex (male vs. female), self-reported race: White, Black, Hispanic or Latino, or other (Middle Eastern, Asian, or Southeast Asian), primary language (English versus non-English), primary insurance status at the time of surgery (Medicare, Medicaid, or private), year of surgery, and SVI score and SVI subtheme scores (socioeconomic status, household composition and disability, minority status and language, and housing type and transportation). The SVI scores were obtained from the Centers for Disease Control and Prevention's website (https://svi.cdc.gov/map.html, (accessed on 1 September 2023)); the year immediately preceding the date of surgery was used as well as patient's domicile at the time of surgery. These scores range from 0–1, with a higher value being indicative of higher vulnerability or deprivation.

Collected clinical, oncological, and operative data included Eastern Cooperative Oncology Group (ECOG) performance status within 30 days of surgery, body mass index (BMI), American Society of Anesthesiologists class, Frankel grade at presentation (D–E vs. A–C), primary cancer (lung, breast, prostate, kidney, thyroid, colorectal, hematologic, or other), modified Bauer score, preoperative Prognostic Nutritional Index (PNI), de novo cancer diagnosis, SINS, emergency-type procedure (performed within 24 h of admission), use of internal fixation, open procedure, number of instrumented vertebrae, and use of transpedicular decompression. The scales used are summarized and referenced in the Supplementary Material Tables S1–S5.

2.4. Primary and Secondary Study Endpoints

The primary endpoint was development of at least one Clavien–Dindo Grade III or IV complication within 30 days of surgery [10]. These are considered major surgical complications and include complications requiring surgical, endoscopic, or radiological intervention (such as epidural hematoma or wound infection requiring revision surgery), or life-threatening complications requiring intensive care unit admission (such as adult respiratory distress syndrome or unplanned intubation) [10]. The secondary endpoint was development of a Clavien–Dindo Grade V complication within 30 days of surgery, which is defined as 30-day mortality.

2.5. Statistical Analysis

All analyses were performed in Stata 16 IC (StataCorp, College Station, TX, USA). An initial data exploration was carried out where distribution of data was assessed using histograms and the Kolmogorov–Smirnov test. A univariable logistic regression analysis was carried out with Clavien–Dindo Grade III or IV complications as the main dependent variable; for the secondary outcome the same analysis was performed with Clavien–Dindo Grade IV complications as the main dependent variable. The included independent variables were age, sex, race (White, Black, Hispanic or Latino, or other), non-English primary language, Medicare primary insurance, Medicaid primary insurance, private primary insurance, year of surgery (2012–2017 or 2018–2023), overall SVI score, socioeconomic status score, household composition and disability score, racial or ethnic group and language score, housing type and transportation score, ECOG performance status, BMI, ASA class, Frankel grade A–C, primary cancer (lung, breast, prostate, kidney, thyroid, colorectal, hematologic, or other), modified Bauer score, preoperative PNI, de novo cancer diagnosis, SINS, emergency-type procedure, use of internal fixation, open procedure, number of instrumented vertebrae, and use of transpedicular decompression. All factors with a p value less than 0.10 were then included in a multivariable stepwise logistic regression analysis with backward elimination. Results are presented as odds ratios (OR) with 95% confidence intervals (CI). Statistical significance was defined as a p value less than 0.05.

3. Results

3.1. Patients' Baseline Data

A total of 165 patients were included in this study (Table 1). The median age of our study population was 63 years (interquartile range [IQR] 54 to 70), and 62% (102 of 165) of patients were men. The race distribution was 18% (n = 29) White, 45% (n = 74) Black, 30% (n = 49) Hispanic or Latino, and 8% (n = 13) other. Non-English was the primary language in 21% (n = 35) of patients. The insurance distribution was as follows: Medicare: 38% (n = 63), Medicaid: 36% (n = 60), and private insurance: 21% (n = 35). The median SVI score was 89.8 (IQR 72.6 to 98.0). The median ECOG performance status was 2 (IQR 1 to 3) and the median ASA Class was 3 (IQR 3 to 3) (Table 2). From the entire group, 21% (35 of 165) of patients presented with Frankel Grade A to C and 32% ($n = 52$) with complete inability to walk. The median modified Bauer score was 2 (1 to 3) and the mean PNI was 42.5 ± 7.7.

Table 1. Sociodemographic, socioeconomic, clinical, oncologic, and operative data of 165 patients.

Parameter	Value
Age in years, median (IQR)	63 (54 to 70)
Male, % (*n*)	61.8 (102)
Race, % (*n*)	
White	17.6 (29)
Black	44.9 (74)
Hispanic/Latino	29.7 (49)
Other	7.8 (13)
Primary language, % (*n*)	
English	78.8 (130)
Non-English	21.2 (35)
Primary insurance, % (*n*)	
Medicare	38.2 (63)
Medicaid	36.4 (60)
Private	21.2 (35)
Year of surgery	
2012–2017	49.7 (82)
2018–2023	50.3 (83)
Social Vulnerability Index, median (IQR)	89.8 (72.6 to 98.0)
SVI subthemes, median (IQR)	
Socioeconomic status	80.4 (56.8 to 93.9)
Household composition and disability	70.1 (44.9 to 86.4)
Minority status and language	91.5 (85.0 to 97.6)
Housing type and transportation	87.6 (73.7 to 95.9)
ECOG performance status, % (*n*)	
0	5.6 (9)
1	36.4 (60)
2	30.3 (50)
3	23.6 (39)
4	4.2 (7)
BMI in kg/m^2, mean ± SD	26.6 ± 5.6
ASA Class, median (IQR)	3 (3 to 3)
Frankel Grade, % (*n*)	
Frankel D–E	78.9 (130)
Frankel A–C	21.1 (35)

Table 1. *Cont.*

Parameter	Value
Primary cancer, % (*n*)	
Breast	15.2 (25)
Lung	15.8 (26)
Prostate	20.0 (33)
Colorectal	4.9 (8)
Kidney	4.9 (8)
Hematologic	20.0 (33)
Other	17.8 (29)
Modified Bauer score, median (IQR)	2 (1 to 3)
Prognostic Nutritional Index, mean ± SD	42.5 ± 7.7
De novo cancer diagnosis, % (*n*)	37.0 (61)
SINS, median (IQR)	11 (8 to 13)
Emergency procedure, % (*n*)	26.0 (43)
Internal fixation	88.5 (146)
Open procedure	73.3 (121)
Number of instrumented levels, median (IQR)	4 (4 to 6)
Transpedicular decompression	55.8 (92)

ECOG = Eastern Cooperative Oncology Group; SINS = Spinal Instability Neoplastic Score.

Table 2. Outcomes by independent risk factor (univariable analysis).

Parameter	Clavien–Dindo Grade III–IV Complication	Odds Ratio with 95% CI	Clavien–Dindo Grade V Complication	Odds Ratio with 9% CI
Increasing Age		0.9 (0.9 to 1.1) $p = 0.52$		1.0 (0.9 to 1.1) $p = 0.21$
Male vs. Female	27% vs. 25%	1.1 (0.5 to 2.2) $p = 0.88$	9% vs. 8%	1.1 (0.4 to 3.5) $p = 0.84$
White vs. Not-White	28% vs. 26%	1.1 (0.5 to 2.7) $p = 0.84$	10% vs. 8%	1.3 (0.3 to 5.0) $p = 0.69$
Black vs. Not-Black	27% vs. 25%	1.1 (0.5 to 2.2) $p = 0.80$	5% vs. 11%	0.5 (0.2 to 1.5) $p = 0.21$
Hispanic/Latino vs. Not Hispanic/Latino	20% vs. 29%	0.6 (0.3 to 1.4) $p = 0.29$	8% vs. 9%	0.9 (0.3 to 2.2) $p = 0.92$
Other race vs. Not Other race	38% vs. 25%	1.9 (0.6 to 6.1) $p = 0.30$	23% vs. 7%	3.9 (0.9 to 16.1) $p = 0.07$ *
Non-English primary language vs. English primary language	17% vs. 28%	0.5 (0.2 to 1.4) $p = 0.18$	9% vs. 8%	1.0 (0.3 to 3.9) $p = 0.98$
Medicare insurance vs. no	24% vs. 27%	0.8 (0.4 to 1.7) $p = 0.61$	8% vs. 9%	0.9 (0.3 to 2.8) $p = 0.84$
Medicaid Insurance vs. no	25% vs. 27%	0.9 (0.4 to 1.9) $p = 0.82$	10% vs. 8%	1.3 (0.4 to 4.1) $p = 0.60$
Private insurance vs. no	29% vs. 25%	1.2 (0.5 to 2.7) $p = 0.70$	6% vs. 9%	0.6 (0.1 to 2.8) $p = 0.51$
Year of surgery 2012–2017 vs. 2018–2023	28% vs. 24%	1.2 (0.6 to 2.4) $p = 0.627$	6% vs. 11%	0.7 (0.4 to 1.3) $p = 0.31$
Increasing SVI		0.8 (0.2 to 3.9) $p = 0.80$		1.1 (0.1 to 13.3) $p = 0.96$
Increasing socioeconomic status vulnerability		0.9 (0.3 to 3.5) $p = 0.93$		1.6 (0.2 to 13.8) $p = 0.69$
Increasing household composition and disability vulnerability		1.1 (0.3 to 4.3) $p = 0.92$		5.0 (0.4 to 58.4) $p = 0.20$
Increasing minority status and language vulnerability		0.6 (0.1 to 5.1) $p = 0.64$		0.5 (0.1 to 12.6) $p = 0.69$

Table 2. *Cont.*

Parameter	Clavien–Dindo Grade III–IV Complication	Odds Ratio with 95% CI	Clavien–Dindo Grade V Complication	Odds Ratio with 9% CI
Increasing housing type and transportation vulnerability		0.9 (0.2 to 5.4) $p = 0.92$		0.9 (0.1 to 14.9) $p = 0.95$
Increasing ECOG performance status		1.8 (1.2 to 2.6) $p = 0.01$ *		2.3 (1.3 to 4.2) $p = 0.01$ *
Increasing BMI		1.0 (0.9 to 1.1) $p = 0.95$		0.8 (0.7 to 0.9) $p = 0.01$ *
Increasing ASA Class		1.4 (0.8 to 2.5) $p = 0.31$		2.2 (0.9 to 5.7) $p = 0.09$ *
Frankel Grade A–C vs. D–E	51% vs. 19%	4.4 (2.0 to 9.8) $p < 0.001$ *	17% vs. 6%	3.2 (1.1 to 9.8) $p = 0.05$ *
Breast cancer vs. no breast cancer	16% vs. 28%	0.5 (0.2 to 1.5) $p = 0.22$	4% vs. 9%	0.4 (0.1 to 3.3) $p = 0.40$
Lung cancer vs. no lung cancer	42% vs. 23%	2.5 (1.1 to 5.9) $p = 0.04$	31% vs. 4%	9.9 (3.1 to 31.7) $p < 0.001$ *
Prostate cancer vs. no prostate cancer	18% vs. 28%	0.6 (0.2 to 1.5) $p = 0.25$	0% vs. 11%	Omitted
Colorectal cancer vs. no colorectal cancer	25% vs. 26%	0.9 (0.2 to 4.9) $p = 0.94$	13% vs. 8%	1.6 (0.2 to 13.9) $p = 0.68$
Kidney cancer vs. no kidney cancer	38% vs. 25%	1.8 (0.4 to 7.7) $p = 0.46$	13% vs. 8%	1.6 (0.2 to 13.9) $p = 0.68$
Hematologic cancer vs. no hematologic cancer	21% vs. 27%	0.7 (0.3 to 1.8) $p = 0.48$	6% vs. 9%	0.6 (0.2 to 3.0) $p = 0.58$
Other cancer vs. no other cancer	34% vs. 24%	1.6 (0.7 to 3.9) $p = 0.26$	4% vs. 10%	0.3 (0.1 to 2.7) $p = 0.31$
Increasing modified Bauer score		0.5 (0.3 to 0.8) $p = 0.001$ *		0.3 (0.2 to 0.6) $p < 0.001$ *
Increasing PNI		0.9 (0.8 to 0.9) $p = 0.005$ *		0.9 (0.8 to 0.9) $p = 0.02$ *
De novo cancer diagnosis vs. no	26% vs. 26%	1.0 (0.5 to 2.1) $p = 0.97$	10% vs. 8%	1.3 (0.4 to 3.9) $p = 0.63$
Increasing SINS		0.9 (0.8 to 0.9) $p = 0.02$ *		1.0 (0.8 to 1.2) $p = 0.97$
Emergency procedure vs. no	40% vs. 21%	2.4 (1.1 to 5.1) $p = 0.02$ *	12% vs. 7%	1.7 (0.5 to 5.2) $p = 0.39$
Internal fixation vs. no	25% vs. 37%	0.6 (0.2 to 1.5) $p = 0.26$	9% vs. 21%	0.3 (0.1 to 0.9) $p = 0.05$ *
Open procedure vs. no	29% vs. 18%	1.8 (0.8 to 4.3) $p = 0.17$	9% vs. 7%	1.4 (0.4 to 5.2) $p = 0.64$
Increasing number of instrumented levels		1.0 (0.8 to 1.3) $p = 0.72$		0.8 (0.5 to 1.2) $p = 0.25$
Transpedicular decompression vs. no	22% vs. 32%	0.6 (0.3 to 1.2) $p = 0.16$	5% vs. 12%	0.4 (0.1 to 1.3) $p = 0.12$

SVI: social vulnerability index; ECOG: Eastern Cooperative Oncology Group; BMI: body mass index; ASA: American Society of Anesthesiologists; PNI: Prognostic Nutritional Index; SINS: spinal instability neoplastic score; * Included in the multivariable model.

3.2. *Univariable Analysis of Factors Associated with Clavien–Dindo Grade III–IV Complications and Grade V Complications*

From the total study group, 26% (43 of 165) of patients developed at least one Clavien–Dindo Grade III or IV complication. These complications included unplanned return to the operating room (n = 12), sepsis (n = 11), pulmonary embolism (n = 9), unplanned intubation (n = 7), adult respiratory distress syndrome (n = 5), meningitis (n = 3), and stroke (n = 2). The rate of Clavien–Dindo Grade V complications was 8.5% (14 of 165). The crude rates of these complications as well as univariable analysis are summarized in Table 2. No sociodemographic or socioeconomic factor was significantly associated with these outcomes on univariable analysis.

3.3. Multivariable Analysis of Factors Associated with Clavien–Dindo Grade III–IV Complications and Grade V Complications

After controlling for ECOG performance status, Frankel Grade A–C, lung cancer, modified Bauer score, PNI, SINS, and emergency procedures (Table 3), independent factors associated with development of at least one Clavien–Dindo Grade III or IV complication were Frankel Grade A–C (OR 6.2, 95% CI 2.4 to 15.5; $p < 0.001$), the modified Bauer score (OR 0.5, 95% CI 0.3 to 0.91; $p = 0.02$), and the PNI (OR 0.9, 95% CI 0.8 to 0.9; $p = 0.02$).

Table 3. Stepwise multivariable logistic regression of factors associated with Clavien–Dindo Grade III–IV Complications or Grade V Complications.

Clavien–Dindo Grave III–IV Complications			
Parameter	**OR**	**95% CI**	***p* Value**
ECOG performance status	1.2	0.8 to 2.0	0.37
Frankel Grade A–C	6.2	2.4 to 15.5	<0.001 *
Lung	0.8	0.2 to 2.8	0.76
Modified Bauer score	0.6	0.4 to 0.9	0.01 *
Prognostic Nutritional Index	0.9	0.8 to 0.9	0.01 *
SINS	0.9	0.8 to 1.0	0.08
Emergency procedure	2.2	0.8 to 6.5	0.15
Clavien–Dindo Grave V Complications			
Parameter	**OR**	**95% CI**	***p* Value**
Other race	6.4	0.7 to 57.8	0.10
ECOG performance status	1.2	0.8 to 2.0	0.37
BMI	0.9	0.7 to 1.0	0.15
ASA Class	1.6	0.4 to 5.8	0.48
Frankel Grade A–C	3.5	0.6 to 20.5	0.17
Lung	5.2	1.1 to 24.5	0.04 *
Modified Bauer score	0.4	0.2 to 0.9	0.03 *
Prognostic Nutritional Index	0.9	0.8 to 0.9	0.04 *
Internal fixation	0.1	0.1 to 0.4	0.01 *

ECOG: Eastern Cooperative Oncology Group; BMI: body mass index; ASA: American Society of Anesthesiologists; SINS: spinal instability neoplastic score; * statistically significant finding.

After controlling for other race, ECOG performance status, BMI, ASA class, Frankel Grade A–C, lung cancer, modified Bauer score, PNI, and internal fixation, independent factors associated with development of a Clavien–Dindo Grade V complication were lung primary cancer (OR 5.2, 95% CI 1.1 to 24.5; $p = 0.04$), modified Bauer score (OR 0.4; 95% CI 0.2 to 0.9; $p = 0.03$), the PNI (OR 0.9, 95% CI 0.8 to 0.9; $p = 0.04$), and use of internal fixation (OR 0.1; 95% CI, 0.1 to 0.4; $p = 0.01$) (Table 3).

4. Discussion

The rate of major complications including perioperative mortality after metastatic spinal tumor surgery is relatively high, estimated at 16–34% [1–4]. While many different factors such as age, multilevel metastases, baseline performance status, frailty, and malnutrition have been shown to be associated with adverse events [1,10,11], data also accounting for other important sociodemographic or socioeconomic data such as race, primary language, and social vulnerability, among others, are limited. In general surgical oncology, disparities in outcomes have predominantly affected minority patients and patients with low socioeconomic status [14]. Black and African-American patients have been shown to have higher risk of adverse events and perioperative mortality across multiple studies [15–17]. Similarly, socially vulnerable patients and patients without private insurance tend to have worse outcomes [18].

The present study sought to examine a cohort of surgical patients and perform an exploratory analysis accounting for many different variables, including sociodemographic, socioeconomic, clinical, oncological, and operative factors and their association with major perioperative morbidity. We found that no single sociodemographic or socioeconomic factor was associated with the development of Clavien–Dindo Grade III or IV complications (major complications) after metastatic spinal tumor surgery. On the other hand, the only clinical factors associated with this endpoint were a preoperative Frankel Grade A–C, the modified Bauer score, and the PNI. Although several other studies have found that race is associated with a higher likelihood of overall complications after oncologic spine surgery [19], a study looking at both minor and major complications found that race was associated with minor, but not major complications, similar to our findings [12]. An institutional series of 328 patients found that race, insurance, and income were not associated with postoperative complications [13]. Likewise, a study examining the impact of insurance status on in-hospital mortality and complications found that after adjusting for acuity of presentation, socioeconomic status, hospital bed size, and hospital teaching status, no difference in outcomes were found [20]. These results suggest that perioperative complications are more likely the result of baseline patient characteristics such as the neurologic exam, extent of disease, and nutritional status, among others.

When examining Clavien–Dindo Grade V complications, we also found that no sociodemographic or socioeconomic factor was associated with this outcome. Short-term mortality, particularly within 30 days, is usually more related to a patient's preoperative functional status, nutritional/inflammatory status, and the development of any perioperative adverse event rather than the primary tumor pathology [8,21,22]. Our findings are consistent, however, with other studies that found that factors such as race, insurance, or social vulnerability were not associated with post-treatment survival on multivariable analysis [19,23,24].

Independent factors associated with both outcomes studied here included the modified Bauer score and the PNI. The former is a composite score that includes primary cancer type as well as extent of disease (assessed by the presence of visceral metastasis and solitary vs. multiple metastatic lesions) and indicates that a patient's baseline extent of disease is perhaps more predictive of the postoperative course as opposed to a particular sociodemographic or socioeconomic parameter [25,26]. Similarly, the PNI is a measure of the nutritional-inflammatory status of a patient and has been found to be associated with outcomes in oncologic spine surgery including postoperative survival and complication occurrence [11,27,28]. While formal research in patients with metastatic spine disease is lacking, nutritional supplementation of cancer patients is a potentially modifiable risk factor that could impact the surgical recovery and tolerability of adjuvant therapy [29,30].

There are several limitations to the study, particularly selection bias. Our study is a single-center experience so results may not be entirely generalizable to other populations. Our study group also consisted of mostly minority and socially vulnerable patients which may not represent other study populations. The lack of an association between sociodemographic or socioeconomic parameters may also be the result of sample size and unmeasured covariates, among others. Nonetheless, over 35 multi-dimensional variables were analyzed in a detailed univariable and multivariable analysis, as opposed to previous studies focused more on comorbidities and surgical parameters as predictors of major perioperative morbidity.

5. Conclusions

The present study sought to examine the association between different multi-dimensional parameters and the development of major complications including 30-day mortality after surgery for metastatic spinal tumors. We found that no sociodemographic or socioeconomic factor predicted these events. On the other hand, preoperative neurologic status, the modified Bauer score, and nutritional status, among others, may be more likely responsible for short-term outcome in this challenging patient population. These findings may prove useful for preoperative risk stratification and future research into potential optimization strategies.

Supplementary Materials: The following supporting information can be downloaded at: https://www.mdpi.com/article/10.3390/cancers16152741/s1. Table S1. Eastern Cooperative Oncology Group (ECOG) Performance Status Scale [1]. Table S2. American Society of Anesthesiologists (ASA) Physical Status Classification System [2]. Table S3. Frankel Classification of Spinal Cord Injury [3]. Table S4. Modified Bauer Score for Prognostic Assessment of Spinal Metastases [4]. Table S5. Spinal Instability Neoplastic Score (SINS) [5]. References [25,31–34] are cited in Supplementary Materials.

Author Contributions: Conceptualization, R.D.l.G.R. and R.Y.; methodology, R.D.l.G.R.; formal analysis, R.D.l.G.R., J.R., A.H.B. and M.K.H.; investigation, All authors; writing—original draft preparation, R.D.l.G.R. and J.R.; writing—review and editing, All authors; supervision, Y.G., S.M., J.H.S. and R.Y. All authors have read and agreed to the published version of the manuscript.

Funding: This research received no external funding.

Institutional Review Board Statement: The study was conducted in accordance with the Declaration of Helsinki, and approved by the Institutional Review Board of Albert Einstein College of Medicine, Bronx, NY, USA (protocol code IRB 2016-6896; 30 September 2016).

Informed Consent Statement: Informed consent was waived given this was a retrospective chart review investigation.

Data Availability Statement: The data presented in this study are available on request from the corresponding author due to privacy concerns.

Conflicts of Interest: The authors declare no conflicts of interest.

References

1. Luksanapruksa, P.; Buchowski, J.M.; Zebala, L.P.; Kepler, C.K.; Singhatanadgige, W.; Bumpass, D.B. Perioperative Complications of Spinal Metastases Surgery. *Clin. Spine Surg.* **2017**, *30*, 4–13. [CrossRef] [PubMed]
2. Boaro, A.; Wells, M.; Chi, J.; Lu, Y.; Smith, T.R.; Groff, M.W.; Zaidi, H. A National Surgical Quality Improvement Program Analysis of Postoperative Major and Minor Complications in Patients with Spinal Metastatic Disease. *World Neurosurg.* **2020**, *140*, e203–e211. [CrossRef] [PubMed]
3. Hussain, I.; Hartley, B.R.; McLaughlin, L.; Reiner, A.S.; Laufer, I.; Bilsky, M.H.; Barzilai, O. Surgery for Metastatic Spinal Disease in Octogenarians and Above: Analysis of 78 Patients. *Glob. Spine J.* **2023**, *13*, 1481–1489. [CrossRef] [PubMed]
4. Park, S.-J.; Lee, C.-S.; Chung, S.-S. Surgical Results of Metastatic Spinal Cord Compression (MSCC) from Non-Small Cell Lung Cancer (NSCLC): Analysis of Functional Outcome, Survival Time, and Complication. *Spine J.* **2016**, *16*, 322–328. [CrossRef] [PubMed]
5. Sarkiss, C.A.; Hersh, E.H.; Ladner, T.R.; Lee, N.; Kothari, P.; Lakomkin, N.; Caridi, J.M. Risk Factors for Thirty-Day Morbidity and Mortality in Extradural Lumbar Spine Tumor Resection. *World Neurosurg.* **2018**, *114*, e1101–e1106. [CrossRef] [PubMed]
6. Paulino Pereira, N.R.; Ogink, P.T.; Groot, O.Q.; Ferrone, M.L.; Hornicek, F.J.; van Dijk, C.N.; Bramer, J.A.M.; Schwab, J.H. Complications and Reoperations after Surgery for 647 Patients with Spine Metastatic Disease. *Spine J.* **2019**, *19*, 144–156. [CrossRef] [PubMed]
7. Szczerba, P. Complications after Surgical Treatment of Spinal Metastases. *Ortop. Traumatol. Rehabil.* **2019**, *21*, 23–31. [CrossRef] [PubMed]
8. Karhade, A.V.; Thio, Q.C.B.S.; Ogink, P.T.; Shah, A.A.; Bono, C.M.; Oh, K.S.; Saylor, P.J.; Schoenfeld, A.J.; Shin, J.H.; Harris, M.B.; et al. Development of Machine Learning Algorithms for Prediction of 30-Day Mortality After Surgery for Spinal Metastasis. *Neurosurgery* **2019**, *85*, E83–E91. [CrossRef] [PubMed]
9. Schoenfeld, A.J.; Le, H.V.; Marjoua, Y.; Leonard, D.A.; Belmont, P.J.; Bono, C.M.; Harris, M.B. Assessing the Utility of a Clinical Prediction Score Regarding 30-Day Morbidity and Mortality Following Metastatic Spinal Surgery: The New England Spinal Metastasis Score (NESMS). *Spine J.* **2016**, *16*, 482–490. [CrossRef] [PubMed]
10. De la Garza Ramos, R.; Goodwin, C.R.; Jain, A.; Abu-Bonsrah, N.; Fisher, C.G.; Bettegowda, C.; Sciubba, D.M. Development of a Metastatic Spinal Tumor Frailty Index (MSTFI) Using a Nationwide Database and Its Association with Inpatient Morbidity, Mortality, and Length of Stay After Spine Surgery. *World Neurosurg.* **2016**, *95*, 548–555.e4. [CrossRef] [PubMed]
11. Rigney, G.H.; Massaad, E.; Kiapour, A.; Razak, S.S.; Duvall, J.B.; Burrows, A.; Khalid, S.I.; De La Garza Ramos, R.; Tobert, D.G.; Williamson, T.; et al. Implication of Nutritional Status for Adverse Outcomes after Surgery for Metastatic Spine Tumors. *J. Neurosurg. Spine* **2023**, *39*, 557–567. [CrossRef] [PubMed]
12. De la Garza Ramos, R.; Choi, J.H.; Naidu, I.; Benton, J.A.; Echt, M.; Yanamadala, V.; Passias, P.G.; Shin, J.H.; Altschul, D.J.; Goodwin, C.R.; et al. Racial Disparities in Perioperative Morbidity Following Oncological Spine Surgery. *Glob. Spine J.* **2023**, *13*, 1194–1199. [CrossRef] [PubMed]

13. Hung, B.; Pennington, Z.; Hersh, A.M.; Schilling, A.; Ehresman, J.; Patel, J.; Antar, A.; Porras, J.L.; Elsamadicy, A.A.; Sciubba, D.M. Impact of Race on Nonroutine Discharge, Length of Stay, and Postoperative Complications after Surgery for Spinal Metastases. *J. Neurosurg. Spine* **2021**, *36*, 678–685. [CrossRef] [PubMed]
14. Nizam, W.; Yeo, H.L.; Obeng-Gyasi, S.; Brock, M.V.; Johnston, F.M. Disparities in Surgical Oncology: Management of Advanced Cancer. *Ann. Surg. Oncol.* **2021**, *28*, 8056–8073. [CrossRef] [PubMed]
15. Akinyemiju, T.; Meng, Q.; Vin-Raviv, N. Race/Ethnicity and Socio-Economic Differences in Colorectal Cancer Surgery Outcomes: Analysis of the Nationwide Inpatient Sample. *BMC Cancer* **2016**, *16*, 715. [CrossRef] [PubMed]
16. Chikovsky, L.; Kutuk, T.; Rubens, M.; Balda, A.N.; Appel, H.; Chuong, M.D.; Kaiser, A.; Hall, M.D.; Contreras, J.; Mehta, M.P.; et al. Racial Disparities in Clinical Presentation, Surgical Procedures, and Hospital Outcomes among Patients with Hepatocellular Carcinoma in the United States. *Cancer Epidemiol.* **2023**, *82*, 102317. [CrossRef] [PubMed]
17. Mets, E.J.; Chouairi, F.K.; Gabrick, K.S.; Avraham, T.; Alperovich, M. Persistent Disparities in Breast Cancer Surgical Outcomes among Hispanic and African American Patients. *Eur. J. Surg. Oncol.* **2019**, *45*, 584–590. [CrossRef] [PubMed]
18. Azap, R.A.; Paredes, A.Z.; Diaz, A.; Hyer, J.M.; Pawlik, T.M. The Association of Neighborhood Social Vulnerability with Surgical Textbook Outcomes among Patients Undergoing Hepatopancreatic Surgery. *Surgery* **2020**, *168*, 868–875. [CrossRef] [PubMed]
19. De la Garza Ramos, R.; Benton, J.A.; Gelfand, Y.; Echt, M.; Flores Rodriguez, J.V.; Yanamadala, V.; Yassari, R. Racial Disparities in Clinical Presentation, Type of Intervention, and in-Hospital Outcomes of Patients with Metastatic Spine Disease: An Analysis of 145,809 Admissions in the United States. *Cancer Epidemiol.* **2020**, *68*, 101792. [CrossRef] [PubMed]
20. Dasenbrock, H.H.; Wolinsky, J.-P.; Sciubba, D.M.; Witham, T.F.; Gokaslan, Z.L.; Bydon, A. The Impact of Insurance Status on Outcomes after Surgery for Spinal Metastases. *Cancer* **2012**, *118*, 4833–4841. [CrossRef] [PubMed]
21. Musharbash, F.N.; Khalifeh, J.M.; Raad, M.; Puvanesarajah, V.; Lee, S.H.; Neuman, B.J.; Kebaish, K.M. Predicting 30-Day Mortality after Surgery for Metastatic Disease of the Spine: The H2-FAILS Score. *Eur. Spine J.* **2023**, *32*, 2513–2520. [CrossRef] [PubMed]
22. Ryvlin, J.; Kim, S.W.; Hamad, M.K.; Fourman, M.S.; Eleswarapu, A.; Murthy, S.G.; Gelfand, Y.; De la Garza Ramos, R.; Yassari, R. The Prognostic Role of Neutrophil-to-Lymphocyte Ratio, Platelet-to-Lymphocyte Ratio, and Systemic Immune-Inflammation Index on Short- and Long-Term Outcome Following Surgery for Spinal Metastases. *J. Neurosurg. Spine* **2024**, *40*, 475–484. [CrossRef] [PubMed]
23. De la Garza Ramos, R.; Javed, K.; Ryvlin, J.; Gelfand, Y.; Murthy, S.; Yassari, R. Are There Racial or Socioeconomic Disparities in Ambulatory Outcome or Survival After Oncologic Spine Surgery for Metastatic Cancer? Results From a Medically Underserved Center. *Clin. Orthop.* **2023**, *481*, 301–307. [CrossRef] [PubMed]
24. Tang, C.; Hess, K.; Bishop, A.J.; Pan, H.Y.; Christensen, E.N.; Yang, J.N.; Tannir, N.; Amini, B.; Tatsui, C.; Rhines, L.; et al. Creation of a Prognostic Index for Spine Metastasis to Stratify Survival in Patients Treated With Spinal Stereotactic Radiosurgery: Secondary Analysis of Mature Prospective Trials. *Int. J. Radiat. Oncol. Biol. Phys.* **2015**, *93*, 118–125. [CrossRef] [PubMed]
25. Leithner, A.; Radl, R.; Gruber, G.; Hochegger, M.; Leithner, K.; Welkerling, H.; Rehak, P.; Windhager, R. Predictive Value of Seven Preoperative Prognostic Scoring Systems for Spinal Metastases. *Eur. Spine J.* **2008**, *17*, 1488–1495. [CrossRef] [PubMed]
26. Goodwin, C.R.; Schoenfeld, A.J.; Abu-Bonsrah, N.A.; Garzon-Muvdi, T.; Sankey, E.W.; Harris, M.B.; Sciubba, D.M. Reliability of a Spinal Metastasis Prognostic Score to Model 1-Year Survival. *Spine J.* **2016**, *16*, 1102–1108. [CrossRef] [PubMed]
27. De la Garza Ramos, R.; Ryvlin, J.; Hamad, M.K.; Fourman, M.S.; Eleswarapu, A.; Gelfand, Y.; Murthy, S.G.; Shin, J.H.; Yassari, R. The Prognostic Nutritional Index (PNI) Is Independently Associated with 90-Day and 12-Month Mortality after Metastatic Spinal Tumor Surgery. *Eur. Spine J.* **2023**, *32*, 4328–4334. [CrossRef] [PubMed]
28. De la Garza Ramos, R.; Ryvlin, J.; Hamad, M.K.; Fourman, M.S.; Gelfand, Y.; Murthy, S.G.; Shin, J.H.; Yassari, R. Predictive Value of Six Nutrition Biomarkers in Oncological Spine Surgery: A Performance Assessment for Prediction of Mortality and Wound Infection. *J. Neurosurg. Spine* **2023**, *39*, 664–670. [CrossRef] [PubMed]
29. Dambrós, B.F.; Kobus, R.A.; da Rosa, R.; Pereira, L.J.; Hinnig, P.d.F.; Di Pietro, P.F.; Kunradi Vieira, F.G. The Effect of Oral Dietary Interventions on Nutritional Status and Treatment Tolerance in Patients with Hematologic Neoplasms Receiving Chemotherapy: A Systematic Review. *Nutr. Rev.* **2023**, nuad161. [CrossRef]
30. Knight, S.R.; Qureshi, A.U.; Drake, T.M.; Lapitan, M.C.M.; Maimbo, M.; Yenli, E.; Tabiri, S.; Ghosh, D.; Kingsley, P.A.; Sundar, S.; et al. The Impact of Preoperative Oral Nutrition Supplementation on Outcomes in Patients Undergoing Gastrointestinal Surgery for Cancer in Low- and Middle-Income Countries: A Systematic Review and Meta-Analysis. *Sci. Rep.* **2022**, *12*, 12456. [CrossRef]
31. Oken, M.M.; Creech, R.H.; Tormey, D.C.; Horton, J.; Davis, T.E.; McFadden, E.T.; Carbone, P.P. Toxicity and Response Criteria of the Eastern Cooperative Oncology Group. *Am. J. Clin. Oncol.* **1982**, *5*, 649–655. [CrossRef] [PubMed]
32. Doyle, D.J.; Hendrix, J.M.; Garmon, E.H. American Society of Anesthesiologists Classification. In *StatPearls*; StatPearls Publishing: Treasure Island, FL, USA, 2024.

33. Frankel, H.L.; Hancock, D.O.; Hyslop, G.; Melzak, J.; Michaelis, L.S.; Ungar, G.H.; Vernon, J.D.; Walsh, J.J. The Value of Postural Reduction in the Initial Management of Closed Injuries of the Spine with Paraplegia and Tetraplegia. I. *Paraplegia* **1969**, *7*, 179–192. [CrossRef] [PubMed]
34. Fisher, C.G.; DiPaola, C.P.; Ryken, T.C.; Bilsky, M.H.; Shaffrey, C.I.; Berven, S.H.; Harrop, J.S.; Fehlings, M.G.; Boriani, S.; Chou, D.; et al. A Novel Classification System for Spinal Instability in Neoplastic Disease: An Evidence-Based Approach and Expert Consensus from the Spine Oncology Study Group. *Spine* **2010**, *35*, E1221–E1229. [CrossRef] [PubMed]

cancers

MDPI

Article

Healthcare Costs and Resource Utilisation of Italian Metastatic Non-Small Cell Lung Cancer Patients

Nicola Gentili [1], William Balzi [1,*], Flavia Foca [2], Valentina Danesi [1], Mattia Altini [3], Angelo Delmonte [4], Giuseppe Bronte [4], Lucio Crinò [4], Nicoletta De Luigi [5], Marita Mariotti [4], Alberto Verlicchi [4], Marco Angelo Burgio [4], Andrea Roncadori [1], Thomas Burke [6] and Ilaria Massa [1]

1 Outcome Research, Healthcare Administration, IRCCS Istituto Romagnolo per lo Studio dei Tumori (IRST) "Dino Amadori", 47014 Meldola, Italy; nicola.gentili@irst.emr.it (N.G.); valentina.danesi@irst.emr.it (V.D.); andrea.roncadori@irst.emr.it (A.R.); ilaria.massa@irst.emr.it (I.M.)

2 Unit of Biostatistics and Clinical Trials, IRCCS Istituto Romagnolo per lo Studio dei Tumori (IRST) "Dino Amadori", 47014 Meldola, Italy; flavia.foca@irst.emr.it

3 Healthcare Administration, Azienda Unità Sanitaria Locale della Romagna, 48121 Ravenna, Italy; mattia.altini@regione.emilia-romagna.it

4 Department of Medical Oncology, IRCCS Istituto Romagnolo per lo Studio dei Tumori (IRST) "Dino Amadori", 47014 Meldola, Italy; angelo.delmonte@irst.emr.it (A.D.); g.bronte@staff.univpm.it (G.B.); lucio.crino@irst.emr.it (L.C.); marita.mariotti@irst.emr.it (M.M.); alberto.verlicchi@irst.emr.it (A.V.); marco.burgio@irst.emr.it (M.A.B.)

5 Ospedale di Stato della Repubblica di San Marino, 47893 San Marino City, San Marino; nicoletta.deluigi@iss.sm

6 MSD Innovation & Development GmbH, 8004 Zurich, Switzerland

* Correspondence: william.balzi@irst.emr.it

Simple Summary: This study aimed to assess the costs and healthcare resource utilization (HCRU) of metastatic non-small cell lung cancer (NSCLC) by biomarker status in the pre- and post-approval of the immuno-oncology agent. The analysis examined healthcare costs and HCRU before and after the local regulatory approval of pembrolizumab as a first-line (1L) treatment. Patients were stratified into mutation-positive and negative/unknown groups according to mutational status. The negative/unknown group was further sub-grouped based on the availability of pembrolizumab at the time of starting 1L treatment. Costs and HCRU were analyzed separately for the 1L treatment and overall disease follow-up across lines of therapy and by groups. The study found that introducing 1L immunotherapy has improved overall survival, but healthcare spending has increased concurrently. Decision-makers may find our results useful in deciding how best to allocate resources for treating metastatic NSCLC in terms of the health–economic model and policy.

Abstract: This study evaluated the economic burden of metastatic non-small cell lung cancer patients before and after the availability of an immuno-oncology (IO) regimen as a first-line (1L) treatment. Patients from 2014 to 2020 were categorized according to mutational status into mutation-positive and negative/unknown groups, which were further divided into pre-1L IO and post-1L IO sub-groups depending on the availability of pembrolizumab monotherapy in 1L. Healthcare costs and HCRU for a 1L treatment and overall follow-up were reported as the mean total and per-month cost per patient by groups. Of 644 patients, 125were mutation-positive and 519 negative/unknown (229 and 290 in pre- and post-1L IO, respectively). The mean total per-patient cost in 1L was lower in pre- (EUR 7804) and post-1L IO (EUR 19,301) than the mutation-positive group (EUR 45,247), persisting throughout overall disease follow-up. However, this difference was less when analyzing monthly costs. Therapy costs were the primary driver in 1L, while hospitalization costs rose during follow-up. In both mutation-positive and post-IO 1L groups, the 1L costs represented a significant portion (70.1% and 66.3%, respectively) of the total costs in the overall follow-up. Pembrolizumab introduction increased expenses but improved survival. Higher hospitalisation and emergency room occupation rates during follow-up reflected worsening clinical conditions of the negative/unknown group than the mutation-positive population.

Keywords: non-small cell lung cancer (NSCLC); immunotherapy; real-world evidence; healthcare resource utilisation (HCRU); costs; economics; administrative databases; Italy

1. Introduction

Globally, lung cancer is the most frequent tumour and the leading cause of cancer-related deaths [1]. In Italy, over 43,900 patients receive a lung cancer diagnosis each year [2]. In particular, non-small cell lung cancer (NSCLC) accounts for approximately 80–85% of all lung cancer diagnoses, with a five-year survival rate of less than 5% for Stage IV disease [3,4]. The high incidence rate of severe disability associated with NSCLC disease is a significant public health issue. Furthermore, the high level of healthcare resource utilisation (HCRU) incurred by NSCLC patients and the high costs of new pharmacological treatment can result in financial pressure for healthcare payers [5,6]. Therefore, the estimate of healthcare costs of NSCLC patients is of great interest nowadays for sound decision-making in the allocation of limited resources to provide the best care in an economically sustainable context. Cost analyses on the management of NSCLC have been examined more and more worldwide, mainly in the USA. However, most papers were limited in assessing the economic value of specific drugs focusing on subgroups of patients with a targetable genetic aberration, or on specific histological subtypes (i.e., squamous or squamous), rather than examining the overall NSCLC category or broader treatment patterns [7–12]. Above all, most studies have been conducted before the approval of newer costly therapies such as immunotherapies, which have changed the overall medical management of metastatic NCSLC in recent years. This new class of medicine has improved clinical outcomes, but healthcare spending has increased concurrently [13–18]. Unfortunately, estimations of the financial burden associated with the management of NSCLC, especially after the approval of new costly therapies such as immune checkpoint inhibitors (ICIs), are lacking in Italy.

Perrone et al. performed one of the first Italian analyses of NSCLC costs in 2004, but the reliability of their findings is now outdated [19]. Another Italian study reported an increase in the economic burden of metastatic NSCLC patients as opposed to previous analyses [20]. A real-world analysis evaluated the management of NSCLC cases diagnosed in the Veneto region in 2015 and 2017 [21]. The study detected a 38% rise in the average overall cost for the 2017 cohort compared to the 2015 cohort due to the introduction of new expensive oncologic drugs for the care of metastatic diseases Likewise, an economic assessment of advanced NSCLC patients treated with either pembrolizumab or tyrosine-kinase inhibitors (TKI) estimated average per-patient healthcare costs of EUR 51,735 and EUR 30,708 during the first year of the first-line (1L) treatment, respectively [22]. A recent cost comparison across Europe showed that the mean per-patient cost related to Italian advanced NSCLC patients who received two or more lines of therapy amounted to EUR 19,317 [23].

Following market access approval by the Italian Medicines Agency, pembrolizumab was authorized in the Emilia–Romagna region in July 2017 as a 1L treatment for metastatic NSCLC patients with a programmed death-ligand 1 (PD-L1) Tumour Proportion Score (TPS) of at least 50% and no targetable mutations. The introduction of immuno-oncology (IO) treatment in the 1L setting has significantly changed the overall medical and economic management of metastatic NSCLC patients. Considering this recent therapeutic innovation, this study evaluated medical costs and the HCRU of metastatic NSCLC before and after the approval of a 1L immunotherapy agent in the Emilia–Romagna region (July 2017).

2. Materials and Methods

2.1. Study Design

This evaluation is an economic addendum analysis of a retro-prospective observational study conducted in IRCCS Istituto Romagnolo per lo studio dei Tumori (IRST) "Dino Amadori" (located in the Emilia–Romagna region), which investigated the clinical outcomes of metastatic NSCLC patients before and after the regional regulatory approval of PD-L1 inhibitors in the 1L setting of NSCLC [24]. In this economic assessment, costs and HCRU were evaluated in the same population reported by Danesi et al., adding the patients with oncogenic driver mutations who were excluded in the previous manuscript [24]. The perspective of the National Healthcare Service (SSN, Servizio Sanitario Nazionale) was adopted while only considering costs sustained by the healthcare payer. Costs and HCRU were expressed as per patient per month (PPPM) and mean total per-patient cost. The analysis was conducted separately for the 1L treatment and overall disease follow-up (FU) across lines of therapy. The first-line period was calculated as the time from the start of the 1L drug administration until the first of the following event: 30 days after the conclusion of the 1L treatment, the start of the second-line therapy, the end of the observational period (December 2020), the death, or the last visit. The overall disease FU period was calculated as the time from the beginning of the 1L drug administration and the end of the observational period (December 2020), the death, or the last visit. The study evaluated costs associated with all–cause hospitalisations, cancer therapies, and outpatient and hospice care. Data on HCRU included the number of ordinary hospitalisations, the relative length of stay (LOS), the number of drug administrations, and outpatient and Emergency Room (ER) admissions. In addition, the LOS of hospice admission was assessed.

2.2. Study Population

Patients included in this economic analysis had the same eligibility criteria as in the previous study [24]: (i) aged ≥18 years (ii) with a confirmed diagnosis of NSCLC presenting with Stage IV or Stage IIIB with a rapidly progressive disease (IIIBrp). These patients also experienced disease progression to Stage IV within six months from the first anticancer treatment without completing both radiotherapy and chemotherapy induction therapy. (iii) Residents of the Emilia–Romagna region (iv) initiated 1L treatment between 1 January 2014 and 30 June 2020 at IRST, and (v) patients were enrolled after signing the informed consent or after death. In comparison to the previous clinical study [24], we excluded patients who died within 30 days of starting 1L treatment to avoid overestimation of costs and HCRU, as well as patients who were enrolled in clinical trials during the study period, because costs were reimbursed by study sponsors. The study subjects were recruited in two phases: before (pre-1L IO) and after (post-1L IO) the approval of pembrolizumab as a 1L treatment in the Emilia–Romagna region in July 2017. The observational period for each patient started at the diagnosis time of Stage IV/IIIBrp and ended with the patient's death or the end of the observational period (December 2020).

2.3. Cohorts Description

The overall population was stratified by mutation status of epidermal growth factor receptor (EGFR) or anaplastic lymphoma kinase (ALK) or receptor tyrosine kinase (ROS1) (EGFR/ALK/ROS1 mutation-positive vs. EGFR/ALK/ROS1 negative or unknown). The patients without oncogenic driver mutations or whose status were unknown were further sub-grouped according to the availability of the first ICI available as 1L monotherapy in the Emilia–Romagna region (pembrolizumab in PD-L1 TPS > 50% metastatic NSCLC) at the date of initiation of 1L systemic anticancer treatment (pre- and post-1L IO, respectively). In short, the medical cost and HCRU were calculated separately for the following patient groups:

1. Mutation-positive with oncogenic driver mutation in EGFR, ALK, or ROS1, regardless of the availability of the first ICI as 1L monotherapy at the date of their 1L starting time.
2. Negative/Unknown without oncogenic driver mutation or unknown status in EGFR, ALK, or ROS1, which was divided into two sub-groups according to the availability of the first ICI as 1L monotherapy:
    - Pre-1L IO included eligible patients who started 1L treatment from January 2014 to June 2017 before the 1L ICI was available in the Emilia–Romagna region;
    - Post-1L IO included eligible patients who started 1L treatment from July 2017 to June 2020 after 1L ICI was available in the Emilia–Romagna region.

2.4. Data Sources

Patients diagnosed with metastatic NSCLC between January 2014 and June 2020 were recruited from the IRST Electronic Health Record (EHR). The clinical dataset was obtained from data registered by physicians in EHR during routine clinical practice. EHR contains visits, routine laboratory examinations, disease assessments, administered drugs, and all the procedures that NSCLC patients could receive in outpatient and inpatient settings. Data on hospitalisation, drug prescriptions, outpatients and ER visits, and hospice care were obtained from multiple administrative databases:

- Hospital Discharge Records (SDO) collects information on hospital admissions, both ordinary (with at least one overnight stay in hospital) and day-hospital stays (admissions without an overnight stay), which was active until April 2016. The SDO collects the start and end date of hospitalisation, the primary diagnosis coded according to the International Classification of Disease, Ninth Revision, Clinical Modification (ICD-9-CM), and the procedures and services provided. The remuneration system is based on the classification of the Diagnosis Related Groups (DRG), which aggregates the activities of each individual diagnosis and defines the reimbursement rate. Under the DRG-based reimbursement system, each hospitalized patient falls into a group of homogeneous diagnostic cases. Therefore, patients with the same DRG value have been allocated the same reimbursement costs, which do not correspond to the total amount of resources used during the hospital stay, but it is an average value of resource utilisation attributable to that DRG [25];
- Outpatient Specialist Assistance Database (ASA) collects individual information on all outpatient visits, clinical tests, and procedures delivered in the outpatient setting. The outpatient costs were estimated based on the assumption that each procedure is reimbursed according to the Regional Healthcare Range of Fees [26]. The ASA costs were calculated by multiplying the unit cost for resource consumption;
- Emergency Room Admissions Database (PS) contained information about any single emergency admission, including procedures, diagnoses, and costs performed during emergency room (ER) admission;
- Electronic Health Records were used to retrieve data on biomarker and gene panel tests.
- Pharmaceutical Databases (FED and AFT–direct hospital administration and territorial pharmacies distribution) coded according to the Anatomical Therapeutic Chemical classification system were used to collect data on drugs administered;
- Hospice Discharge Records contain the main information about any single hospice admission;
- Registry of Mortality (REM) of the Emilia–Romagna region was used to retrieve data on vital status.

The assignment of a patient identification code to all Emilia–Romagna inhabitants, regardless of admission setting (inpatient or outpatient), is an enabled deterministic record linkage among these various databases.

2.5. Outcome Measures

Costs and HCRU associated with the 1L therapy and the overall disease FU were estimated separately for the three groups of patients. A mean per-patient total and monthly costs were estimated for the following categories:

- Ordinary hospitalization refers to costs of all-cause hospitalization (with at least one overnight stay in hospital), except inpatient stays for therapy administration (identified by code 410);
- Cancer therapy included costs of dispensed drugs, ordinary hospitalization, and day-hospital service for therapy administration (Code 410), and the costs associated with the outpatient setting of drug administration (Code 99.25), medical visits, and blood draws performed before each drug administration;

- Outpatient procedures included costs associated with FU visits, diagnostic exams, biomarker and gene panel tests, laboratory tests, and day-hospital admissions (with code different from 410) performed in the outpatient setting;
- Hospice included all costs associated with the hospice admission.

For HCRU, we collected the number and LOS of ordinary all-cause hospitalizations except for therapy administration (Code 410), the number of drug administrations (ordinary and day-hospital admission with Code 410, and outpatient visits with Code 99.25), the number of outpatient visits (except access, which reported Code 99.25), the LOS of hospice care, and the number of all-cause ER admissions.

2.6. Statistical Analysis

Categorical data were presented as frequencies and percentages, while continuous data were summarized using median and minimum–maximum values for patient demographic and treatment characteristics. Mean PPPM was reported for HCRU and costs, considering the period of 1L treatment and the overall disease FU across the lines of treatments. Mean total cost and HCRU per patient were also reported, as well as the percentile distribution to better observe the data distribution. All the analyses were conducted using SAS 9.4 software (SAS Institute, Cary, NC, USA).

3. Results

3.1. Patient Characteristics

A total of 644 patients were considered according to the study inclusion/exclusion criteria. We identified 125 patients with oncogenic driver mutations (EGFR, ALK, or ROS1 mutation-positive group) and 519 without mutations or unknown status (EGFR, ALK, or ROS1 negative/unknown group). The negative/unknown population was split into pre-1L IO (N = 229) and post-1L IO (N = 290) sub-groups. Patient demographic and clinical characteristics are summarized for each group in Table 1.

Most patients were over 70, with a median age of 70.6 (min–max: 35.7–89.9). In both pre- and post-1L IO groups, the majority of patients were males ($\geq$65.1%). An opposite pattern was observed in the mutation-positive group, where females were 69.9%. Most patients in the negative/unknown group were smokers, with a similar proportion in pre- (94.8%) and post-1L IO (92.6%). Conversely, the number of "never" (50.9%) and "ever" (49.1%) smokers was similar in the mutation-positive group. A slight difference in ECOG (Eastern Cooperative Oncology Group) Performance Status (PS) at IIIBrp/IV stage diagnosis was observed between the mutation-positive and negative/unknown groups. The predominant histology was adenocarcinoma, in particular, in the mutation-positive group (96.0%), with a comparable proportion in pre- (75.6%) and post-1L IO (78.2%). Among the known metastatic sites, the contralateral lung was the most prevalent metastasis location in all three cohorts, accounting for more than one-third of patients.

3.2. Treatment Patterns

All 644 patients who met the study's criteria received a 1L treatment. Due to the poor prognosis, only 37.4% and 11.2% of patients received second- and third-line treatment, respectively. Only 3.7% of patients received additional treatment beyond the third-line treatment (Supplementary Tables S1 and S2).

In the mutation-positive cohort, 103 patients (82.4%) were treated with 1L targeted therapy according to their mutation status, while 17 (13.6%) and five (4.0%) patients received multi- and single-agent chemotherapy, respectively (Table 2).

In the negative/unknown cohort, multi-agent was the most common 1L regimen in pre- (67.7%) and post-1L IO (49.0%). In pre-1L IO, 74 patients (32.3%) were treated with single-agent therapy. In comparison, in post-1L IO, the 1L treatment most utilized after multi-agent chemotherapy was the PD-1/PD-L1 inhibitor single-agent pembrolizumab administrated to 67 patients (23.1%). Only 19 patients (6.5%) received pembrolizumab in combination with chemotherapy. The median duration of the 1L treatment was 10.1 months (min–max: 1.0–67.0) for the mutation-positive group, and 2.7 (min–max: 1.0–49.7) and and 3.8 (min–max: 1.0–41.2) months for the negative/unknown cohort in pre- and post-1L IO, respectively. The median duration of overall FU across lines of therapy was 17.5 months (min–max: 1.6–76.8) for the mutation-positive group, and 5.8 (min–max: 1.0–78.9) and 8.3 (min–max: 1.0–41.3) months for the negative/unknown cohort in pre- and post-1L IO, respectively.

Table 1. Baseline demographic and clinical characteristics for mutation-positive patients with oncogenic driver mutations (EGFR, ALK, and ROS1 mutations) and patients without mutations (EGFR, ALK, and ROS1 negative or unknown), which were presented in two separate subgroups (pre- and post-1L IO).

	EGFR, ALK, or ROS1 Mutation-Positive Patients	EGFR, ALK, or ROS1 Negative/Unknown patients	
Characteristics	**N = 125 (%)**	**Pre-1L IO N = 229 (%)**	**Post-1L IO N = 290 (%)**
IIIBrp/IV stage			
IIIBrp	2 (2.6)	10 (4.4)	6 (2.1)
IV	123 (98.4)	219 (95.6)	284 (97.9)
Age at IIIBrp/IV stage diagnosis			
<70 years	69 (55.2)	118 (51.5)	124 (42.8)
70–74 years	18 (14.4)	52 (22.7)	67 (23.1)
75–79 years	13 (10.4)	35 (15.3)	70 (24.1)
80–84 years	18 (14.4)	22 (9.6)	20 (6.9)
≥85 years	7 (5.6)	2 (0.9)	9 (3.1)
Gender			
Female	87 (69.6)	80 (34.9)	93 (32.1)
Male	38 (30.4)	149 (65.1)	197 (67.9)
Race			
White	123 (98.4)	228 (99.6)	290 (100.0)
Other	2 (1.6)	1 (0.4)	0 (0.0)
Smoking history			
Never	57 (50.9)	9 (5.2)	17 (7.4)
Ever	55 (49.1)	165 (94.8)	212 (92.6)
Unknown	13	55	61
Year smoked			
≤20 years	7 (17.5)	9 (6.9)	17 (13.1)
>20 years	33 (82.5)	122 (93.1)	112 (86.9)
Unknown	40	131	129
Packs/year			
≤20 packs/years	14 (37.8)	11 (8.9)	20 (15.9)
>20 packs/years	23 (62.2)	113 (91.1)	106 (84.1)
Unknown	88	105	164
ECOG PS at IIIBrp/IV stage diagnosis			
0	26 (22.6)	37 (17.0)	42 (15.2)
1	67 (58.3)	143 (65.6)	186 (67.1)
≥2	22 (19.1)	38 (17.4)	49 (17.7)
Unknown	10	11	13
Histology			
Squamous cell	1 (0.8)	37 (16.4)	57 (20.0)
Non-squamous cell	121 (96.8)	172 (76.4)	223 (78.2)
Adenocarcinoma	*120 (96.0)*	*170 (75.6)*	*223 (78.2)*
Large cell carcinoma	*1 (0.8)*	*2 (0.8)*	*0 (0.0)*
Other	3 (2.4)	16 (7.2)	5 (1.8)
Unknown	0	4	5
Location of metastases			
Bone	41 (32.8)	80 (34.9)	79 (27.2)
Lymph nodes	37 (29.6)	49 (21.4)	78 (26.9)
Brain	30 (24.0)	35 (15.3)	49 (16.9)
Liver	14 (11.2)	23 (10.0)	26 (9.0)
Pleura	25 (20.0)	30 (13.1)	44 (15.2)
Contralateral lung	49 (39.2)	77 (33.6)	99 (34.1)
Other	15 (12.0)	67 (29.2)	45 (15.5)
Missing/Unknown	0	3	5

Table 2. First-line (1L) treatments administered by mutation status. The negative/unknown cohort was further grouped based on the 1L immune checkpoint inhibitor monotherapy availability at 1L starting time (pre-and post-1L IO).

	EGFR, ALK, or ROS1 Mutation-Positive Patients	EGFR, ALK, or ROS1 Negative/Unknown Patients	
First-line (1L) Therapies	***N* = 125 (%)**	**Pre-1L IO *N* = 229 (%)**	**Post-1L IO *N* = 290 (%)**
Multi-agent chemotherapy	17 (13.6)	155 (67.7)	142 (49.0)
Gemcitabine + Platin	5 (4.0)	67 (29.3)	90 (31.0)
Pemetrexed +/− Platin	12 (9.6)	83 (36.2)	43 (14.9)
Paclitaxel + Carboplatin	—	5 (2.2)	9 (3.1)
Single-agent chemotherapy	5 (4.0)	74 (32.3)	62 (21.4)
Gemcitabine	4 (3.2)	42 (18.4)	30 (10.3)
Vinorelbine	1 (0.8)	28 (12.2)	31 (10.7)
Docetaxel	—	4 (1.7)	1 (0.4)
Targeted therapy	103 (82.4)	0 (0.0)	0 (0.0)
Afatinib	23 (18.4)	—	—
Alectinib	7 (5.6)	—	—
Crizotinib	7 (5.6)	—	—
Erlotinib	10 (8.0)	—	—
Gefitinib	37 (29.6)	—	—
Osimertinib	19 (15.2)	—	—
PD-1/PD-L1 inhibitor single agent	—	—	67 (23.1)
Pembrolizumab	—	—	67 (23.1)
PD-1/PDL1 inhibitor + chemotherapy	—	—	19 (6.5)

3.3. Healthcare Costs

The mean total per-patient cost associated with 1L treatment in the mutation-positive group amounted to EUR 45,247, which resulted in a mean per-patient per-month cost (PPPM) of EUR 3814 (Table 3).

For the negative/unknown group, the mean total per-patient cost was lower, ranging from EUR 7804 in pre-IO 1L to EUR 19,301 in post-IO 1L, or EUR 3381 and EUR 3464 per-patient per-month cost, respectively (Table 3). The main cost driver was associated with cancer therapy, accounting for about 76.5% (EUR 34,597) and 64.9% (EUR 12,517) in the mutation-positive and post-1L IO groups, respectively. The higher costs associated with patients treated in the pre-1L IO group were mainly driven by cancer therapy (EUR 2790) and hospitalization (EUR 2789), representing 35.8% and 35.7% of the overall cost, respectively. The hospitalization expenditure associated with the negative/unknown group was remarkably high, especially in pre-1L IO. Regarding the outpatient procedures, the mean total per-patient cost ranged from a maximum of EUR 5967 in the mutation-positive group to a minimum of EUR 1988 in the pre-IO 1L group. However, when the PPPM spending was analyzed, the trend of the outpatient cost was the opposite, resulting in a monthly cost of EUR 573 for the mutation-positive group and EUR 576 and EUR 741 for pre- and post-IO 1L, respectively. The lowest costs were associated with hospice visits across all groups.

The mean total per-patient cost associated with the overall disease FU varied from EUR 70,985 in the mutation-positive group to EUR 19,649 and EUR 29,111 in pre- and post-IO 1L (Table 4).

Table 3. Costs related to the 1L treatment are reported in euros (€) as mean per patient per month (PPPM) and other descriptive statistics, grouped by mutation status. The negative/unknown cohort was further sub-grouped based on 1L starting time in pre- and post-1L IO.

1L Costs	EGFR, ALK, or ROS1 Mutation-Positive Patients							EGFR, ALK, or ROS1 Negative/Unknown Patients Pre-1L IO							EGFR, ALK, or ROS1 Negative/Unknown Patients Post-1L IO						
	Mean PPPM € (%)	Mean Cost € (%)	Percentiles of the Costs Distribution					Mean PPPM € (%)	Mean Cost € (%)	Percentiles of the Costs Distribution					Mean PPPM € (%)	Mean Cost € (%)	Percentiles of the Costs Distribution				
			10%	25%	50%	75%	90%			10%	25%	50%	75%	90%			10%	25%	50%	75%	90%
Hospitalization	575 (15.1)	4415 (9.7)	0	0	1471	7500	13,297	1233 (37.2)	2789 (35.7)	0	0	0	4161	8405	1154 (33.3)	3181 (16.5)	0	0	0	4332	8799
Cancer therapy	2583 (67.7)	34,597 (76.5)	4771	9892	24,730	49,689	82,893	1398 (42.1)	2790 (35.8)	750	1340	3500	6340	10,542	1510 (43.6)	12,517 (64.9)	507	957	2331	14,711	36,119
Outpatient procedures	573 (15.0)	5967 (13.2)	1355	2443	4593	7617	11,726	576 (17.4)	1988 (25.5)	19	547	1309	2347	4070	741 (21.4)	3403 (17.6)	750	1455	2461	4163	7087
Hospice	83 (2.2)	268 (0.6)	0	0	0	0	0	111 (3.3)	237 (3.0)	0	0	0	0	0	59 (1.7)	200 (1.0)	0	0	0	0	0
Total cost	3814 (100.0)	45,247 (100.0)	8707	16,657	37,878	60,276	91,313	3318 (100.0)	7804 (100.0)	2939	5254	7641	13,283	17,852	3464 (100.0)	19,301 (100.0)	2846	5067	10,249	24,317	47,118

Table 4. Costs related to the overall disease follow-up (from the start of 1L treatment until the end, last visit, or death) were reported in PPPM (€) and other descriptive statistics, grouped by mutation status. The negative/unknown cohort was further sub-grouped based on 1L starting time in pre- and post-1L IO.

Overall Costs	EGFR, ALK, or ROS1 Mutation-Positive Patients							EGFR, ALK, or ROS1 Negative/Unknown Patients Pre-1L IO							EGFR, ALK, or ROS1 Negative/Unknown Patients Post-1L IO						
	Mean PPPM € (%)	Mean Cost € (%)	Percentiles of the Costs Distribution					Mean PPPM € (%)	Mean Cost € (%)	Percentiles of the Costs Distribution					Mean PPPM € (%)	Mean Cost € (%)	Percentiles of the Costs Distribution				
			10%	25%	50%	75%	90%			10%	25%	50%	75%	90%			10%	25%	50%	75%	90%
Hospitalization	631 (17.2)	7290 (10.2)	0	0	4508	12,116	17,241	1376 (45.2)	6926 (35.2)	0	1758	4161	9230	16,204	1179 (36.4)	6413 (22.1)	0	0	4161	9129	17,863
Cancer therapy	2414 (65.7)	53,895 (75.9)	6739	15,588	35,140	62,606	132,707	914 (30.0)	7187 (36.6)	800	1760	4186	8877	14,216	1333 (41.2)	16,424 (56.4)	546	1445	6204	21,917	44,745
Outpatient procedures	484 (13.2)	8556 (12.1)	2276	4196	7256	11,123	16,905	458 (15.0)	3834 (19.5)	122	778	2125	4533	8788	571 (17.6)	5475 (18.8)	1147	2010	3752	7753	12,065
Hospice	144 (3.9)	1244 (1.8)	0	0	0	394	5516	298 (9.8)	1702 (8.7)	0	0	0	1576	4985	155 (4.8)	799 (2.7)	0	0	0	197	2659
Total cost	3673 (100.0)	70,985 (100.0)	15,311	33,562	56,055	81,266	152,708	3046 (100.0)	19,649 (100.0)	5505	8721	14,815	23,794	35,389	3238 (100.0)	29,111 (100.0)	5408	10,572	20,978	38,490	60,314

It was remarkable that the expenditures associated with the 1L of treatment accounted for 63.7% and 66.3% of the total costs associated with the overall disease FU in the mutation-positive and post-IO 1L groups, respectively. Conversely, the mean per-patient total cost related to the 1L treatment of pre-IO 1L patients represented not even half (39.7%) of the total cost associated with the overall disease FU. Compared with the 1L treatment, even if the mean total per-patient cost of cancer therapy increased, a modest decrease in monthly expenditures was observed in drugs and outpatient visits across groups during overall disease follow-up (Tables 3 and 4). Conversely, monthly costs related to hospitalization and hospice stays increased during the overall disease follow-up (Tables 3 and 4).

In the pre-1L IO group, the monthly ordinary hospitalization cost (45.2%) exceeded that of drug therapy, becoming the primary cost driver during the overall disease follow-up (Table 4).

As in the 1L treatment, the cost associated with hospice continued to have a low budget impact on overall cost in all cohorts (Tables 3 and 4).

3.4. HCRU

HCRU reported as the mean total number per person and PPPM showed low hospitalization in 1L and overall disease follow-up for all groups. However, both negative cohorts had fewer inpatient admissions than the mutation-positive group. The total LOS was similar across groups. The average length of hospitalization was between 6 and 8 days in 1L treatment (with a monthly hospitalization range of 0.1–0.3 days), and between 14 and 16 days during overall disease follow-up (monthly hospitalization range of 1.2–3.3 days) (Tables 5 and 6).

The total number of cancer therapy administrations in the mutation-positive group varied from 17.4 in 1L treatment to 28.4 in overall disease follow-up (Tables 5 and 6). Among negative/unknown patients, the total mean number of pharmacological treatments ranged from 16.2 to 13.6 in 1L and between 20.5 and 21.4 in overall disease follow-up (Tables 5 and 6). The findings showed a marked difference in negative/unknown cohorts, where the mean PPPM number of cancer therapy administrations nearly doubled during 1L treatment in the pre-IO 1L group (4.8) compared to the post-IO 1L group (2.5). The same trend was observed throughout the entire disease follow-up, even if the gap narrowed (pre 2.94 vs. post 2.1).

Outpatient visits accounted for one of the greatest HCRU proportions in each group during 1L and the entire disease FU (Tables 5 and 6). The mean number of total outpatient visits was much larger in the mutation-positive population than in the negative groups. However, focusing on HCRU per patient per month, the number of outpatient visits was similar across groups in 1L and entire disease FU (between 2.1 and 2.9).

We noticed hospice stay was short during 1L among all groups, increasing during overall disease FU, especially in pre-1L IO negative patients (Tables 5 and 6).

The rate of ER visits was relatively low but higher in the negative/unknown pre-IO 1L group in overall disease follow-up (Tables 5 and 6).

Table 5. Healthcare resources utilization (HCRU) related to the 1L line of treatment was reported as PPPM (€) and other descriptive statistics, grouped by mutation status. The negative/unknown cohort was further sub-grouped based on 1L starting time in pre- and post-1L IO.

1L HCRU	EGFR, ALK, or ROS1 Mutation-Positive Patients							EGFR, ALK, or ROS1 Negative/Unknown Patients Pre-1L IO							EGFR, ALK, or ROS1 Negative/Unknown Patients Post-1L IO						
	PPPM	Mean HCRU	Percentiles of HCRU Distribution					PPPM	Mean HCRU	Percentiles of HCRU Distribution					PPPM	Mean HCRU	Percentiles of HCRU Distribution				
			10%	25%	50%	75%	90%			10%	25%	50%	75%	90%			10%	25%	50%	75%	90%
Number of Hospitalization	0.1	1.0	0.0	0.0	1.0	1.0	3.0	0.27	0.6	0.0	0	0.0	1.0	2.0	0.3	0.8	0.0	0.0	0.0	1.0	2.0
Hospitalization LOS	1.0	6.9	0.0	0.0	2.0	10.0	21.0	3.24	6.7	0.0	0.0	0.0	9.0	20.0	3.1	8.0	0.0	0.0	0.0	13.0	22.5
Number of cancer therapy administrations	1.9	17.4	0.0 *	3.0	15.0	28.0	37.0	4.75	16.20	1.0	1.6	12.0	23.0	34.0	2.5	13.6	3.0	6.0	9.0	17.0	28.0
Number of outpatients visit	2.4	27.2	6.0	10.0	20.0	38.0	55.0	2.33	8.2	1.0	2.0	5.0	11.0	18.0	2.9	13.7	4.0	5.0	9.0	16.0	27.5
Hospice LOS	0.4	1.3	0.0	0.0	0.0	0.0	0.0	0.53	1.2	0.0	0.0	0.0	0.0	0.0	0.3	1.0	0.0	0.0	0	0.0	0.0
ER admissions	0.2	1.2	0.0	0.0	1.0	2.0	4.0	0.37	1.1	0.0	0.0	1.0	2.0	3.0	0.4	1.0	0.0	0.0	1.0	2.0	3.0

* HCRUs associated with 1L cancer therapy administrations were not detected for 14 mutation-positive patients treated during the abolition of day-hospital stays (April 2016).

Table 6. Healthcare resources utilization (HCRU) related to the overall disease follow-up (from the start of 1L treatment until the end, last visit, or death) was reported as PPPM (€) and other descriptive statistics, grouped by mutation status. The negative/unknown cohort was further sub-grouped based on 1L starting time in pre- and post-1L IO.

Overall HCRU	EGFR, ALK, or ROS1 Mutation-Positive Patients							EGFR, ALK, or ROS1 Negative/Unknown Patients Pre-1L IO							EGFR, ALK, or ROS1 Negative/Unknown Patients Post-1L IO						
	PPPM	Mean HCRU	Percentiles of HCRU Distribution					PPPM	Mean HCRU	Percentiles of HCRU Distribution					PPPM	Mean HCRU	Percentiles of HCRU Distribution				
			10%	25%	50%	75%	90%			10%	25%	50%	75%	90%			10%	25%	50%	75%	90%
Number of Hospitalization	0.2	1.7	0.0	0.0	1.0	3.0	4.0	0.33	1.7	0.0	1.0	1.0	2.0	4.0	0.3	1.6	0.0	0.0	1.0	2.0	4.0
Hospitalization LOS	1.2	14.0	0.0	0.0	9.0	22.0	36.0	3.34	14.9	0.0	2.0	10.0	21.0	33.0	3.1	15.5	0.0	0.0	9.0	23.0	39.0
Number of cancer therapy administrations	1.4	28.4	2.0	10.0	24.0	37.0	68.0	2.94	20.5	1.0	6.0	15.0	26.0	41.0	2.1	21.4	4.0	7.0	15.0	29.0	48.5
Number of outpatients visit	2.2	40.5	10.0	18.0	32.0	54.0	90.0	2.10	18.8	1.0	3.0	10.0	23.0	44.0	2.4	22.9	4.0	9.0	15.5	32.0	49.5
Hospice LOS	0.7	6.1	0.0	0.0	0.0	2.0	27.0	1.48	8.5	0.0	0.0	0.0	8.0	25.0	0.8	4.0	0.0	0.0	0.0	2.0	13.0
ER admissions	0.1	1.9	0.0	0.0	1.0	3.0	5.0	0.33	2.0	0.0	1.0	1.0	3.0	4.0	0.3	1.6	0.0	0.0	1.0	2.0	3.5

4. Discussion

The current study provided a real-world data analysis on the costs and HCRU of managing metastatic NSCLC in pre- and post-approval of IO therapy in the 1L setting. The analysis was conducted to investigate the costs and HCRU according to the mutational status of patients: patients with oncogenic driver mutations and patients without mutations or unknown status. Negative/unknown patients were further grouped in pre-1L IO and post-1L IO; that is, before and after the availability of the first ICI as 1L therapy in the Emilia–Romagna region (pembrolizumab in PD-L1 TPS $\geq$ 50%). Costs and HCRU were assessed as mean total per-patient and per-month costs separately for the 1L therapy and the overall disease follow-up across lines of therapy.

Although NSCLC disease is a significant public health issue regarding economic burden, little is known about trends in the cost of NSCLC management in Italy. To the best of our knowledge, this economic assessment of metastatic NSCLC disease is one of the few Italian studies conducted after the introduction of new ICIs, and that includes a resource-utilization analysis. Our study showed that the higher mean total per-patient costs were associated with the mutation-positive group, followed by post-1L IO and pre-1L IO in 1L treatment and overall disease FU. The differences in the clinical pathways and, more in general, in the approach to the disease among these three groups concern the use of different drugs, the duration of treatment, and the survival gain, which are the most responsible for this remarkable cost difference. Despite the high prices of new drugs, the cost difference was less pronounced among groups when PPPM costs were analyzed. This is because PPPM was not affected by treatment duration or prolonged survival as the mean total per-patient cost.

The findings showed that the growth in cancer drug prices was exceeded by more than half of the overall cancer spending. The high prices of these new cancer drugs influence current and future spending. However, these high prices may be legitimized if drugs may prolong survival and improve quality of life.

Most HCRU categories, such as hospital admissions for pharmacological treatment or outpatient services, decreased with the course of the disease. In contrast, other items, such as hospitalizations and hospice visits, grew over time.

It is not surprising that the costs sustained by the National Health Service for the treatment of metastatic NSCLC were mainly driven by oncological therapies, followed by hospitalizations and outpatient health services. This pattern is coherent with previous Italian investigations [20,22]. Due to patients' worsening clinical conditions, hospitalization costs associated with the total disease FU become the most significant component of total costs in pre-1L IO. A large discrepancy in findings exists with the study of Migliorino et al., who reported a mean total PPPM halved from our 1L and total disease FU costs [20]. However, these disparities can be explained by the fact that these kinds of studies are sensitive to the period in which the studies are conducted, and the fact that the study of Migliorino was conducted in 2012, more than 10 years ago. Conversely, more similar to our findings are the results estimated by Buja et al. [21], even if their study population included only 52.07% of Stage IV NSCLC cases; it is also known that the cost associated with NSCLC disease increases as the disease progresses [27]. However, the reported total PPPM cost ranged from EUR 2601 for NSCLC patients diagnosed in 2015 to EUR 3611 for patients diagnosed in 2017 after adopting new drugs for metastatic patients [27]. Our findings on cancer therapy, in particular, for negative/unknown patients, are in line with costs estimated by Piantedosi et al., who reported a pharmaceutical expenditure per patient per month of EUR 1942 for mutation-positive populations and EUR 1316 for negative/unknown mutational status populations [28].

In line with the findings of a multinational investigation that included Italy [29], the most common setting for resource use was the outpatient context. Our study findings related to monthly HCRU showed that mutation-positive patients with oncogenic driver mutations (EGFR, ALK, or ROS1 mutations) seem to have a lower risk of hospitalization and ER visits than the negative/unknown population. However, further investigations are required.

The introduction of new agents in clinical practices increased oncological therapy costs associated with mutation-positive and post-1L IO cohorts. The mean per-patient total cost associated with post-1L IO is higher than those of pre-1L IO (+€ 11,497 in 1L). However, when we considered the mean per patient per month (PPPM), the findings were similar (+EUR 81 in 1L) due to a cost dilution for improving survival. Therefore, the availability of pembrolizumab in the 1L setting has increased the mean per-patient total cost, but it has demonstrated superior survival benefit, increasing the median overall survival from 6.2 months in pre-1L IO to 8.9 months in post-1L IO as documented by Danesi et al. [24]. This observation is consistent with the greater survival rate reported by previous studies on the efficacy of costly drugs included in updated NSCLC clinical pathways [30,31].

Our study has several limitations. First, the analysis collected data at the hospital level and did not capture potential costs for home care. This cost may be relevant, especially in the late phases of the disease, contributing to a healthcare cost increase. Moreover, indirect costs such as caregiver burden and lost workplace productivity are not evaluated. The strength of this study is the inclusion of an HCRU analysis based on detailed real-world data, which is scarce in previous Italian studies.

5. Conclusions

The current analysis provides real-world data on the cost and HCRU of NSCLC from the National Health Service perspective. The results demonstrate that the mutation-positive group has the highest costs, followed by the post-1L IO population and, lastly, the pre-1L IO population. This discrepancy in cost can be attributed to the introduction of new expensive anticancer treatments and the extension of survivability in mutation-positive and post-1L IO patients. The economic burden of mutation-positive and post-1L IO is extremely high during the first line of therapy, compared to the following treatment lines. However, when PPPM expenses are examined, the cost disparity across groups is less noticeable.

Our results confirmed that introducing 1L immunotherapy has improved overall survival, but healthcare spending has increased concurrently with anticancer treatments and hospitalization accounting for a considerable portion of total expenses. The follow-up data revealed that the negative/unknown group had worsening clinical conditions compared to the mutation-positive population, as evidenced by a higher rate of hospitalisation and ER visits.

This study is one of the first Italian analyses that covered detailed cost and HCRU data among metastatic NSCLC. In this context, real-world evidence is becoming increasingly significant, allowing for a better understanding of the cost-effectiveness of various therapeutic alternatives. Nonetheless, our findings are purely descriptive, and the data provided here may help in informing decision-makers to determine resource allocation in treating metastatic NSCLC regarding the health-economic model and policy.

Supplementary Materials: The following supporting information can be downloaded at: https://www.mdpi.com/article/10.3390/cancers16030592/s1, Table S1: Second-line treatments administered by mutation status; Table S2: Third-line treatments administered by mutation status.

Author Contributions: Authors I.M., T.B., V.D., A.D., F.F., L.C. and M.A. were involved in the conception and design of the study. N.G. and W.B. contributed to the collection and assembly of data. F.F. led statistical analysis. A.R. contributed to statistical analysis. V.D., I.M., T.B., N.G. and W.B. contributed to data analysis and interpretation, G.B., A.V. and M.A.B. contributed to collecting informed consents. Authors N.D.L. and M.M. manually reviewed unstructured data on EHR. V.D. drafted the manuscript, supervised by I.M., T.B. and F.F. All authors have read and agreed to the published version of the manuscript.

Funding: This research was sponsored by Merck & Co. Inc., Rahway, NJ, USA, who provided financial support for the study and was involved in the study design (grant number L1P1652).

Institutional Review Board Statement: This study was approved by the Ethics Committee of IRST IRCCS Area Vasta CEROM (approval number 8574).

Informed Consent Statement: Informed consent was obtained from all subjects involved in the study.

Data Availability Statement: The raw data presented in this study are available at a reasonable request from the corresponding author.

Conflicts of Interest: The author T.B. is an employee of Merck &Co. Inc, the sponsor of this study and manuscript. All remaining authors have declared no conflict of interest.

References

1. Sung, H.; Ferlay, J.; Siegel, R.L.; Laversanne, M.; Soerjomataram, I.; Jemal, A.; Bray, F. Global Cancer Statistics 2020: GLOBOCAN Estimates of Incidence and Mortality Worldwide for 36 Cancers in 185 Countries. *CA Cancer J. Clin.* **2021**, *71*, 209–249. [CrossRef]
2. I Numeri del Cancro in Italia 2022. Available online: https://www.aiom.it/i-numeri-del-cancro-in-italia/ (accessed on 28 February 2023).
3. Breathnach, O.S.; Freidlin, B.; Conley, B.; Green, M.R.; Johnson, D.H.; Gandara, D.R.; O'Connell, M.; Shepherd, F.A.; Johnson, B.E. Twenty-two years of phase III trials for patients with advanced non-small-cell lung cancer: Sobering results. *J. Clin. Oncol.* **2001**, *19*, 1734–1742. [CrossRef]
4. Arbour, K.C.; Riely, G.J. Systemic Therapy for Locally Advanced and Metastatic Non-Small Cell Lung Cancer: A Review. *JAMA* **2019**, *322*, 764–774. [CrossRef]
5. Luengo-Fernandez, R.; Leal, J.; Gray, A.; Sullivan, R. Economic burden of cancer across the European Union: A population-based cost analysis. *Lancet Oncol.* **2013**, *14*, 1165–1174. [CrossRef]
6. Vergnenègre, A.; Chouaïd, C. Review of economic analyses of treatment for non-small-cell lung cancer (NSCLC). *Expert. Rev. Pharmacoecon. Outcomes Res.* **2018**, *18*, 519–528. [CrossRef]
7. Wong, W.B.; Wu, N.; Yang, E.; Davies, J.; Chae, Y.K. Real-World Clinical and Economic Outcomes and the Role of Bevacizumab in Patients with Non-Small-Cell Lung Cancer With Liver Metastases. *J. Oncol. Pract.* **2019**, *15*, e878–e887. [CrossRef]
8. Nesline, M.K.; Knight, T.; Colman, S.; Patel, K. Economic Burden of Checkpoint Inhibitor Immunotherapy for the Treatment of Non-Small Cell Lung Cancer in US Clinical Practice. *Clin. Ther.* **2020**, *42*, 1682–1689. [CrossRef]
9. Lin, H.M.; Pan, X.; Hou, P.; Huang, H.; Wu, Y.; Ren, K.; Jahanzeb, M. Economic burden in patients with ALK + non-small cell lung cancer, with or without brain metastases, receiving second-line anaplastic lymphoma kinase (ALK) inhibitors. *J. Med. Econ.* **2020**, *23*, 894–901. [CrossRef] [PubMed]
10. Chai, Q.; Shen, Y.; Du, J.; Zhu, J.; Wu, B. Economic burden of patients with advanced non-small-cell lung cancer receiving nivolumab versus chemotherapy in China. *Immunotherapy* **2020**, *12*, 245–254. [CrossRef] [PubMed]
11. Chouaid, C.; Monnet, I.; Robinet, G.; Perol, M.; Fournel, P.; Vergnenegre, A. Economic impact of gefitinib for refractory non-small-cell lung cancer: A Markov model-based analysis. *Curr. Med. Res. Opin.* **2007**, *23*, 1509–1515. [CrossRef] [PubMed]
12. Vera-Llonch, M.; Weycker, D.; Glass, A.; Gao, S.; Borker, R.; Barber, B.; Oster, G. Healthcare costs in patients with metastatic lung cancer receiving chemotherapy. *BMC Health Serv. Res.* **2011**, *11*, 305. [CrossRef]
13. Verma, V.; Sprave, T.; Haque, W.; Simone, C.B.; Chang, J.Y.; Welsh, J.W.; Thomas, C.R., Jr. A systematic review of the cost and cost-effectiveness studies of immune checkpoint inhibitors. *J. Immunother. Cancer* **2018**, *6*, 128. [CrossRef] [PubMed]
14. Huang, M.; Lopes, G.D.L.; Insinga, R.P.; Burke, T.; Ejzykowicz, F.; Zhang, Y.; Feliciano, J.L. Cost-effectiveness of pembrolizumab versus chemotherapy as first-line treatment in PD-L1-positive advanced non-small-cell lung cancer in the USA. *Immunotherapy* **2019**, *11*, 1463–1478. [CrossRef] [PubMed]
15. Huang, M.; Lou, Y.; Pellissier, J.; Burke, T.; Liu, F.X.; Xu, R.; Velcheti, V. Cost Effectiveness of Pembrolizumab vs. Standard-of-Care Chemotherapy as First-Line Treatment for Metastatic NSCLC that Expresses High Levels of PD-L1 in the United States. *Pharmacoeconomics* **2017**, *35*, 831–844. [CrossRef]
16. Bhadhuri, A.; Insinga, R.; Guggisberg, P.; Panje, C.; Schwenkglenks, M. Cost effectiveness of pembrolizumab vs. chemotherapy as first-line treatment for metastatic NSCLC that expresses high levels of PD-L1 in Switzerland. *Swiss Med. Wkly.* **2019**, *149*, w20170. [CrossRef] [PubMed]
17. Barbier, M.C.; Pardo, E.; Panje, C.M.; Gautschi, O.; Lupatsch, J.E.; Swiss Group for Clinical Cancer Research (SAKK). A cost-effectiveness analysis of pembrolizumab with or without chemotherapy for the treatment of patients with metastatic, non-squamous non-small cell lung cancer and high PD-L1 expression in Switzerland. *Eur. J. Health Econ.* **2021**, *22*, 669–677. [CrossRef] [PubMed]
18. Chouaid, C.; Bensimon, L.; Clay, E.; Millier, A.; Levy-Bachelot, L.; Huang, M.; Levy, P. Cost-effectiveness analysis of pembrolizumab versus standard-of-care chemotherapy for first-line treatment of PD-L1 positive (>50%) metastatic squamous and non-squamous non-small cell lung cancer in France. *Lung Cancer* **2019**, *127*, 44–52. [CrossRef] [PubMed]
19. Perrone, F.; Benelli, G.; Lopatriello, S.; Portalone, L.; Salvati, F.; Zorat, P.; Negrini, C. Cost of non-small cell lung cancer in Italy. Results of the longitudinal study ALCEA (Advanced Lung Cancer Economic Assessment). 2004 ASCO Annual meeting. *J. Clin. Oncol.* **2004**, *22*, 8265–8865. [CrossRef]

20. Migliorino, M.R.; Santo, A.; Romano, G.; Cortinovis, D.; Galetta, D.; Alabiso, O.; Cartenì, G.; Vari, S.; Fasola, G.; Pazzola, A.; et al. Economic burden of patients affected by non-small cell lung cancer (NSCLC): The LIFE study. *J. Cancer Res. Clin. Oncol.* **2017**, *143*, 783–791. [CrossRef]
21. Buja, A.; Pasello, G.; De Luca, G.; Bortolami, A.; Zorzi, M.; Rea, F.; Pinato, C.; Dal Cin, A.; De Polo, A.; Schiavon, M.; et al. Non-Small-Cell Lung Cancer: Real-World Cost Consequence Analysis. *JCO Oncol. Pract.* **2021**, *17*, e1085–e1093. [CrossRef]
22. Franchi, M.; Cortinovis, D.; Corrao, G. Treatment Patterns, Clinical Outcomes and Healthcare Costs of Advanced Non-Small Cell Lung Cancer: A Real-World Evaluation in Italy. *Cancers* **2021**, *13*, 3809. [CrossRef]
23. Verleger, K.; Penrod, J.R.; Daumont, M.M.; Solem, C.; Luo, L.; Macahilig, C.; Hertel, N. Costs and cost drivers associated with non-small-cell lung cancer patients who received two or more lines of therapy in Europe. *Clinicoecon. Outcomes Res.* **2020**, *12*, 22–33. [CrossRef]
24. Danesi, V.; Massa, I.; Foca, F.; Delmonte, A.; Crinò, L.; Bronte, G.; Ragonesi, M.; Maltoni, R.; Manunta, S.; Cravero, P.; et al. Real-World Outcomes and Treatments Patterns Prior and after the Introduction of First-Line Immunotherapy for the Treatment of Metastatic Non-Small Cell Lung Cancer. *Cancers* **2022**, *14*, 4481. [CrossRef]
25. Giunta della Regione Emilia Romagna, Delibera n.1673/2014. Determinazione delle Tariffe per Prestazioni di Assistenza Ospedaliera in Strutture Pubbliche e Private Accreditate della Regione Emilia-Romagna Applicabili a Decorrere dall' 01/01/2014. Available online: https://salute.regione.emilia-romagna.it/siseps/sanita/sdo/files/DGR_1673_2014.pdf/@@download/file/DGR_1673_2014.pdf (accessed on 1 February 2023).
26. Regione Emilia-Romagna. Nomenclatore Tariffario Specialistica Ambulatoriale, 6 April 2018. 2018. Available online: https://salute.regione.emilia-romagna.it/specialistica-ambulatoriale/nomenclatore-tariffario-regionale (accessed on 1 February 2023).
27. Wood, R.; Taylor-Stokes, G.; Lees, M.; Chirita, O. Cost Burden Associated with Advanced Non-Small Cell Lung Cancer (A-NSCLC): Impact of Disease Stage. *BMC Cancer* **2017**, *20*, PA427. [CrossRef]
28. Piantedosi, F.; Cerisoli, R.; Battiloro, C.; Andreozzi, F.; Vitiello, F.; Gilli, M.; De Marino, V.; Letizia, A.; Bianco, A.; Caprice, I.; et al. Treatments of Advanced Non-Small Cell Lung Cancer (NSCLC) in an Italian Center: Drug Utilization and the Treatment Costs of Innovative Drugs. *Farmeconomia Health Econ. Ther. Pathways* **2019**, *20*, 27–41. [CrossRef]
29. Lee, D.H.; Isobe, H.; Wirtz, H.; Aleixo, S.B.; Parente, P.; De Marinis, F.; Huang, M.; Arunachalam, A.; Kothari, S.; Cao, X.; et al. Health care resource use among patients with advanced non-small cell lung cancer: The PIvOTAL retrospective observational study. *BMC Health Serv. Res.* **2018**, *18*, 147. [CrossRef] [PubMed]
30. Reck, M.; Rodríguez-Abreu, D.; Robinson, A.G.; Hui, R.; Csőszi, T.; Fülöp, A.; Gottfried, M.; Peled, N.; Tafreshi, A.; Cuffe, S.; et al. Pembrolizumab versus Chemotherapy for PD-L1-Positive Non-Small-Cell Lung Cancer. *N. Engl. J. Med.* **2016**, *375*, 1823–1833. [CrossRef] [PubMed]
31. Mok, T.S.K.; Wu, Y.L.; Kudaba, I.; Kowalski, D.M.; Cho, B.C.; Turna, H.Z.; Castro, G., Jr.; Srimuninnimit, V.; Laktionov, K.K.; Bondarenko, I.; et al. KEYNOTE-042 Investigators. Pembrolizumab versus chemotherapy for previously untreated, PD-L1-expressing, locally advanced or metastatic non-small-cell lung cancer (KEYNOTE-042): A randomised, open-label, controlled, phase 3 trial. *Lancet* **2019**, *393*, 1819–1830. [CrossRef] [PubMed]

cancers

MDPI

Article

Machine Learning as a Tool for Early Detection: A Focus on Late-Stage Colorectal Cancer across Socioeconomic Spectrums

Hadiza Galadima [1,*], Rexford Anson-Dwamena [1], Ashley Johnson [1], Ghalib Bello [2], Georges Adunlin [3] and James Blando [1]

1 School of Community and Environmental Health, Old Dominion University, Norfolk, VA 23529, USA; ranso002@odu.edu (R.A.-D.); ajohn239@odu.edu (A.J.); jblando@odu.edu (J.B.)
2 Department of Environmental Medicine & Public Health, Icahn School of Medicine at Mount Sinai, New York, NY 10029, USA; ghalibbello@gmail.com
3 Department of Pharmaceutical, Social and Administrative Sciences, Samford University, Birmingham, AL 35229, USA; gadunlin@samford.edu
* Correspondence: hgaladim@odu.edu; Tel.: +1-757-683-7084

Simple Summary: This research explores the potential of machine learning (ML) to predict late-stage colorectal cancer (CRC) diagnoses. The focus is on understanding how socioeconomic and regional factors affect cancer care, particularly in detecting CRC at an advanced stage. We aim to merge data on social determinants of health with individual demographics to uncover patterns indicating higher CRC risk. We compared various ML models, such as decision trees, random forest, and gradient boosting to find the most effective tool for this task. The goal is to utilize artificial intelligence (AI) for early, more accurate CRC detection, which can lead to better treatment outcomes. This study promises to significantly contribute to cancer research, potentially leading to more personalized and efficient healthcare strategies that could ultimately save lives.

Abstract: Purpose: To assess the efficacy of various machine learning (ML) algorithms in predicting late-stage colorectal cancer (CRC) diagnoses against the backdrop of socio-economic and regional healthcare disparities. Methods: An innovative theoretical framework was developed to integrate individual- and census tract-level social determinants of health (SDOH) with sociodemographic factors. A comparative analysis of the ML models was conducted using key performance metrics such as AUC-ROC to evaluate their predictive accuracy. Spatio-temporal analysis was used to identify disparities in late-stage CRC diagnosis probabilities. Results: Gradient boosting emerged as the superior model, with the top predictors for late-stage CRC diagnosis being anatomic site, year of diagnosis, age, proximity to superfund sites, and primary payer. Spatio-temporal clusters highlighted geographic areas with a statistically significant high probability of late-stage diagnoses, emphasizing the need for targeted healthcare interventions. Conclusions: This research underlines the potential of ML in enhancing the prognostic predictions in oncology, particularly in CRC. The gradient boosting model, with its robust performance, holds promise for deployment in healthcare systems to aid early detection and formulate localized cancer prevention strategies. The study's methodology demonstrates a significant step toward utilizing AI in public health to mitigate disparities and improve cancer care outcomes.

Keywords: socioeconomic disparity; cancer care; predictive modeling; machine learning; AI; social determinants of health in oncology; spatial analysis; precision care

1. Introduction

Colorectal cancer (CRC) represents one of the most prevalent malignancies globally [1], standing as the third most commonly diagnosed cancer in both men and women and the third leading cause of cancer-related deaths in the United States in 2023 [2]. Overall, the incidence of CRC is declining among adults in the U.S., influenced by multiple factors. Increased adherence to CRC screening plays a crucial role in early detection, resulting in higher curability rates and improved survival rates [2–7]. Additionally, factors such as dietary improvements and lifestyle changes also contribute to lower incidence by preventing cancer occurrence [8,9]. However, despite advancements in detection methods and treatment modalities to reduce the overall incidence of advanced-stage CRC, it remains a significant public health challenge owing to its substantial mortality rates [2,10]. Comprehensive understanding and awareness of its risk factors, prevention strategies, and early symptoms are essential in combating its progression and ensuring timely medical intervention.

Literature has recognized a combination of genetic, environmental, and lifestyle factors plays a contributory role in CRC etiology [11]. Several demographic variables are related to CRC health outcomes, disparity, and mortality, including sex, age, race/ethnicity, and others. These demographic variables have also been proposed as factors influencing the determination of disease progression at diagnosis, ultimately impacting treatment decisions and plans of care. Several studies have also highlighted the lifelong effects on health that social determinants of health (SDOHs)—defined as the "conditions in which people are born, grow, live, work, and age" [12]—and their interactions with non-modifiable factors can have [13,14]. However, such studies tend to focus on elucidating the effect-modifying role of one factor at a time, even though other factors may be involved. A reason for this approach may be the scarcity of analytical tools (due to analytical complexity) for properly accounting for the complex interaction patterns that exist among several potential cancer factors. A more comprehensive approach to describing and evaluating how multi-level factors affect cancer health outcomes require a clear emphasis on how multiple factors at different levels interact with one another. One promising approach to this problem is machine learning. While there are well-established 'traditional' statistical methods to predict cancer-risk outcomes based on several potential risk factors, many of these methods are not optimal for accurately delineating complex non-linear relationships that might exist between many risk factors and an outcome of interest. Machine learning (ML) techniques allow for an agnostic, data-driven approach to map out potentially complex relationships that are difficult to specify analytically (e.g., in the form of a regression-type equation).

1.1. Machine Learning Approaches in Predicting Cancer Outcomes—A Literature Review

Machine learning (ML) is a rapidly evolving field within biomedical research, particularly in oncology. It leverages the vast amount of data collected from various health platforms to enhance the precision of cancer diagnoses [15,16]. At its core, ML involves the use of algorithms and statistical techniques to analyze and learn from data patterns [17–19]. In the context of cancer research, ML techniques often utilize rich gene expression datasets and integrate various risk factors to create predictive models [20–22]. For instance, in a study by Hornbrook et al, ML integrated demographic factors such as gender and age with clinical metrics, such as blood count to predict early colorectal cancer [23]. Following a similar trajectory, numerous studies have successfully employed ML to integrate clinical parameters such as tumor grade, blood indices, gender, smoking history, and age, leading to accurate predictions of bone metastases in thyroid cancer patients [24]. Similar factors have been instrumental in predicting the probability of advanced colorectal neoplasia in asymptomatic adults using deep learning model [25]. There is a growing repository of ML models constructed on data sourced from cancer databases such as the surveillance, epidemiology, and end results (SEER) Program (https://seer.cancer.gov/), which utilize predictors encompassing tumor attributes, demographic characteristics, and clinical characteristics, to forecast metrics such as mortality and survivorship across a range of cancers including oral, endometrial, and lung cancers [26–30].

Recent advancements in ML, particularly methods such as artificial neural networks (ANN) and deep learning, have showcased promising results. They have been pivotal in estimating the likelihood of cancers such as lung and colorectal spreading further. These techniques integrate both clinical and demographic data for their predictions [31,32].

Moreover, ML models have been meticulously curated to classify patients based on their susceptibility to cancer development, disease stage, and potential treatment outcomes, employing data from varied sources such as electronic health record (EHR) and SEER [33–35].

Furthermore, certain studies have explored the complex interplay between different variables using ML techniques. A prime example would be the study by Levitsky et al., which employed patient-reported data within an ML framework, aiming to discern how varying factors might collaboratively influence the prediction of lung cancer onset [36]. In summation, machine learning, with its innovative approaches, emerges as an invaluable tool in contemporary medical research that could significantly enhance conventional methods of predicting cancer outcomes.

1.2. Role of Social Determinants of Health in Cancer Research

In line with population and public health research, increasingly, social determinants of health (SDOHs), at the time of diagnosis or study enrollment are collected in epidemiologic studies of cancer that enable a comprehensive analysis of cancer risk factors [37–40]. While population-based cancer registries play a crucial role in monitoring cancer trends, they may not comprehensively capture all incidences of cancer. Additionally, limitations in the collection of variables for hypothesis-driven research within these registries can potentially introduce bias into the results [41–43]. For example, information on patient insurance status, patient comorbidities, and active follow-up of patients are inconsistently available. Cancer data can be improved when used in combination with other secondary databases containing social determinants of health to increase our understanding of the underlying causes of cancer health disparities [43,44].

The influence of SDOH, neighborhood and environmental attributes on cancer-related outcomes such as mortality, survivorship, and stage at diagnosis has been increasingly recognized in the scientific community. Health care accessibility, represented by factors such as the presence or absence of a primary care physician and insurance status, holds substantial sway over cancer screening rates and subsequent outcomes. For instance, residing in neighborhoods characterized by high levels of racial and ethnic segregation has been associated with low cancer screening rates and detrimental health outcomes [45,46]. Notably, a lack of insurance coverage has been linked to poorer health outcomes [47–52]. Socioeconomic elements, including financial insecurity, poverty, low-income status, and employment conditions, also exert a significant impact on cancer-related health metrics [45,48,52–54]. In addition, adverse social and educational determinants such as high social vulnerability and limited educational attainment have been correlated with negative outcomes in cancer screening and overall health [45,55].

In addition to these established factors, other variables have emerged as potentially relevant based on authoritative recommendations. Korn et al. proposed a systematic review protocol to compile variables related to SDOH constructs for cancer screening and outcomes. These include variables such as food insecurity, housing, language and literacy skills, transportation, affordability, incarceration, and more [56]. These SDOH constructs were identified and organized based on established frameworks and definitions, providing a comprehensive view of the complex interplay between SDOH and cancer outcomes.

Through these studies, it becomes evident that SDOH are not merely peripheral elements but integral components that significantly modulate cancer outcomes. This evidence emphasizes the need for a more holistic approach to cancer research and treatment, one that encompasses the complex interplay of these determinants.

1.3. Study Purpose

The purpose of this study is to explore the advanced capabilities of machine learning (ML) and artificial intelligence (AI) in predicting late-stage colorectal cancer (CRC) diagnoses, within the broader context of addressing socioeconomic and regional disparities in cancer care. By integrating individual- and census tract-level social determinants of health (SDOHs) with sociodemographic factors, the study aims to identify patterns that may signal a higher risk of late-stage CRC, which is characterized here as diagnoses made at regional stage or with distant metastasis/systemic disease. Central to the research is the comparative analysis of a suite of ML models—including penalized lasso logistic regression, decision tree, random forest, gradient boosting, and SVM classifier—to evaluate their predictive prowess and ensure the most effective algorithm is deployed for this critical healthcare challenge. This approach, which focuses on prognostic predictions using ML algorithms, is a crucial element in cancer care, offering potential for early detection and improved treatment outcomes. The study's ultimate goal is to harness the power of AI to generate precise, population-level predictions, thereby contributing significantly to the field of cancer care and management.

2. Materials and Methods

2.1. Study Design and Setting

This study uses an ecological design to examine CRC outcomes for the period 2000 to 2020 in men and women aged 18 years of age and older residing in the state of Virginia. The chosen study setting offers a distinct structure for exploring CRC since it represents a significant health issue in Virginia, where 26 counties have been recognized as having the highest colorectal cancer mortality rates in the country [57–59].

2.2. Theoretical Framework

This study introduces an innovative theoretical framework, the adaptive predictive framework for cancer outcomes (APF-CO) in Figure 1, that synergistically merges elements from the social-ecological model [60], the healthy people 2030 model [61], and the Kaiser Foundation's framework on social determinants of health (SDOHs) [62]. Designed to foster a nuanced understanding of cancer outcomes, this integrative framework serves as a substrate for employing machine learning algorithms to predict cancer outcomes effectively.

In this multifaceted approach, we combine both clinical variables and SDOH to construct a more holistic understanding of cancer outcomes. The framework is structured around several key categories that span individual and societal determinants of health: healthcare access, socio-economic status, diet and physical activity, educational attainment, environmental factors, neighborhood characteristics, social and community support, clinical metrics, treatment options, demographic attributes, and health behaviors.

To add depth and context to our framework, these categories are strategically mapped across four levels of influence as outlined in the social-ecological model: individual, interpersonal, organizational, and community. The intention behind this mapping is to illustrate that variables from these categories are not isolated entities but interact dynamically across different layers of the social fabric. This facilitates a comprehensive understanding of how such complex interactions can exert a cascading influence on cancer outcomes.

By amalgamating a wealth of variables, drawn from diverse yet interconnected domains, this modified theoretical framework offers an enriched, layered perspective. The ultimate goal is to capitalize on machine-learning methodologies to decipher the intricate web of determinants, thereby offering predictive understandings that are both accurate and encompassing. This unprecedented approach, incorporating an expansive database that combines traditional cancer registry data with metrics related to SDOH, sets the stage for ground-breaking advancements in predictive oncology.

2.3. Data Sources

The primary data for this project i.e., cancer cases specific to CRC are obtained from the Virginia Cancer Registry (VCR) [63]. The data include information on patient demographic characteristics, residential locations, as well as histological and clinical characteristics, among other information. Census tracts-level social determinants of health include data from the U.S. Census Bureau's 2019 American Community Survey 5-year estimates (2015–2019) [64], and from the mySidewalk health data [65]. mySidewalk includes more than 6000 preloaded community-level indicators from more than 50 trusted sources for the entire country; these include data from the National Neighborhood Data Archive (NaNDA), the Health Resources and Services Administration (HRSA), the Centers for Disease Control (CDC), the Environmental Protection Agency (EPA) National Air Toxics Assessment, etc. [65]. These datasets are merged with the VCR dataset based on the patient's residential census tract at time of diagnosis as a common identifier.

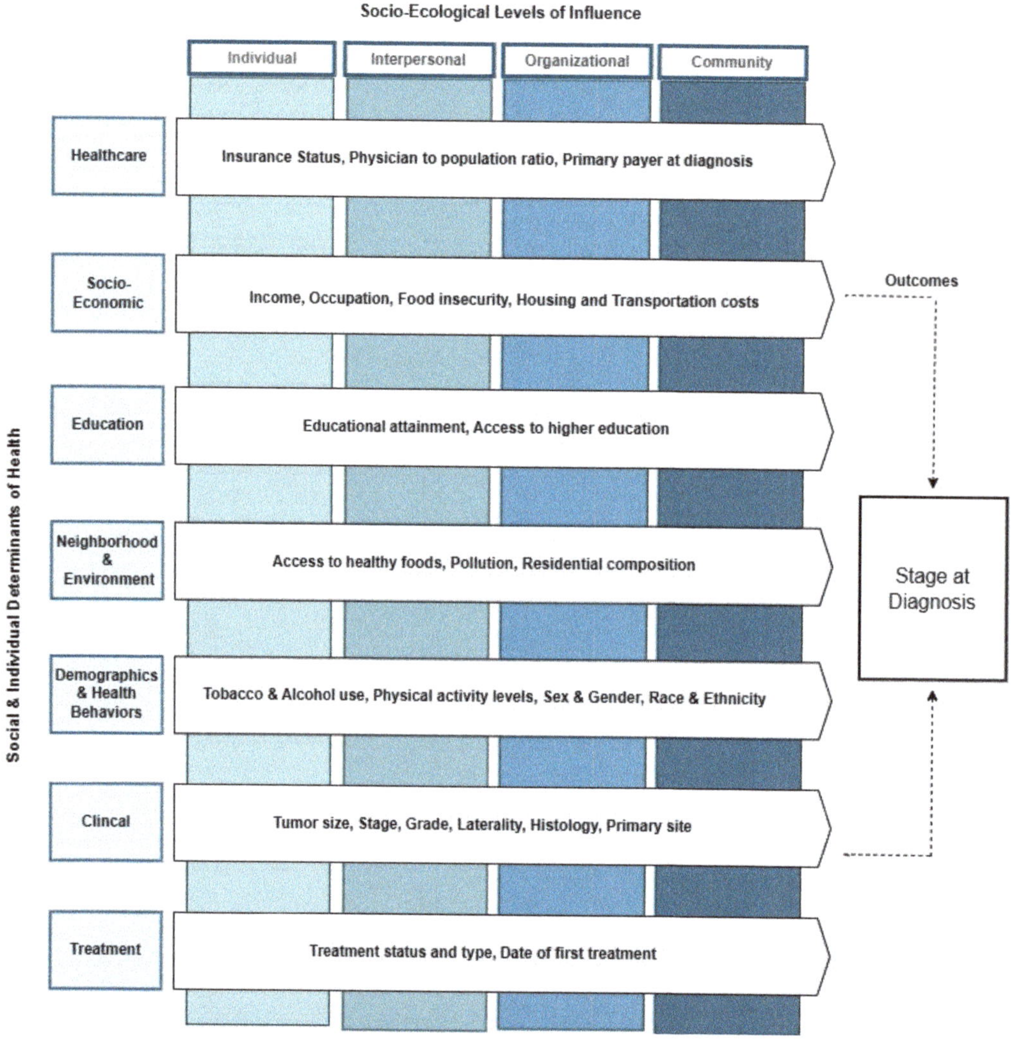

Figure 1. Adaptive predictive framework for cancer outcomes (APF-CO).

2.4. Study Population

Individuals aged 18 to 89, residing in Virginia between 2000 and 2020, and who were diagnosed with primary and secondary CRC were selected for the analysis. The CRC cases were identified using the following International Classification of Disease, 10th revision, Clinical Modification (ICD-10-CM) codes: C18.0-C18.9, C19.9, and C20. Cases with missing or invalid residential information at diagnosis were excluded.

2.5. Data Collection and Variables Definitions

Individual-level Variables: Baseline characteristics were obtained from the VCR. They include patient demographic characteristics (age at diagnosis, sex, patient race and ethnicity, marital status), year of CRC diagnosis, primary payer at diagnosis, residential location (county, zip code, census tract); clinical characteristics such as tumor stage at the time of diagnosis, tumor characteristics, primary tumor site, histologic type, grade, laterality, and treatment information. Previous studies have shown individual factors that have been associated with adverse cancer outcomes include age, gender, race and ethnicity [66,67]. Important individual clinical factors include tumor size and thickness, tumor grade, histology, stage at diagnosis, lymph node count and location, and treatment types [68–71].

Neighborhood Social Determinant of Health Measures: The neighborhood SDOH variables used in this study are summarized in Figure 1. They include socioeconomic, racial, and geographic disparities (urban vs. rural). It has been shown that there is a higher incidence and risk of adverse CRC outcomes amongst rural populations when compared to urban populations [52,72,73].

Outcome Measure: The primary outcome of interest is a binary variable representing the stage of CRC at diagnosis (late-stage vs. early stage). We defined "late" stage as all CRC diagnoses recorded at regional stage (regional by direct extension, regional lymph nodes only, and regional by both extension and lymph nodes) and distant metastasis/systemic disease. We defined 'early' stage as all CRC diagnoses recorded as 'localized' and in situ [70].

2.6. Data Linkage and Management

The integration of the cancer registry data and the social determinants of health (SDOH) information from census tracts was pivotal in constructing a comprehensive dataset that not only highlights individual cancer outcomes but also provides an invaluable lens into their potential interplays with socio-economic determinants at the micro-geographic level. The primary dataset from the cancer registry contained specific residence information for each patient. These residence data served as a key attribute for the data linkage.

Initially, we accessed a comprehensive dataset from a 20-year-long cancer registry, revealing 74,921 documented CRC cases. Using the ArcGIS platform, a majority of the cancer cases were geocoded based on patients' residence information, translating them to specific geographic co-ordinates. As a result, 74,435 records (99.35% of the total cases) were perfectly georeferenced into their respective census tracts. For the 0.65% (486 records) that were not initially georeferenced, the Missouri Census Data Center's (MCDC) "apportioned" population weight methodology was employed. This method, available on the MCDC's online platform [74], employs patients' zip codes to transition or "crosswalk" these cases into designated census tracts. The procedure involves assigning a case to the census tract with the highest population percentage from the given zip code, resulting in the zip code-census tract crosswalk methodology. From the 486 records processed using MCDC, 454 were successfully matched, and only 32 records (0.04% of the total sample) remained un-georeferenced.

The culmination of the linkage process yielded a unified dataset, encompassing 87 features and a total of 74,921 rows. Rigorous data management protocols were meticulously applied post-integration to address any missing values, discrepancies, or inconsistencies that might have emerged during the merger. Specifically, an initial assessment revealed that 75 features had missing values. To ensure data quality, columns with more than 90% missing values were dropped, and missing values in numerical features were imputed with median values, ensuring minimal impact on data distribution, while categorical features were filled with a placeholder string 'unknown', preserving the original structure without introducing bias. Rows lacking the crucial 'stage at diagnosis' data were also removed, resulting in a refined dataset of 41,839 samples and 86 features. This rigorous approach enhanced the dataset's analytical robustness and reliability.

2.7. An Overview of Machine Learning Techniques in Predicting Cancer Outcomes

Lasso Logistic Regression, a variant of logistic regression, is a statistical method used for modeling the probability of a binary outcome based on multiple predictor variables. This method, ideal for handling high-dimensional data, simplifies the model by reducing the coefficients of less significant predictors. More specifically, this method reduces the impact of less significant variables by shrinking their coefficients towards zero, thus simplifying the model and enhancing interpretability [75–77].

Decision trees is a machine learning algorithm used for both classification and regression tasks. This algorithm operates by sorting instances based on their feature values through a process known as recursive binary partitioning. Each node in a decision tree represents a specific feature, and each branch represents a decision path based on feature values that leads to the next node [78,79]. They function through a sequence of binary decisions: for example, in our context of 86 features, if a feature value X_k is less than or equal to threshold S, the tree follows the left branch; otherwise, it follows the right. This process continues recursively until a leaf node, representing the final decision, is reached. The process of node selection and thresholds determination ('S') is determined through optimization techniques, making decision trees highly adaptable to specific datasets.

Random forest is an ensemble learning method. It operates by constructing a multitude of decision trees during the training phase. For classification tasks, the random forest model predicts the output class by employing a majority voting system across all the decision trees, where each tree votes for a class, and the class receiving the most votes becomes the model's prediction. For regression tasks, it aggregates the predictions of individual trees by calculating their mean. Unlike a single decision tree, random forest reduces the risk of overfitting and increases prediction accuracy by combining the predictions of numerous trees [79,80].

Gradient Boosting is a powerful machine learning technique used in both regression and classification problems. It operates by training decision trees iteratively [81]. Each subsequent tree in a gradient-boosted model focuses more on observations that previous trees predicted inaccurately, essentially placing higher weight on these errors. This error-correcting approach allows gradient boosting to continuously improve its predictions throughout the training process [79]. The emphasis in gradient boosting is on improving accuracy and reducing bias through iterative refinement, making it particularly effective in complex predictive tasks such as cancer diagnosis and prognosis.

Support Vector Machines (SVMs) are supervised learning models that analyze data and recognize patterns. They are used for classification and regression analysis. In scenarios where data are linearly separable, SVMs employ a linear approach to establish a hyperplane that best divides the data into distinct classes [82]. However, given the complexity and non-linear relationships often present in medical datasets, including those related to cancer, the use of SVMs with non-linear kernels is recommended. These non-linear kernels enable the delineation of intricate decision boundaries and are more adept at handling high-dimensional data.

2.8. Statistical Analyses

The cancer registry and population census data were merged to integrate records from both sources. Patients' characteristics between early- and late-stage diagnosis were compared in a bivariate analysis using chi-square tests for categorical variables and *t*-tests for continuous variables. Similarly, *t*-tests were utilized to compare the SDOH characteristics at the census tract levels.

In the exploratory data analysis phase, several machine learning models from the scikit-learn library to predict late-stage cancer diagnosis were used. This array included lasso logistic regression, employing L1 regularization with the 'saga' solver; decision tree; random forest; gradient boosting; and a variant of support vector machine (SVM), specifically the SGD (stochastic gradient descent) classifier with hinge loss function. Notably, this method serves as a computationally efficient approximation of SVMs, leveraging stochastic gradient descent for optimization in high-volume data scenarios. The random forest model was configured with its default number of tree estimators, while the gradient boosting classifier utilized Scikit-learn's default settings. These default hyperparameter settings were chosen for an initial broad assessment. Each model was configured to address class imbalance using class weights.

To minimize overfitting and rigorously evaluate the performance of the models, a 5-fold cross-validation approach was used. This approach involved splitting the data into five distinct subsets or 'folds'. In each iteration, four folds were used for training while the remaining fold served as the validation set. This process was repeated five times, ensuring each fold was used for validation once. By doing so, this method offers a more comprehensive assessment of a model's performance across different data subsets, reducing biases and providing an indication of its generalization capabilities. Performance metrics including ROC-AUC, accuracy, sensitivity, and specificity were computed, capturing different aspects of model efficacy. Additionally, for a comprehensive geographical analysis, the best-performing model, based on these metrics, was used to estimate late-stage cancer probabilities across various census tracts in Virginia, employing spatial–temporal analysis for visualizing and identifying significant clusters over time.

All data management and spatial analyses were conducted using SAS and ArcGIS, respectively, with Python and Scikit-learn serving as the primary tools for machine learning model fitting and evaluation. The level of significance was set at $p < 0.05$, ensuring statistical rigor in our findings.

3. Results

3.1. Baseline Characteristics

Baseline characteristics between early-stage ((42.74%) and late-stage (57.26%) diagnosis are summarized in Table 1. Patients diagnosed at an early stage had a slightly higher mean age (66.72 years) than those diagnosed at a late stage (65.85 years, $p < 0.0001$). A significantly greater proportion of patients aged 40–49 were diagnosed at late stage ($p < 0.0001$). Concerning race and ethnicity, there were slight variations, with Hispanics and NH Asians being marginally overrepresented in the late diagnosis group ($p = 0.005$).

Table 1. Selected baseline characteristics by stage of diagnosis status.

Patient Characteristics	Early n = 17,884 (42.74%)	Late n = 23,955 (57.26%)	
	Frequency (%) or Mean (SE)	Frequency (%) or Mean (SE)	p-Value
Age at Diagnosis			<0.0001
Age in years, Mean (SE)	66.72 (0.1)	65.85 (0.1)	
Age Group			<0.0001
18–39	471 (2.63%)	790 (3.30%)	
40–49	1262 (7.06%)	2288 (9.55%)	
50–64	5678 (31.75%)	7578 (31.63%)	
65+	10,473 (58.56%)	13,299 (55.52%)	
Race & Ethnicity			0.005
NH White	12,263 (68.67%)	16,305 (68.19%)	
NH Black	3263 (18.27%)	4279 (17.89%)	
Hispanic	1786 (10.00%)	2517 (10.53%)	
NH Asian	440 (2.46%)	702 (2.94%)	
NH Pacific Islander	68 (0.38%)	74 (0.31%)	
Unknown/Not Documented	39 (0.22%)	35 (0.15%)	

Table 1. *Cont.*

Patient Characteristics	Early n = 17,884 (42.74%)	Late n = 23,955 (57.26%)	
	Frequency (%) or Mean (SE)	Frequency (%) or Mean (SE)	p-Value
Marital Status at Diagnosis			<0.0001
Married	9578 (57.00%)	11,935 (53.95%)	
Unmarried	6523 (38.82%)	9437 (42.66%)	
Unknown	702 (4.18%)	752 (3.40%)	
Primary Payer at Diagnosis			<0.0001
Medicaid	284 (1.70%)	636 (2.83%)	
Medicare	9267 (55.52%)	11,762 (52.28%)	
Private Insurance	6124 (36.69%)	8295 (36.87%)	
Military	601 (3.60%)	680 (3.02%)	
Indian/Public Health Service	2 (0.01%)	1 (0.00%)	
Self-pay/Uninsured	413 (2.47%)	1122 (4.99%)	
Year of Diagnosis			<0.0001
2000–2004	5346 (29.89%)	7242 (30.23%)	
2005–2009	4836 (27.04%)	5882 (24.55%)	
2010–2014	3763 (21.04%)	4917 (20.53%)	
2015–2019	3821 (21.37%)	5705 (23.82%)	
2020	118 (0.66%)	209 (0.87%)	
Stage of disease at diagnosis			<0.0001
In Situ	2594 (14.50%)	0 (0.00%)	
Localized	15,290 (85.50%)	0 (0.00%)	
Regional	0 (0.00%)	16,005 (66.81%)	
Distant	0 (0.00%)	7950 (33.19%)	
Not Staged/Unknown	0 (0.00%)	0 (0.00%)	
Primary Site			<0.0001
Colon	12,521 (70.01%)	17,645 (73.66%)	
Rectum	5363 (29.99%)	6310 (26.34%)	
Grade			<0.0001
Grade I	3421 (19.13%)	2390 (9.98%)	
Grade II	8589 (48.03%)	13,067 (54.55%)	
Grade III	1069 (5.98%)	4162 (17.37%)	
Grade IV	194 (1.08%)	570 (2.38%)	
T-cell	1 (0.01%)	1 (0.00%)	
B-cell	89 (0.50%)	92 (0.38%)	
NK Cell	1 (0.01%)	0 (0.00%)	
Unknown Grade	4520 (25.27%)	3673 (15.33%)	
Treatment Status			<0.0001
No treatment given	351 (4.54%)	711 (6.54%)	
Treatment given	7256 (93.88%)	10,044 (92.44%)	

Table 1. *Cont.*

Patient Characteristics	Early $n = 17{,}884$ (42.74%)	Late $n = 23{,}955$ (57.26%)	
	Frequency (%) or Mean (SE)	Frequency (%) or Mean (SE)	*p*-Value
Active surveillance (watchful waiting)	17 (0.22%)	5 (0.05%)	
Unknown if treatment was given	105 (1.36%)	106 (0.98%)	
Days between date of initial diagnosis and date first course of treatment			0.2142
Time Lag, Mean (SE)	9.93 (1.97)	13.67 (2.28)	
Surgery			<0.0001
Yes	16,627 (92.97%)	19,698 (82.23%)	
No	1077 (6.02%)	4060 (16.95%)	
Unknown	180 (1.01%)	197 (0.82%)	
Chemotherapy			<0.0001
Yes	1835 (10.26%)	13,276 (55.42%)	
No	15,575 (87.09%)	10,330 (43.12%)	
Unknown	474 (2.65%)	349 (1.46%)	
Radiation Therapy			<0.0001
Yes	1384 (7.75%)	4063 (16.97%)	
No	15,541 (86.98%)	18,717 (78.19%)	
Unknown	943 (5.28%)	1157 (4.83%)	
Vital Status			<0.0001
Dead	7275 (40.68%)	14,859 (62.03%)	
Alive	10,609 (59.32%)	9096 (37.97%)	

Marital status significantly affected the stage at diagnosis. Married individuals were more frequently diagnosed early, while a larger percentage of unmarried patients were diagnosed at late stage ($p < 0.0001$). The primary payer at diagnosis showed that Medicaid beneficiaries and the self-pay/uninsured group were more prone to late stage ($p < 0.0001$). The year of diagnosis revealed temporal differences in staging. For instance, the period between 2015 and 2019 saw a surge in late diagnoses ($p < 0.0001$). The stage of the disease at diagnosis was as expected, with in situ and localized stages in the early diagnosis group, contrasted by regional and distant stages in the late group.

Primary site analysis showed that colon diagnoses were more predominant in the late diagnosis group, whereas rectum diagnoses leaned towards the early diagnosis group ($p < 0.0001$). Regarding disease grade, early diagnoses had a greater proportion of Grade I, while late diagnoses were rich in Grade II and III cases ($p < 0.0001$).

Treatment patterns displayed notable differences between the groups. Surgery was more common in the early diagnosis group, whereas chemotherapy and radiation therapy were more prevalent in the late diagnosis group ($p < 0.0001$). The vital status highlighted a concerning trend, with a majority (62.03%) of the late diagnosis group succumbing to the disease, in comparison to 40.68% in the early diagnosis group ($p < 0.0001$). Detailed information on the baseline characteristics can be found in the Supplementary Content in Table S1: Baseline Characteristics by Stage of Diagnosis Status.

3.2. Census Tracts Characteristics by Stage at Diagnosis

The bivariate analysis of census tract SDOH characteristics and stage at diagnosis, displayed in Table 2, reveals some intriguing disparities between early- (42.74%) and late-stage (57.26%) patients. Access to healthcare, socio-economic status, education, lifestyle behaviors, ethnicity, and environmental exposure all display certain associations with the stage of diagnosis. Key differences include a higher percentages of uninsured individuals, less routine check-ups, and lower access to healthy food in tracts with late-stage patients. Socio-economic factors such as lower household income, higher expenditure on transportation, and less workforce participation also correlate with late-stage diagnoses. Educationally, those areas tend to have more people with less than high school education, but fewer with some college education but no degree. Interestingly, areas with late-stage diagnoses also recorded higher levels of binge drinking and a higher Hispanic population percentage. Environmental exposure factors, including slightly elevated diesel particulate matter levels and more prevalent underground storage tanks, were also more common in areas with late-stage diagnoses. These findings suggest that a range of socioeconomic, behavioral, and environmental factors may influence the stage at which patients are diagnosed with cancer. Detailed information on the census tracts characteristics can be found in the Supplementary Content in Table S2: Neighborhood Census Tracts Characteristics by Stage of Diagnosis Status.

3.3. Results of the Predictive Machine Learning Models

Table 3 presents the performance metrics from the cross-validation of five different machine-learning models to predict CRC late-stage diagnosis. In the comparative analysis of the ML models, the gradient boosting model exhibited superior performance with the highest ROC-AUC score of 0.8549, indicating a strong capability in distinguishing between late-stage and non-late-stage CRC diagnoses. It also achieved the highest prediction accuracy at 77.25%, suggesting it is the most reliable model for correct predictions among those tested. In terms of sensitivity, which measures the correct identification of actual late-stage CRC cases, the lasso logistic regression model was the most proficient, with a sensitivity score of 0.7405.

The random forest model, despite its highest specificity (80.72%), fell short in sensitivity (56.40%), indicating a tendency to miss a significant number of late-stage cases. This could be a critical drawback in medical diagnostics where failing to identify late-stage disease could have dire consequences. On the other hand, the decision tree and SVM (SGD classifier) models showed a balance between sensitivity and specificity but lagged in overall accuracy and exhibited low ROC-AUC scores of 0.7298 and 0.7006, respectively, suggesting they might not be as effective for this particular diagnostic challenge.

In conclusion, the gradient boosting stands out as the most promising model, offering a particularly robust approach for this prediction task.

3.4. Performance of the Best ML Predictive Model

To validate the performance of our gradient boosting model (GBM), which has proven to be the most performant in predicting late-stage colorectal cancer, we conducted a single-run evaluation. This involved partitioning our dataset into an 80–20 split, where 20% constituted the testing set. The model was recalibrated on the training set, then we applied it to the test set to compute critical metrics. The Receiver Operating Characteristic (ROC) curve, depicted in Figure 2, was generated, resulting in an Area Under Curve (AUC) of 0.86—a strong indicator of the model's discriminative power. To refine the model's predictive precision, an optimal decision threshold was calculated at 0.446, which improved the model's sensitivity to 79.54% and specificity to 75.92%, thereby balancing the trade-off between detecting actual cases and avoiding false alarms. Furthermore, the calibration curve, illustrated in Figure 3, was derived from this evaluation, showcasing a close alignment between predicted probabilities and actual outcomes, further confirming the model's reliability. These measures collectively confirm the robustness of the gradient boosting model as a reliable tool for clinical prognostic applications.

Table 2. Selected neighborhood census tracts characteristics by stage of diagnosis status.

Census Tract Characteristics	Early n = 17,884 (42.74%)	Late n = 23,955 (57.26%)	
	Mean (SE)	Mean (SE)	p-Value
Access to Healthcare			
Percent Uninsured	7.816 (0.04)	7.9552 (0.04)	0.0085
Doctor Checkup in Past Year Among Adults (2020)	76.7273 (2.98)	76.5405 (3.03)	<0.0001
Doctor Checkup in Past Year Among Adults (2020)	76.7273 (2.98)	76.5405 (3.03)	<0.0001
Population with a Disability (2017–2021)	13.2833 (0.05)	13.1551 (0.04)	0.0372
Socio Economic			
% Spent on Housing & Transportation	53.5814 (0.06)	53.2928 (0.05)	0.0003
%Spent on Housing	26.0618 (0.01)	26.0798 (0.01)	0.2533
% Spent on Transportation	27.5196 (0.06)	27.213 (0.06)	0.0003
Employment Access Index (2016)	20,613.6 (177)	21,241.2 (158)	0.0082
Labor Force Participation Rate (2017–2021)	63.3817 (0.08)	63.6564 (0.07)	0.0093
Median Household Income (2017–2021)	82,806.2 (326.1)	83,742.1 (285.2)	0.0311
% Pop with Access to Healthy Food	0.7214 (0.002)	0.7144 (0.001)	0.0088
Educational Attainment			
Less than High school education	9.8888 (0.05)	10.027 (0.05)	0.0446
Educational Attainment—Some College No Degree (2017–2021)	8.1371 (0.03)	8.0137 (0.02)	0.0005
Behaviors			
Binge Drinking Among Adults (2020)	15.3011 (0.02)	15.3652 (0.01)	0.0017
Race and Ethnicity			
White per capita	0.633 (0.002)	0.6335 (0.002)	0.8212
Black per capita	0.2003 (0.002)	0.1952 (0.001)	0.0141
Asian per capita	0.0483 (0.006)	0.0495 (0.005)	0.0987
Hispanic per capita	0.0789 (0)	0.0821 (0)	0.0008
Environmental Exposures			
Air Quality: Respiratory Hazard Index (2014)	0.4039 (0.005)	0.4051 (0.004)	0.0707
Diesel Particulate Matter Environmental Justice Index (2021)	14.1463 (0.1)	14.398 (0.09)	0.0501
Diesel Particulate Matter Level in Air (2021)	0.2206 (0.008)	0.224 (0.007)	0.0026
Underground Storage Tanks (2021)	5.044 (0.05)	5.2027 (0.04)	0.0114
Population Weighted Density	3359.9 (43.17)	3546.9 (39.87)	0.0015

Table 3. Results of machine learning model evaluation for late-stage diagnosis prediction.

Model	ROC-AUC	Overall Prediction Accuracy	Sensitivity	Specificity
Lasso (Penalized Logistic Regression)	0.7864	0.7159	0.7405	0.6975
Decision Tree	0.7006	0.7068	0.6580	0.7432
Random Forest	0.7554	0.7032	0.5640	0.8072
Gradient Boosting	0.8549	0.7725	0.7263	0.8070
SVM (SGD Classifier)	0.7298	0.6760	0.6793	0.6735

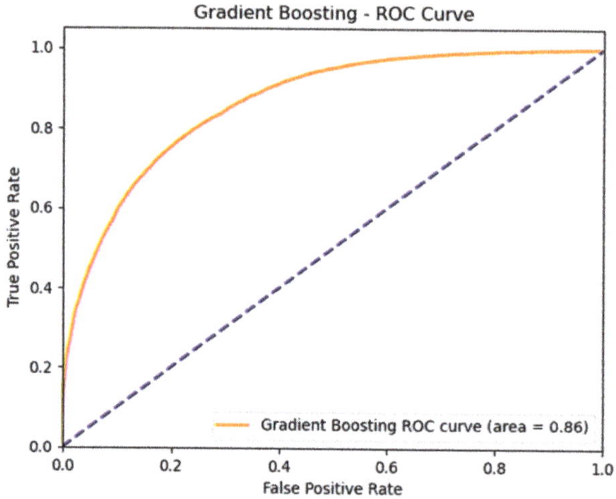

Figure 2. ROC curve from the GBM *. * GBM: Gradient Boosting Model.

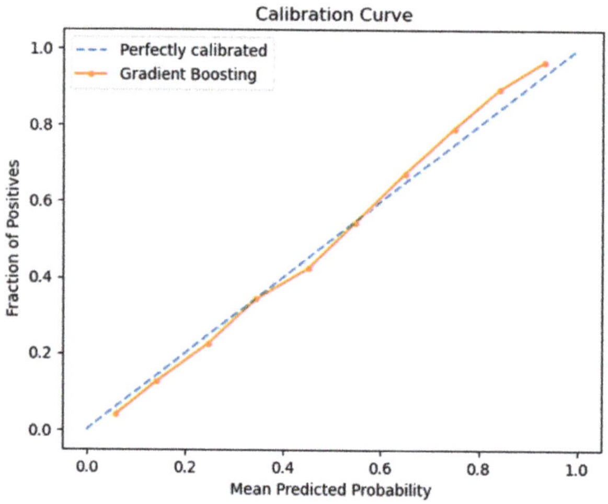

Figure 3. Calibration curve from the GBM *. * GBM: Gradient Boosting Model.

3.5. Feature Importance

The feature importance scores from the gradient boosting model, displayed in Figure 4, are indicative of the relative contribution of each predictor to the model's performance for making predictions. These scores are calculated based on how much each feature contributes to reducing the model's loss function across all the trees in the ensemble. Each feature's score is a sum of the reduction in the loss attributed to that feature across all trees in the model.

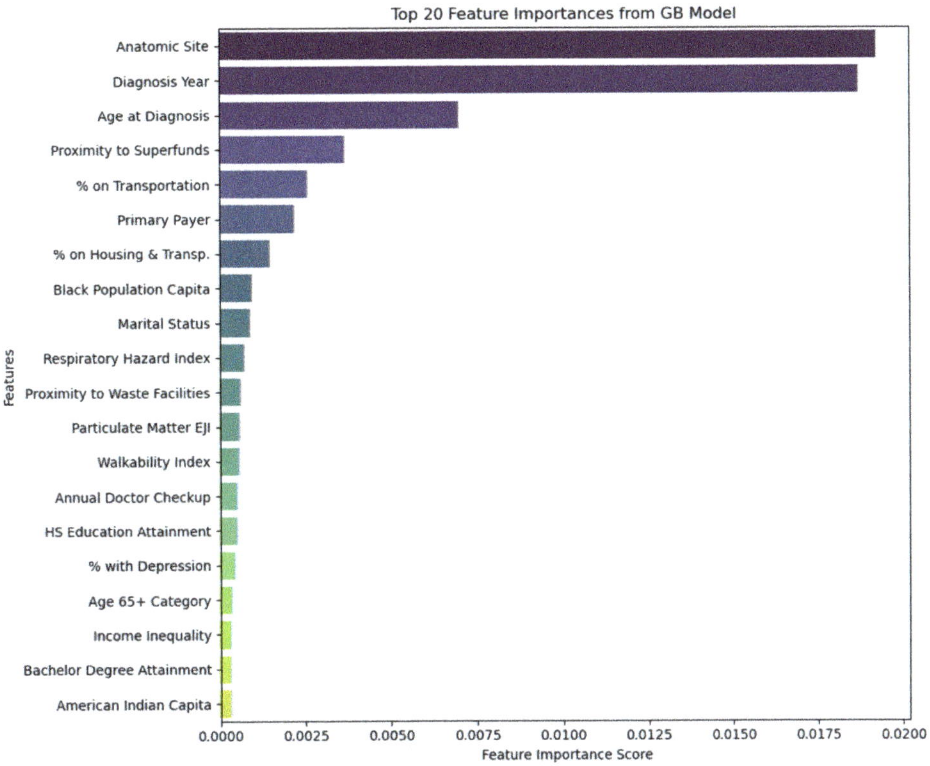

Figure 4. Feature importance for the gradient boosting model.

The anatomic site exhibits the highest importance with an importance score of 0.019238. This signifies that the location of the cancer within the body significantly impacts the stage at diagnosis. The year of diagnosis follows with an importance score of 0.018704, reflecting how advancements or changes in diagnostic methods over time may affect late-stage diagnosis rates. Notably, specific years, such as 2015 and 2016, have been highlighted due to an increased demand for screening [83,84] and the potential delays in diagnosis [85] which can impact the stage at which CRC is identified. Age at diagnosis is also a crucial factor, with an importance score of 0.007015. It is worth noting that age has been established as a significant factor influencing the stage at which CRC is diagnosed [54,70]. Environmental factors such as proximity to superfund sites, though less impactful, still provide meaningful predictive power, suggesting a potential link between environmental factors and disease progression. Socioeconomic factors such as expenditures on transportation and housing, along with the primary payer, are also amongst the top predictors, hinting at the socioeconomic dimensions of healthcare access and outcomes. Social factors such as marital status may reflect the impact of support networks on health, while 'black per capita' indicates the potential influence of racial factors and disparities on late-stage diagnosis. Environmental quality indices, including respiratory hazard index and proximity to pollution and waste facilities, alongside health behaviors such as regular checkups and mental health status represented by the percentage with depression, show lower but non-negligible influence. Overall, it is important to note that these importance scores are not indicative of causation or statistical significance. These scores assist in emphasizing the multifaceted nature of cancer diagnosis stages, influenced by a blend of medical, environmental, socioeconomic, and behavioral factors.

3.6. Results of the Spatio-Temporal Analysis

A preliminary examination of the spatial distribution of anticipated probabilities at the census tract level as displayed in Figure 5, indicates that the greatest likelihood for late stage is observed inside a rural crescent spanning from the Appalachia Mountains to southwest Virginia and in northern Virginia. The analysis presented in Figure 6 highlights several hotspots of late-stage CRC diagnosis across Virginia. Deep red tracts in the southwestern counties, including Lee, Scott, Buchanan, and Tazewell, are predominantly within rural settings and are marked by significant challenges related to socio-economic and healthcare access, potentially contributing to delayed CRC diagnoses. Historically, these areas were heavily reliant on coal mining, which served as a major source of employment and played a significant role in mitigating poverty. However, the decline of the coal industry has not only led to economic challenges but also left a legacy of health exposures for former coal miners. In the western and central regions of Virginia, counties such as Rockingham, Augusta, Albemarle, Amherst, Bedford, and Campbell, exhibit hotspots despite their mixed rural–suburban landscapes and generally favorable socio-economic conditions and healthcare access. Notably, these counties are also characterized by a significant retiree population, suggesting that the age demographic, with a larger proportion of elderly residents, could be influencing the incidence of CRC. Interestingly, northern Virginia, represented by Fairfax County, also emerges as a hotspot highlighting the multifaceted nature of healthcare access and utilization. This county, while boasting a higher socio-economic status (SES), has its own set of challenges that come with affluence, such as increased traffic and resultant air quality concerns. The presence of hotspots across varied socio-economic landscapes underscores the complex interrelation of factors influencing late-stage CRC diagnoses and emphasizes the need for region-specific interventions.

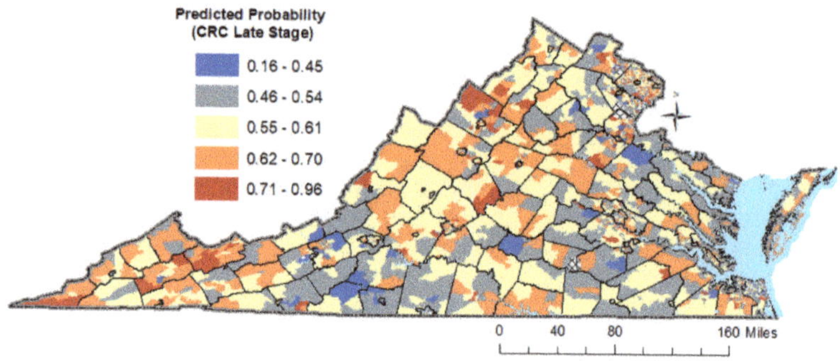

Figure 5. Predicted probability for CRC late stage in Virginia by census tract.

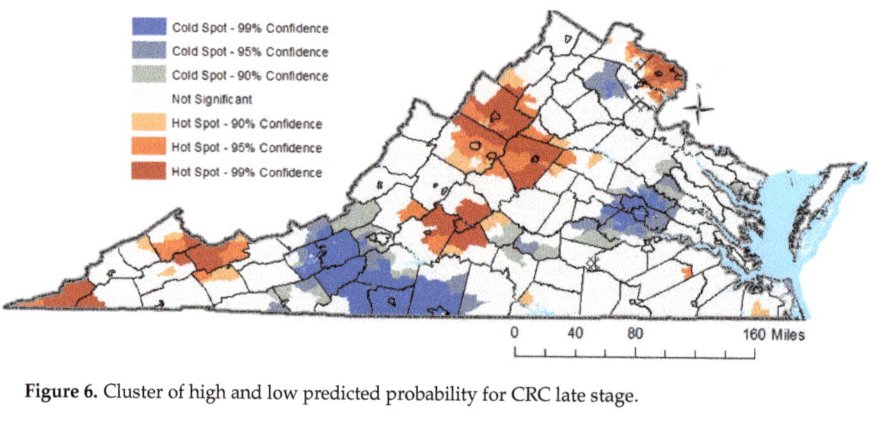

Figure 6. Cluster of high and low predicted probability for CRC late stage.

4. Discussion

In this work, we presented a ML framework for predicting CRC outcomes. More specifically, the study incorporates an ML model along with spatial accessibility measurement to highlight the spatial disparities in the probability of a late-stage CRC diagnosis based on an array of social determinants of health variables, drawn from diverse yet interconnected domains. The study also introduced an innovative theoretical framework, integrating a wealth of SDOH variables to cancer registry data with a primary emphasis on its generalizability and potential for reuse to predict cancer outcomes using ML techniques. After rigorous data preprocessing, we evaluated the performance of five distinct machine-learning algorithms using the ROC-AUC and other metrics. Notably, the gradient boosting model achieved a superior ability to predict late-stage diagnosis. In contrast to previous studies that predominantly focused on validating machine-learning techniques for predicting cancer diagnoses within the general population, our research extends beyond the validation of the gradient boosting model. We specifically targeted high-risk demographic cohorts and conducted an exhaustive analysis of social determinants of health.

According to our gradient boosting model, the top five contributors to the diagnosis of late-stage CRC, ranked in order of importance, are anatomic site, year of diagnosis, age at diagnosis, proximity to superfund sites, and payer at the time of diagnosis. These findings offer a novel perspective for examining the hierarchy of significance among contributors to late-stage CRC diagnosis when utilizing national data. At a more comprehensive level, encompassing all 20 contributors pinpointed by the gradient boosting model, the factors contributing to the prediction of late-stage CRC diagnosis is ascribed to the intricate interplay among individual-level, community-level, and environmental factors. These results align with established literature, where each of these contributors has previously been recognized as a potential risk factor for late-stage CRC diagnosis [54,86,87]. It goes without saying that the gradient boosting model accurately discerned the key drivers of late-stage CRC diagnosis, marking the initial crucial phase in the development of targeted intervention strategies to enhance outcomes in CRC.

The gradient boosting model has become increasingly instrumental in oncology, offering a multifaceted approach to cancer research, diagnosis, treatment, and prognosis. This powerful algorithm leverages ensemble learning to enhance the accuracy of predictive models and has proven particularly valuable in various facets of cancer management. Gradient boosting finds notable applications in predicting cancer risk, [88] survival, [89,90] and diagnosis stages, as well as assisting in cancer classification [91,92]. The capacity of the gradient boosting model to integrate diverse data sources and discern intricate patterns has proven transformative in advancing the understanding of cancer and improving patient outcomes.

Historical space–time analysis of cancer data has typically entailed examining aggregated data to detect patterns in order to understand how areas with varying levels of risk evolve over time [93,94]. In this study, we also identified spatio-temporal clusters of high and low predicted probability for late-stage CRC. Using the census tract as the unit, the analyses identified about 10 statistically significant clusters in Virginia. The spatio-temporal analysis facilitated the refinement of estimates related to area-level factors and established risk factors for CRC, including their interactive dynamics. Furthermore, this analysis yielded tangible, location-specific evidence that can guide targeted intervention strategies.

5. Limitations

Since the gradient boosting model employed in this study adopts a data-driven approach, the model's performance and predictive capabilities are contingent upon the availability and quality of the data. For example, previous literature has identified several SDOHs that have been associated with poor CRC health outcomes that were unable to be obtained. Some of these include social isolation, neighborhood disadvantage/deprivation, health literacy, and transportation options [45,54,95,96]. Data were analyzed from a single state cancer registry. To further determine and verify the robustness and broad applicability of the results, national cancer databases such as the surveillance, epidemiology, and end results should be analyzed. Regarding the aforementioned limitations, we intend to further investigate them in subsequent studies. Finally, in these analyses default hyperparameter settings were chosen from Scikit-learn for an initial broad assessment, with future work planned to fine-tune these parameters using techniques such as GridSearchCV or RandomizedSearchCV for optimized performance.

6. Conclusions

In conclusion, this study has not only showcased the advanced capabilities of machine learning algorithms in predicting late-stage colorectal cancer but also underscored the critical role of spatial accessibility measurements in understanding the disparities in late-stage CRC diagnosis. The spatio-temporal analysis implemented here is particularly instrumental, revealing statistically significant clusters of late-stage CRC diagnoses that necessitate focused public health strategies. These strategies are vital in addressing the observed disparities, reducing the incidence of late-stage CRC, and moving towards the eradication of health inequities. The study's multifaceted ML approach, with gradient boosting leading the way, has not only validated its predictive accuracy but also illuminated the path for future research to fortify and refine these predictive models, with the ultimate aim of enhancing cancer care and management across diverse populations.

Supplementary Materials: The following supporting information can be downloaded at: https://www.mdpi.com/article/10.3390/cancers16030540/s1, Table S1: Baseline Characteristics by Stage of Diagnosis Status; Table S2: Neighborhood Census Tracts Characteristics by Stage of Diagnosis Status.

Author Contributions: Conceptualization, H.G., R.A.-D., A.J., G.B., G.A. and J.B.; methodology, H.G., G.B. and R.A.-D.; software, H.G. and R.A.-D.; validation, H.G. and G.B.; formal analysis, H.G.; investigation, H.G.; data curation, H.G.; writing—original draft preparation, H.G., R.A.-D., A.J., G.B., G.A. and J.B.; writing—review and editing, H.G., R.A.-D., A.J., G.B., G.A. and J.B.; visualization, H.G. and R.A.-D.; supervision, H.G.; funding acquisition, H.G. All authors have read and agreed to the published version of the manuscript.

Funding: This research was funded by the School of Public Health Initiatives (SPHI) grant from Old Dominion University, project number 300852-011 awarded to Hadiza Galadima.

Institutional Review Board Statement: The study was conducted in accordance with the Declaration of Helsinki and approved by the Human Subjects Review Committee of the Old Dominion University (protocol code [1993954-1] and approved on 5 January 2023).

Informed Consent Statement: Not applicable.

Data Availability Statement: Data are contained within the article and Supplementary Materials.

Acknowledgments: The authors would like to express their gratitude to the Virginia Department of Health and the Virginia Cancer Registry for their invaluable assistance in data acquisition.

Conflicts of Interest: The authors declare no conflicts of interest.

References

1. Bray, F.; Ferlay, J.; Soerjomataram, I.; Siegel, R.L.; Torre, L.A.; Jemal, A. Global cancer statistics 2018: GLOBOCAN estimates of incidence and mortality worldwide for 36 cancers in 185 countries. *CA Cancer J. Clin.* **2018**, *68*, 394–424. [CrossRef]
2. Siegel, R.L.; Miller, K.D.; Wagle, N.S.; Jemal, A. Cancer statistics, 2023. *CA Cancer J. Clin.* **2023**, *73*, 17–48. [CrossRef]
3. Moyer, V.A.; US Preventive Services Task Force. Screening for prostate cancer: US Preventive Services Task Force recommendation statement. *Ann. Intern. Med.* **2012**, *157*, 120–134. [CrossRef]
4. Zauber, A.G. The impact of screening on colorectal cancer mortality and incidence: Has it really made a difference? *Dig. Dis. Sci.* **2015**, *60*, 681–691. [CrossRef]
5. Zauber, A.G.; Winawer, S.J.; O'Brien, M.J.; Lansdorp-Vogelaar, I.; van Ballegooijen, M.; Hankey, B.F.; Shi, W.; Bond, J.H.; Schapiro, M.; Panish, J.F. Colonoscopic polypectomy and long-term prevention of colorectal-cancer deaths. *N. Engl. J. Med.* **2012**, *366*, 687–696. [CrossRef] [PubMed]
6. Siegel, R.L.; Fedewa, S.A.; Anderson, W.F.; Miller, K.D.; Ma, J.; Rosenberg, P.S.; Jemal, A. Colorectal cancer incidence patterns in the United States, 1974–2013. *JNCI J. Natl. Cancer Inst.* **2017**, *109*, djw322. [CrossRef] [PubMed]

7. Levin, B.; Lieberman, D.A.; McFarland, B.; Andrews, K.S.; Brooks, D.; Bond, J.; Dash, C.; Giardiello, F.M.; Glick, S.; Johnson, D. Screening and surveillance for the early detection of colorectal cancer and adenomatous polyps, 2008: A joint guideline from the American Cancer Society, the US Multi-Society Task Force on Colorectal Cancer, and the American College of Radiology. *Gastroenterology* **2008**, *134*, 1570–1595. [CrossRef] [PubMed]
8. Kushi, L.H.; Doyle, C.; McCullough, M.; Rock, C.L.; Demark-Wahnefried, W.; Bandera, E.V.; Gapstur, S.; Patel, A.V.; Andrews, K.; Gansler, T. American Cancer Society Guidelines on nutrition and physical activity for cancer prevention: Reducing the risk of cancer with healthy food choices and physical activity. *CA Cancer J. Clin.* **2012**, *62*, 30–67. [CrossRef]
9. Rawla, P.; Sunkara, T.; Barsouk, A. Epidemiology of colorectal cancer: Incidence, mortality, survival, and risk factors. *Gastroenterol. Rev.* **2019**, *14*, 89–103. [CrossRef] [PubMed]
10. Arnold, M.; Sierra, M.S.; Laversanne, M.; Soerjomataram, I.; Jemal, A.; Bray, F. Global patterns and trends in colorectal cancer incidence and mortality. *Gut* **2017**, *66*, 683–691. [CrossRef] [PubMed]
11. Jasperson, K.W.; Tuohy, T.M.; Neklason, D.W.; Burt, R.W. Hereditary and familial colon cancer. *Gastroenterology* **2010**, *138*, 2044–2058. [CrossRef]
12. Commission on Social Determinants of Health. *Closing the Gap in a Generation: Health Equity through Action on the Social Determinants of Health: Final Report of the Commission on Social Determinants of Health*; World Health Organization: Geneva, Switzerland, 2008.
13. Braveman, P.; Gottlieb, L. The social determinants of health: It's time to consider the causes of the causes. *Public Health Rep.* **2014**, *129*, 19–31. [CrossRef]
14. Pinheiro, L.C.; Reshetnyak, E.; Akinyemiju, T.; Phillips, E.; Safford, M.M. Social determinants of health and cancer mortality in the Reasons for Geographic and Racial Differences in Stroke (REGARDS) cohort study. *Cancer* **2022**, *128*, 122–130. [CrossRef]
15. Yu, K.-H.; Beam, A.L.; Kohane, I.S. Artificial intelligence in healthcare. *Nat. Biomed. Eng.* **2018**, *2*, 719–731. [CrossRef]
16. Chen, M.; Decary, M. *Artificial Intelligence in Healthcare: An Essential Guide for Health Leaders*; SAGE Publications: Los Angeles, CA, USA, 2020; pp. 10–18.
17. Silva, T.C.; Zhao, L. *Machine Learning in Complex Networks*; Springer: Berlin/Heidelberg, Germany, 2016.
18. Hastie, T.; Tibshirani, R.; Friedman, J.H.; Friedman, J.H. *The Elements of Statistical Learning: Data Mining, Inference, and Prediction*; Springer: Berlin/Heidelberg, Germany, 2009; Volume 2.
19. Alpaydin, E. *Introduction to Machine Learning*; MIT Press: Cambridge, MA, USA, 2020.
20. Fakoor, R.; Ladhak, F.; Nazi, A.; Huber, M. *Using Deep Learning to Enhance Cancer Diagnosis and Classification*; ACM: New York, NY, USA, 2013; pp. 3937–3949.
21. Aliferis, C.F.; Tsamardinos, I.; Massion, P.P.; Statnikov, A.R.; Fananapazir, N.; Hardin, D.P. Machine Learning Models for Classification of Lung Cancer and Selection of Genomic Markers Using Array Gene Expression Data. In Proceedings of the FLAIRS Conference, St. Augustine, FL, USA, 12–14 May 2003; pp. 67–71.
22. Passos, I.C.; Mwangi, B.; Kapczinski, F. Big data analytics and machine learning: 2015 and beyond. *Lancet Psychiatry* **2016**, *3*, 13–15. [CrossRef] [PubMed]
23. Hornbrook, M.C.; Goshen, R.; Choman, E.; O'Keeffe-Rosetti, M.; Kinar, Y.; Liles, E.G.; Rust, K.C. Early colorectal cancer detected by machine learning model using gender, age, and complete blood count data. *Dig. Dis. Sci.* **2017**, *62*, 2719–2727. [CrossRef] [PubMed]
24. Liu, W.C.; Li, Z.Q.; Luo, Z.W.; Liao, W.J.; Liu, Z.L.; Liu, J.M. Machine learning for the prediction of bone metastasis in patients with newly diagnosed thyroid cancer. *Cancer Med.* **2021**, *10*, 2802–2811. [CrossRef] [PubMed]
25. Yang, H.J.; Cho, C.W.; Jang, J.; Kim, S.S.; Ahn, K.S.; Park, S.K.; Park, D.I. Application of deep learning to predict advanced neoplasia using big clinical data in colorectal cancer screening of asymptomatic adults. *Korean J. Intern. Med.* **2021**, *36*, 845–856. [CrossRef] [PubMed]
26. Gupta, S.; Tran, T.; Luo, W.; Phung, D.; Kennedy, R.L.; Broad, A.; Campbell, D.; Kipp, D.; Singh, M.; Khasraw, M.; et al. Machine-learning prediction of cancer survival: A retrospective study using electronic administrative records and a cancer registry. *BMJ Open* **2014**, *4*, e004007. [CrossRef] [PubMed]
27. Hung, M.; Park, J.; Hon, E.S.; Bounsanga, J.; Moazzami, S.; Ruiz-Negrón, B.; Wang, D. Artificial intelligence in dentistry: Harnessing big data to predict oral cancer survival. *World J. Clin. Oncol.* **2020**, *11*, 918–934. [CrossRef]
28. Manz, C.R.; Chen, J.; Liu, M.; Chivers, C.; Regli, S.H.; Braun, J.; Draugelis, M.; Hanson, C.W.; Shulman, L.N.; Schuchter, L.M.; et al. Validation of a Machine Learning Algorithm to Predict 180-Day Mortality for Outpatients with Cancer. *JAMA Oncol.* **2020**, *6*, 1723–1730. [CrossRef]
29. Lynch, C.M.; Abdollahi, B.; Fuqua, J.D.; de Carlo, A.R.; Bartholomai, J.A.; Balgemann, R.N.; van Berkel, V.H.; Frieboes, H.B. Prediction of lung cancer patient survival via supervised machine learning classification techniques. *Int. J. Med. Inform.* **2017**, *108*, 1–8. [CrossRef]
30. Praiss, A.M.; Huang, Y.; St Clair, C.M.; Tergas, A.I.; Melamed, A.; Khoury-Collado, F.; Hou, J.Y.; Hu, J.; Hur, C.; Hershman, D.L.; et al. Using machine learning to create prognostic systems for endometrial cancer. *Gynecol. Oncol.* **2020**, *159*, 744–750. [CrossRef]
31. Kudo, S.E.; Ichimasa, K.; Villard, B.; Mori, Y.; Misawa, M.; Saito, S.; Hotta, K.; Saito, Y.; Matsuda, T.; Yamada, K.; et al. Artificial Intelligence System to Determine Risk of T1 Colorectal Cancer Metastasis to Lymph Node. *Gastroenterology* **2021**, *160*, 1075–1084. [CrossRef] [PubMed]

32. She, Y.; Jin, Z.; Wu, J.; Deng, J.; Zhang, L.; Su, H.; Jiang, G.; Liu, H.; Xie, D.; Cao, N.; et al. Development and Validation of a Deep Learning Model for Non-Small Cell Lung Cancer Survival. *JAMA Netw. Open* **2020**, *3*, e205842. [CrossRef] [PubMed]
33. Bergquist, S.L.; Brooks, G.A.; Keating, N.L.; Landrum, M.B.; Rose, S. Classifying Lung Cancer Severity with Ensemble Machine Learning in Health Care Claims Data. *Proc. Mach. Learn. Res.* **2017**, *68*, 25–38. [PubMed]
34. Wang, R.; Weng, Y.; Zhou, Z.; Chen, L.; Hao, H.; Wang, J. Multi-objective ensemble deep learning using electronic health records to predict outcomes after lung cancer radiotherapy. *Phys. Med. Biol.* **2019**, *64*, 245005. [CrossRef]
35. Nartowt, B.J.; Hart, G.R.; Muhammad, W.; Liang, Y.; Stark, G.F.; Deng, J. Robust Machine Learning for Colorectal Cancer Risk Prediction and Stratification. *Front. Big Data* **2020**, *3*, 6. [CrossRef]
36. Levitsky, A.; Pernemalm, M.; Bernhardson, B.M.; Forshed, J.; Kölbeck, K.; Olin, M.; Henriksson, R.; Lehtiö, J.; Tishelman, C.; Eriksson, L.E. Early symptoms and sensations as predictors of lung cancer: A machine learning multivariate model. *Sci. Rep.* **2019**, *9*, 16504. [CrossRef] [PubMed]
37. Council, N.R. *Analysis of Cancer Risks in Populations Near Nuclear Facilities: Phase 1*; National Academies Press: Cambridge, MA, USA, 2012.
38. Elena, J.W.; Travis, L.B.; Simonds, N.I.; Ambrosone, C.B.; Ballard-Barbash, R.; Bhatia, S.; Cerhan, J.R.; Hartge, P.; Heist, R.S.; Kushi, L.H. Leveraging epidemiology and clinical studies of cancer outcomes: Recommendations and opportunities for translational research. *J. Natl. Cancer Inst.* **2013**, *105*, 85–94. [CrossRef] [PubMed]
39. Rodgers, K.M.; Udesky, J.O.; Rudel, R.A.; Brody, J.G. Environmental chemicals and breast cancer: An updated review of epidemiological literature informed by biological mechanisms. *Environ. Res.* **2018**, *160*, 152–182. [CrossRef]
40. Patel, C.J.; Kerr, J.; Thomas, D.C.; Mukherjee, B.; Ritz, B.; Chatterjee, N.; Jankowska, M.; Madan, J.; Karagas, M.R.; McAllister, K.A. Opportunities and challenges for environmental exposure assessment in population-based studies. *Cancer Epidemiol. Prev. Biomark.* **2017**, *26*, 1370–1380. [CrossRef]
41. McClish, D.; Penberthy, L. Using Medicare data to estimate the number of cases missed by a cancer registry: A 3-source capture-recapture model. *Med. Care* **2004**, *42*, 1111–1116. [CrossRef]
42. Izquierdo, J.N.; Schoenbach, V.J. The potential and limitations of data from population-based state cancer registries. *Am. J. Public Health* **2000**, *90*, 695. [PubMed]
43. McClure, L.A.; Miller, E.A.; Tannenbaum, S.L.; Hernandez, M.N.; MacKinnon, J.A.; He, Y.; LeBlanc, W.G.; Lee, D.J. Linking the National Health Interview Survey with the Florida Cancer Data System: A Pilot Study. *J. Regist. Manag.* **2016**, *43*, 16.
44. Sugarman, J.R.; Holliday, M.; Ross, A.; Castorina, J.; Hui, Y. Improving American Indian cancer data in the Washington State Cancer Registry using linkages with the Indian Health Service and tribal records. *Cancer Interdiscip. Int. J. Am. Cancer Soc.* **1996**, *78*, 1564–1568.
45. Coughlin, S.S. Social determinants of breast cancer risk, stage, and survival. *Breast Cancer Res. Treat.* **2019**, *177*, 537–548. [CrossRef] [PubMed]
46. Buehler, J.W.; Castro, J.C.; Cohen, S.; Zhao, Y.; Melly, S.; Moore, K. Personal and Neighborhood Attributes Associated with Cervical and Colorectal Cancer Screening in an Urban African American Population. *Prev. Chronic Dis.* **2019**, *16*, E118. [CrossRef] [PubMed]
47. Shariff-Marco, S.; Breen, N.; Stinchcomb, D.G.; Klabunde, C.N. Multilevel predictors of colorectal cancer screening use in California. *Am. J. Manag. Care* **2013**, *19*, 205–216.
48. Mitchell, J.A.; Watkins, D.C.; Modlin, C.S., Jr. Social Determinants Associated with Colorectal Cancer Screening in an Urban Community Sample of African-American Men. *J. Mens. Health* **2013**, *10*, 14–21. [CrossRef] [PubMed]
49. Leech, M.M.; Weiss, J.E.; Markey, C.; Loehrer, A.P. Influence of Race, Insurance, Rurality, and Socioeconomic Status on Equity of Lung and Colorectal Cancer Care. *Ann. Surg. Oncol.* **2022**, *29*, 3630–3639. [CrossRef] [PubMed]
50. Tawk, R.; Abner, A.; Ashford, A.; Brown, C.P. Differences in Colorectal Cancer Outcomes by Race and Insurance. *Int. J. Environ. Res. Public Health* **2015**, *13*, 48. [CrossRef] [PubMed]
51. Balan, N.; Petrie, B.A.; Chen, K.T. Racial Disparities in Colorectal Cancer Care for Black Patients: Barriers and Solutions. *Am. Surg.* **2022**, *88*, 2823–2830. [CrossRef]
52. Salem, M.E.; Puccini, A.; Trufan, S.J.; Sha, W.; Kadakia, K.C.; Hartley, M.L.; Musselwhite, L.W.; Symanowski, J.T.; Hwang, J.J.; Raghavan, D. Impact of Sociodemographic Disparities and Insurance Status on Survival of Patients with Early-Onset Colorectal Cancer. *Oncologist* **2021**, *26*, e1730–e1741. [CrossRef] [PubMed]
53. Warren Andersen, S.; Blot, W.J.; Lipworth, L.; Steinwandel, M.; Murff, H.J.; Zheng, W. Association of Race and Socioeconomic Status with Colorectal Cancer Screening, Colorectal Cancer Risk, and Mortality in Southern US Adults. *JAMA Netw. Open* **2019**, *2*, e1917995. [CrossRef] [PubMed]
54. Coughlin, S.S. Social determinants of colorectal cancer risk, stage, and survival: A systematic review. *Int. J. Color. Dis.* **2020**, *35*, 985–995. [CrossRef]
55. Bauer, C.; Zhang, K.; Xiao, Q.; Lu, J.; Hong, Y.R.; Suk, R. County-Level Social Vulnerability and Breast, Cervical, and Colorectal Cancer Screening Rates in the US, 2018. *JAMA Netw. Open* **2022**, *5*, e2233429. [CrossRef]
56. Korn, A.R.; Walsh-Bailey, C.; Pilar, M.; Sandler, B.; Bhattacharjee, P.; Moore, W.T.; Brownson, R.C.; Emmons, K.M.; Oh, A.Y. Social determinants of health and cancer screening implementation and outcomes in the USA: A systematic review protocol. *Syst. Rev.* **2022**, *11*, 117. [CrossRef]

57. Siegel, R.L.; Sahar, L.; Robbins, A.; Jemal, A. Where Can Colorectal Cancer Screening Interventions Have the Most Impact? Where Can Colorectal Cancer Screening Have the Most Impact? *Cancer Epidemiol. Biomark. Prev.* **2015**, *24*, 1151–1156. [CrossRef] [PubMed]
58. Rogers, C.R.; Moore, J.X.; Qeadan, F.; Gu, L.Y.; Huntington, M.S.; Holowatyj, A.N. Examining factors underlying geographic disparities in early-onset colorectal cancer survival among men in the United States. *Am. J. Cancer Res.* **2020**, *10*, 1592–1607. [PubMed]
59. Kuo, T.-M.; Meyer, A.M.; Baggett, C.D.; Olshan, A.F. Examining determinants of geographic variation in colorectal cancer mortality in North Carolina: A spatial analysis approach. *Cancer Epidemiol.* **2019**, *59*, 8–14. [CrossRef]
60. Centers for Disease Control and Prevention. *The Social-Ecological Model: A Framework for Prevention*; Centers for Disease Control and Prevention: Atlanta, GE, USA, 2015. Available online: https://www.cdc.gov/violenceprevention/about/social-ecologicalmodel.html (accessed on 30 August 2023).
61. US Department of Health and Human Services; Office of Disease Prevention and Health Promotion. Healthy People 2030. 2021. Available online: https://health.gov/healthypeople/objectives-and-data/social-determinants-health (accessed on 30 August 2023).
62. Artiga, S.; Hinton, E. *Beyond Health Care: The Role of Social Determinants in Promoting Health and Health Equity*; Kaiser Family Foundation: San Francisco, CA, USA, 2018; Volume 10.
63. Health, V.D.o. Virginia Cancer Registry (VCR)—Data. Available online: https://www.vdh.virginia.gov/virginia-cancer-registry/data/ (accessed on 1 May 2023).
64. United States Census Bureau. *2015–2019 American Community Survey 5-Year Estimates*; US Department of Commerce: Washington, DC, USA, 2019.
65. mySidewalk. Data Is for the People. Available online: https://www.mysidewalk.com/ (accessed on 28 November 2023).
66. Cui, W.; Finkelstein, J. Using EHR Data to Identify Social Determinants of Health Affecting Disparities in Cancer Survival. *Stud. Health Technol. Inform.* **2022**, *290*, 967–971. [CrossRef]
67. Gehlert, S.; Hudson, D.; Sacks, T. A Critical Theoretical Approach to Cancer Disparities: Breast Cancer and the Social Determinants of Health. *Front. Public Health* **2021**, *9*, 674736. [CrossRef]
68. Yu, Y.; Carey, M.; Pollett, W.; Green, J.; Dicks, E.; Parfrey, P.; Yilmaz, Y.E.; Savas, S. The long-term survival characteristics of a cohort of colorectal cancer patients and baseline variables associated with survival outcomes with or without time-varying effects. *BMC Med.* **2019**, *17*, 150. [CrossRef]
69. He, Z.; Zhang, J.; Yuan, X.; Xi, J.; Liu, Z.; Zhang, Y. Stratification of Breast Cancer by Integrating Gene Expression Data and Clinical Variables. *Molecules* **2019**, *24*, 631. [CrossRef]
70. Galadima, H.I.; Adunlin, G.; Hughes, M.S.; Cropp, C.D.; Lucero, L.; Akpinar-Elci, M. Racial disparities and treatment trends among young-onset colorectal cancer patients: An analysis of a hospital cancer registry. *Cancer Epidemiol.* **2021**, *72*, 101911. [CrossRef]
71. Harvey, V.M.; Enos, C.W.; Chen, J.T.; Galadima, H.; Eschbach, K. The Role of Neighborhood Characteristics in Late Stage Melanoma Diagnosis among Hispanic Men in California, Texas, and Florida, 1996–2012. *J. Cancer Epidemiol.* **2017**, *2017*, 8418904. [CrossRef] [PubMed]
72. Zahnd, W.E.; Gomez, S.L.; Steck, S.E.; Brown, M.J.; Ganai, S.; Zhang, J.; Arp Adams, S.; Berger, F.G.; Eberth, J.M. Rural-urban and racial/ethnic trends and disparities in early-onset and average-onset colorectal cancer. *Cancer* **2021**, *127*, 239–248. [CrossRef] [PubMed]
73. Abualkhair, W.H.; Zhou, M.; Ochoa, C.O.; Lacayo, L.; Murphy, C.; Wu, X.C.; Karlitz, J.J. Geographic and intra-racial disparities in early-onset colorectal cancer in the SEER 18 registries of the United States. *Cancer Med.* **2020**, *9*, 9150–9159. [CrossRef] [PubMed]
74. Missouri Census Data Center. MABLE/Geocorr: Geographic Correspondence Engine. 2018. Available online: https://mcdc.missouri.edu/applications/geocorr.html (accessed on 3 May 2023).
75. Hosmer, D.W., Jr.; Lemeshow, S.; Sturdivant, R.X. *Applied Logistic Regression*; John Wiley & Sons: Hoboken, NJ, USA, 2013; Volume 398.
76. Rafique, R.; Islam, S.R.; Kazi, J.U. Machine learning in the prediction of cancer therapy. *Comput. Struct. Biotechnol. J.* **2021**, *19*, 4003–4017. [CrossRef] [PubMed]
77. Wang, X.; Bo, D.; Shi, C.; Fan, S.; Ye, Y.; Philip, S.Y. A survey on heterogeneous graph embedding: Methods, techniques, applications and sources. *IEEE Trans. Big Data* **2022**, *9*, 415–436. [CrossRef]
78. Quinlan, J.R. Induction of decision trees. *Mach. Learn.* **1986**, *1*, 81–106. [CrossRef]
79. Bertsimas, D.; Wiberg, H. Machine learning in oncology: Methods, applications, and challenges. *JCO Clin. Cancer Inform.* **2020**, *4*, CCI.20.00072. [CrossRef] [PubMed]
80. Breiman, L. Random forests. *Mach. Learn.* **2001**, *45*, 5–32. [CrossRef]
81. Friedman, J.H. Greedy function approximation: A gradient boosting machine. *Ann. Stat.* **2001**, *29*, 1189–1232. [CrossRef]
82. Cortes, C.; Vapnik, V. Support-vector networks. *Mach. Learn.* **1995**, *20*, 273–297. [CrossRef]
83. Levin, T.R.; Corley, D.A.; Jensen, C.D.; Schottinger, J.E.; Quinn, V.P.; Zauber, A.G.; Lee, J.K.; Zhao, W.K.; Udaltsova, N.; Ghai, N.R. Effects of organized colorectal cancer screening on cancer incidence and mortality in a large community-based population. *Gastroenterology* **2018**, *155*, 1383–1391.e1385. [CrossRef] [PubMed]

84. Shapiro, J.A.; Soman, A.V.; Berkowitz, Z.; Fedewa, S.A.; Sabatino, S.A.; de Moor, J.S.; Clarke, T.C.; Doria-Rose, V.P.; Breslau, E.S.; Jemal, A. Screening for colorectal cancer in the United States: Correlates and time trends by type of test. *Cancer Epidemiol. Biomark. Prev.* **2021**, *30*, 1554–1565. [CrossRef]
85. Hubers, J.; Sonnenberg, A.; Gopal, D.; Weiss, J.; Holobyn, T.; Soni, A. Trends in wait time for colorectal cancer screening and diagnosis 2013–2016. *Clin. Transl. Gastroenterol.* **2020**, *11*, e00113. [CrossRef]
86. Demb, J.; Earles, A.; Martínez, M.E.; Bustamante, R.; Bryant, A.K.; Murphy, J.D.; Liu, L.; Gupta, S. Risk factors for colorectal cancer significantly vary by anatomic site. *BMJ Open Gastroenterol.* **2019**, *6*, e000313. [CrossRef]
87. Parikh-Patel, A.; Bates, J.H.; Campleman, S. Colorectal cancer stage at diagnosis by socioeconomic and urban/rural status in California, 1988–2000. *Cancer* **2006**, *107*, 1189–1195. [CrossRef] [PubMed]
88. Li, Y.; Zou, Z.; Gao, Z.; Wang, Y.; Xiao, M.; Xu, C.; Jiang, G.; Wang, H.; Jin, L.; Wang, J. Prediction of lung cancer risk in Chinese population with genetic-environment factor using extreme gradient boosting. *Cancer Med.* **2022**, *11*, 4469–4478. [CrossRef] [PubMed]
89. Bibault, J.-E.; Chang, D.T.; Xing, L. Development and validation of a model to predict survival in colorectal cancer using a gradient-boosted machine. *Gut* **2021**, *70*, 884–889. [CrossRef] [PubMed]
90. Chen, Y.; Jia, Z.; Mercola, D.; Xie, X. A gradient boosting algorithm for survival analysis via direct optimization of concordance index. *Comput. Math. Methods Med.* **2013**, *2013*, 873595. [CrossRef] [PubMed]
91. Aryal, S.; Paudel, B.; Aryal, S.; Paudel, B. Supervised classification using gradient boosting machine: Wisconsin breast cancer dataset. *Int. J. Sci. Res. Eng. Trends* **2020**, *6*, 1887–1892.
92. Vo, D.M.; Nguyen, N.-Q.; Lee, S.-W. Classification of breast cancer histology images using incremental boosting convolution networks. *Inf. Sci.* **2019**, *482*, 123–138. [CrossRef]
93. Liu, B.; Zhu, L.; Zou, J.; Chen, H.-S.; Miller, K.D.; Jemal, A.; Siegel, R.L.; Feuer, E.J. Updated methodology for projecting US-and state-level cancer counts for the current calendar year: Part I: Spatio-temporal modeling for cancer incidence. *Cancer Epidemiol. Biomark. Prev.* **2021**, *30*, 1620–1626. [CrossRef]
94. Guo, Y.; Zeng, H.; Zheng, R.; Li, S.; Barnett, A.G.; Zhang, S.; Zou, X.; Huxley, R.; Chen, W.; Williams, G. The association between lung cancer incidence and ambient air pollution in China: A spatiotemporal analysis. *Environ. Res.* **2016**, *144*, 60–65. [CrossRef]
95. Brady, L.A.; Tumiel-Berhalter, L.M.; Schad, L.A.; Bentham, A.; Vitale, K.; Norton, A.; Noronha, G.; Swanger, C.; Morley, C.P. Increasing Breast, Cervical, and Colorectal Cancer Screenings: A Qualitative Assessment of Barriers and Promoters in Safety-Net Practices. *J. Patient Cent. Res. Rev.* **2021**, *8*, 323–330. [CrossRef]
96. Choy, A.M.; Lebwohl, B.; Krigel, A. Impact of social determinants of health on colorectal cancer screening and surveillance in the COVID reopening phase. *Eur. J. Gastroenterol. Hepatol.* **2022**, *34*, 739–743. [CrossRef]

cancers

MDPI

Review

Sleep and Cancer

Courtney M. Vaughn [1] and Bradley V. Vaughn [2,*]

1 Department of Pediatrics, Division of Pediatric Hematology and Oncology, Washington University School of Medicine, St. Louis, MO 63110, USA; cmvaughn@wustl.edu
2 Department of Neurology, Division of Sleep Medicine, University of North Carolina, Chapel Hill, NC 27599, USA
* Correspondence: vaughnb@neurology.unc.edu

Simple Summary: Over two-thirds of patients with cancer have an issue with their sleep, and some research indicates that sleep may impact the development and progression of cancer. The aim of this review is to highlight the current information on sleep issues, such as sleep duration, sleep disruption, and sleep disorders, and the development and progression of cancer, as well as the impact of cancer on sleep. This article outlines the common sleep complaints in patients with cancer and discusses a logical approach and treatment options for sleep issues in patients with cancer.

Abstract: Background/Objectives: Sleep issues are common in the general population, and these problems occur even more frequently for people with cancer. Sleep problems may pre-exist a patient's cancer diagnosis, and there is a growing interest in understanding the impact of sleep on cancer development and progression. Sleep disorders may impact cancer through altered metabolism, impacts on immune response, and alterations in hormones and gene expression. Sleep disorders may also arise after, or be aggravated by, an individual's cancer and cancer treatment. Treating a person with cancer's sleep disorder may help improve their healing, mental health, cognition, and overall resilience. **Methods:** Studies examining a variety of aspects of the relationship between sleep and cancer were found by searching the National Library of Medicine and characterized by their specific information provided on the relationship between sleep and cancer. **Results:** This review article summarizes our current understanding of the complex inter-relationship between sleep and cancer, the underlying mechanisms that create these connections, and the methods and impact of treating sleep issues in cancer patients. The article also outlines an approach to sleep complaints for clinicians caring for patients with cancer. **Conclusions:** Significant research is still needed to understand the full relationship between sleep disorders and cancer. The impact of sleep issues on cancer and of cancer on sleep appears to be specific to the tissue and the molecular type of cancer. The treatment of sleep disorders is multimodal, and offers a promising avenue to improve the health and quality of life of cancer patients.

Keywords: sleep; sleep disorders; sleep disruption; cancer; insomnia; excessive sleepiness

1. Introduction

1.1. What Is Sleep?

Sleep is a normal dynamic physiological state, which is characterized by the decreased responsiveness of the central nervous system to the environment. During this state, several brain and body functions occur that are important in the maintenance of organs and maximizing performance. Sleep is regulated, in part, by the accumulation of byproducts from neuronal and somatic activity, the homeostatic drive, and by an individual's circadian rhythm that helps with timing of sleep periods and coordinating other cycles [1]. A variety of substances constitute the homeostatic drive; these substances increase during the wake period. These substances include, but are not limited to, inflammatory-related molecules such as adenosine, galanin, oleamide, cytokines, and tumor necrosis factor, as well as other byproducts of cellular activity. The circadian rhythm is a recurrent transcription-translation loop that creates a clock of approximately 24 h that regulates multiple physiological cycles. The control of these multiple cycles is in an attempt to optimize our preparedness for recurring physiological events and save energy when these processes are not needed. Although we think of sleep as one of these events, many processes are governed by a circadian rhythm, and over 20% of our genes are transcribed in a circadian fashion. From a sleep–wake viewpoint, the main function of the circadian rhythm is to promote our ability to be awake. The circadian drive typically builds through the day to remain awake and offset the promotion of sleep by the homeostatic drive. These two major drivers help explain the timing of sleep and the length of sleep through what is known as the two process model [2]. In this model, the circadian drive promotes wakefulness through the day, while at the same time, the homeostatic drive builds up as a chemical capacitor to promote sleep (Figure 1). Once the homeostatic drive is above the circadian drive to be awake, the person feels sleepy. Through the night, the substances comprising the homeostatic drive are metabolized and reprocessed via the mechanisms in sleep. By morning, the homeostatic drive to sleep dips below the circadian drive to be awake, and the person awakens [2].

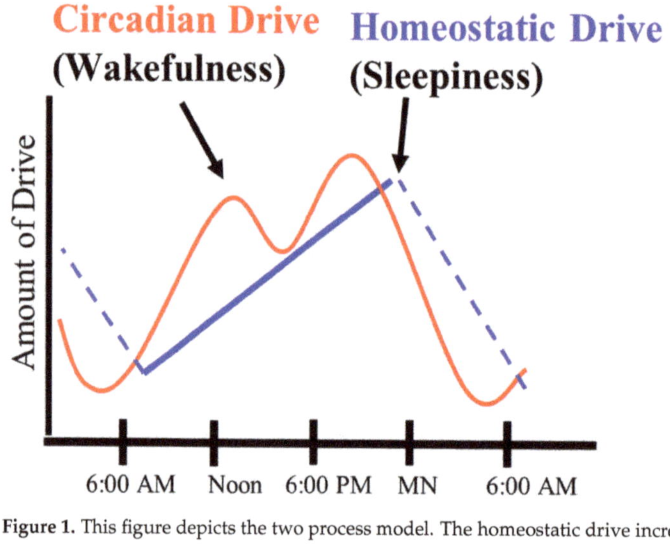

Figure 1. This figure depicts the two process model. The homeostatic drive increases as a result of activity while awake and then is metabolized during sleep. This drive increases the drive for sleep. The circadian drive also increases through the day and opposes the homeostatic drive by promoting wakefulness. The circadian rhythm is accentuated by light, activity, food, and social interaction during the waking period.

Sleep may be contextually thought of as one state, but comprises multiple different states. Sleep is typically subdivided into non-rapid eye movement (NREM) sleep and rapid eye movement (REM) sleep [3]. NREM sleep is also subdivided into Stages N1, N2, and N3, which are associated with a gradual decrease in responsiveness to the environment and isolate the cerebral cortex from sensory inputs for processes such as replenishing neurotransmitters and energy stores, synaptic pruning, and processing flushing of waste products. Some of these functions also occur in REM sleep. We associate this state with dreaming and emotional processing. REM sleep is also thought to have important secondary effects on the immune system, autonomic system regulation, and the processing of emotions [4].

1.2. What Is Cancer?

Cancer is a collection of diseases linked by the characteristics of the uncontrolled growth of abnormal cells. According to the World Health Organization, approximately one in five individuals will develop cancer in their lifetime, and there are an estimated 20 million new cancer cases diagnosed and 9.7 million deaths related to cancer each year [5]. According to the American Cancer Society, more than 2 million people are diagnosed with cancer in the United States annually. As therapies have improved, the growing population of cancer survivors is estimated to be over 18 million people. These patients will require evaluation for and management of the sequelae of their disease and treatment [6]. While the different kinds of cancer share the commonality of uncontrolled cellular growth, the underlying triggers and downstream effects are unique. Any organ system can develop cancer. Additionally, cancer cells can spread to other organs, either through local invasion or by metastasis. Some of the cellular processes that allow for the spread of the cancer appear to be linked to sleep and the circadian rhythm. Significant debate exists as to the impact of sleep on cancer risk and progression, with many important scientific findings supporting either a correlation or no impact [7,8]. Even though some generalizations may be made regarding cancer, it is important to realize that the interplay of sleep and cancer is likely specific to the tissue and molecular subtype of cancer based on the underlying molecular and physiological processes of each cancer type. Although this makes generalizations difficult, the overarching conclusion is that cancer may have unique interactions with sleep. In understanding the impact of sleep on cancer, it is also important to acknowledge that sleep is strongly intertwined with additional processes that have been independently studied for their effect on cancer, such as circadian rhythm and melatonin secretion. While sleep and circadian rhythms are heavily linked, they are two separate processes. This article will touch briefly on some aspects of the circadian rhythm; however, we will mostly focus on the interaction of sleep and cancer.

Sleep offers an opportunity to broaden our understanding of cancer in the light of understanding the influence of both the states of wake and sleep on normal and aberrant cellular and organ function. Understanding sleep also promotes a better understanding of the influence of these states on the treatment of cancer and the interaction on the body as a whole. In addition to illuminating vulnerabilities, studying sleep offers the opportunity for new paradigms in therapy and improvements in the quality of life for patients with cancer.

2. Influence of Sleep on Developing Cancer

2.1. Sleep Duration and Cancer Risk

Sleep provides a vital period for several regulatory functions; understanding the impact of sleep duration and disruption on these regulatory functions may enlighten us to the role of sleep duration in the risk of the developing of cancer. Some cancers appear to have a possible relation to sleep duration (Table 1); however, this association is complex and numerous studies addressing this question have reached different conclusions. Longer sleep length may increase the risk for cancer. In a study of the UK Biobank and breast cancer, Richmond found a 1.19 weighted odds ratio in favor of developing breast cancer for each hour of sleep longer than 8 h and a mild protective effect of sleep for less than 7 h [9]. Other studies show an association between longer sleep duration and cancer; for example, there is an association between a sleep duration more than 9 h and a higher risk of colorectal and liver cancer and a sleep duration greater than 10 h and lung cancer [10–12]. In contrast, Verksalo et al. described a lower incidence of breast cancer in individuals who had longer sleep duration in a prospective study [13]. Kakizaki also found an increased risk of development of breast cancer in women who slept less than 6 h a day. Two studies studying this same question could not determine a relationship between sleep duration and breast cancer [14–16]. Zhou et al. also found that short sleep duration was associated with an increased risk of cancer of the lung, by 16% [17]. Short sleep duration may also increase the risk of colorectal and other cancers [18]. In a long-term follow-up study involving sleep duration, Gapstur et al. found a correlation between shorter sleep duration and the development of prostate cancer [19], and Sigurdardottir et al. also found that sleep disruption and a shorter sleep duration are correlated with an increased risk of the development of prostate cancer in older males [20]. Alternatively, Lu, using a meta-analysis of 10 studies, did not find a statistically significant relationship of short or long sleep duration with an increased overall risk of cancer, but trends were noted for short sleep with the development of prostate cancer, thyroid cancer, and ovarian cancer, and long sleep duration with colorectal cancer [21]. An umbrella review of this topic also supports the conclusion that the impact of sleep duration on carcinogenesis appears to be tissue-specific [20]. This conclusion is also supported by a study by Li et al. which supported both an increased risk of 21% for long sleep duration and colorectal cancer, and a trend for skin cancer with short sleep duration. The fact that the impact of sleep duration appears to be tissue-specific raises questions as to the association being more related to specific underlying physiological pathways intrinsic to each tissue type, or whether the relationship is based on the response of each tissue type to the impact of sleep on more systemic control mechanisms, such as the immune system [22,23]. Evidence from animal data supports a role for sleep restriction in carcinogenesis. One study found that sleep restriction increased polyp development in mice with a genetic predisposition to form intestinal neoplasms [24]. These studies suggest that sleep duration may play a role in the development of some cancers or may exacerbate a pre-existing abnormality, making cancer more likely. These studies also do not give us an understanding of the role that each stage of sleep may play in cancer development. We currently lack any knowledge of the contribution of specific sleep stages (NREM, REM) and perturbations therein as it relates to carcinogenesis.

Table 1. Cancer types associated with sleep issues.

Sleep Issue	Cancers Found in Association	Sources
Prolonged Sleep Duration	Breast cancer, colorectal cancer, liver cancer, lung cancer	[9–12]
Shortened Sleep Duration	Breast cancer, lung cancer, colorectal cancer, prostate cancer, skin cancer	[14,17–20]
Insomnia	Breast cancer, lung cancer, thyroid cancer, oral cancer, prostate cancer	[17,20,25–28]
Obstructive Sleep Apnea	Breast cancer, prostate cancer, nasal cancer, melanoma, bladder cancer, lung cancer, liver cancer, cervical cancer, kidney cancer, uterine cancer, colorectal cancer	[29–33]
Parasomnias	Breast cancer, oral cancer	[30]
Hypersomnia	Gastric cancer, head and neck cancer	[34]

2.2. *Sleep Disorders and Cancer Development*

Beyond sleep duration, other sleep disturbances and disorders may impact cancer risk (Table 1). Fang et al. used a nationwide, nested case–control study to determine that, through complex mechanisms, sleep disorders may increase cancer risk [30]. Some of this risk may be tissue-specific, but also dependent upon the type of sleep disruption. Zhou et al. found, in a meta-analysis of 11 studies including over 460,000 participants, that sleep disruption increased the overall risk of cancer [17]. Assessing multiple studies, the increased risk of any cancer attributable to sleep disturbances is, at most, a small increase. By exploring this relationship for individual tumor types, we may be able to better understand the impact of sleep disruption on cancer and the mechanism of this relationship. When specifically looking at breast cancer, the hazard ratio increased to 2.38 for women who endorsed insomnia, characterized as non-restorative sleep, difficulty initiating sleep, or difficulty maintaining sleep in a study from Norway of 33,332 women [25]. Yap et al. also found in a meta-review that the presence OSA increased the risk of developing breast cancer by 36% [29].

Each sleep disorder may influence different molecular processes, and thus the effect of sleep disorders on cancer may be more specific to the type of sleep disruption and tumor type (Table 1). For example, in their meta-analysis, Zhou et al. more specifically found that insomnia was associated with an increased risk of lung cancer with an odds ratio of 1.11, but sleep apnea did not appear to increase the risk of lung cancer [17]. Likewise, Shi et al. performed a meta-analysis with over 570,000 subjects, and found a 24% increase in the risk of cancer in those with the complaint of insomnia, with a higher risk of cancer in women. Shi et al. also found that the highest associated risk for patients with insomnia was developing thyroid cancer [26]. A similar connection was noted by Chui et al., in a study looking at insomnia and breast cancer risk [27]. An increased risk of breast cancer and oral cancer was also described in 43,585 patients with insomnia who used hypnotics [28]. While additional studies have sought to answer this same question, this association was not replicable. For example, an additional study of 110,011 women did not find a link between insomnia and breast cancer [35]. This pattern of conflicting evidence has also been seen for prostate cancer. One Icelandic cohort of 2102 senior men over a 5-year follow-up showed that those endorsing difficulties initiating and maintaining sleep had a 70% higher risk of prostate cancer [20]. Yet, several other studies were unable to confirm this link in prostate cancer. Some of these discrepancies may be based on how insomnia is defined and diagnosed in each study. This potential risk of insomnia and cancer raised questions as to the possibility of the influence of insomnia on hormonal regulation, melatonin, and the immune system (Figure 2). Insomnia in patients with coexisting depression, are known to have elevated the thyroid-stimulating hormone (TSH), as sleep is noted to normally suppress this hormone [36]. Therefore, the increase in TSH could increase the incidence of thyroid cancer in some individuals. Melatonin also decreases in some insomnia patients, and is noted to have an impact on checking cell proliferation, slowing mitotic processes, and influencing the immune mechanisms. Insomnia itself has been linked to changes in inflammation and immune function, which are all plausible pathways by which insomnia may increase the likelihood of the development of cancer [37].

Other types of sleep disorders may increase the risk of some cancers. In addition to individuals with insomnia, Fang et al. found that patients with parasomnias have an increased risk of breast cancer and a significant increase in risk of oral cancers [30]. Fang et al. also described that subjects with obstructive sleep apnea (OSA) had a higher risk of breast, prostate, and nasal cancer. Using OSA as the model for sleep disruption, Gozal et al. found hazard ratios ranging from 1.07 to 1.41 in several types of cancer in individuals with OSA [31]. Although the overall risk of cancer in individuals with OSA was not found to be elevated, individuals with OSA were noted to have a significantly increased incidence of several types of cancer, including melanoma, bladder, lung, liver, cervix, and kidney. In a study involving approximately 20,000 subjects, Marriott et al found that nocturnal hypoxemia was independently associated with cancer, and OSA severity was associated with increased incidence of cancer, but the latter was felt to be related to other coexisting risks [38]. Thus, they concluded that OSA was not an independent risk factor for cancer. Sillah et al. described an association between OSA and an increased risk of breast cancer, uterine cancer, melanoma, and renal cancer based on a population of 34,402 participants [32]. In a study of 163 participants, the incidence of colorectal neoplasia on colonoscopy was three times higher in participants who had polysomnogram verified OSA than participants who did not have sleep disordered breathing [32,33]. Sleep apnea has been postulated to have several pathophysiological cascades, triggering a multitude of mechanisms that could lead to possible increases in the incidence of cancer (Figure 2). The expression of the hypoxia-inducible factor is altered by OSA [39]. The hypoxia-inducible factor regulates processes that help protect cells in the setting of prolonged hypoxemia, but also impact cell cycle and growth. The relatively rapid cycle of hypoxia and recovery clearly influences the cell metabolism, inflammatory and immune response [40]. Similarly, the oxidative stress of sleep apnea may induce changes in DNA and RNA stability [41]. The link of sleep apnea and cancer is very complex and many confounding variables exist, such as obesity [42]. These studies, however, suggest that the potential link between sleep and cancer may depend upon the specific pathways that are interrupted, and that sleep itself may have an impact on stabilizing cell growth and inhibiting carcinogenesis. Therefore, understanding the link between sleep disruption and downstream secondary effects, resulting in mechanistic and microenvironmental changes, is key to understanding the impact of sleep disorders on the development and progression of cancer.

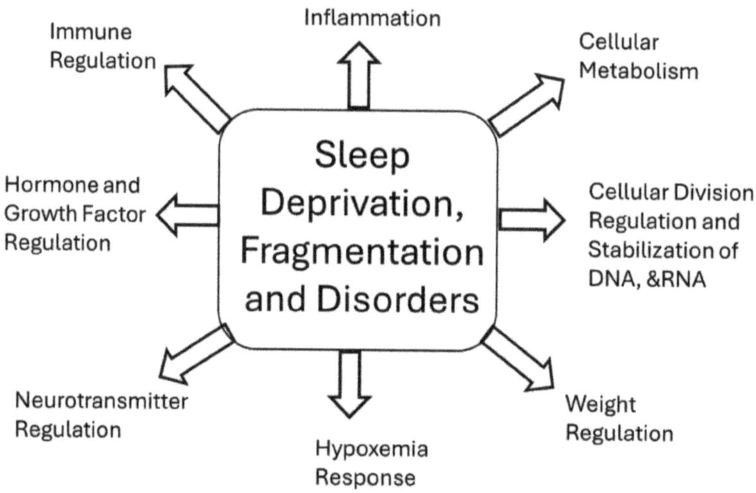

Figure 2. This diagram demonstrates the variety of mechanisms by which sleep, sleep disruption, and sleep disorders may influence cancer development and progression.

Hypersomnia disorders may also increase the risk for cancer. Higher incidences of head and neck and gastric tumors were found in women with narcolepsy [34]. The mechanisms proposed that could underly the impact of narcolepsy on cancer risk are related to the immune response or the loss of orexin [34]. Narcolepsy with cataplexy (narcolepsy type 1) results from the loss of neurons that produce orexin. Orexin is relevant to narcolepsy as it appears to help stabilize the wake state. However, orexin also has proposed systemic roles, notably including that it may regulate apoptosis through the Orexin1R receptor. This receptor has been found to be expressed in some colorectal and pancreatic tumors, indicating a potential vulnerability of these tumors to orexin [43]. When tumors are subjected to orexin A in vivo or in vitro, there is a significant reduction in tumor size [44]. Interestingly, a dual orexin receptor antagonist, almorexant, with a similar ability to orexin A, also causes apoptosis in pancreatic cancer cells, raising interesting implications for therapy [45]. Thus, it is conceivable that the loss of orexin in narcolepsy could prevent the inhibition of aberrant cell growth. This connection supports the possibility that some forms of sleep disorders, such as narcolepsy, may give additional clues to specific tissue regulation.

These studies suggest that individuals with insomnia, hypersomnia, parasomnia, or OSA may have a higher risk of developing cancer. The link of sleep disruption to cancer may be confounded by changes in immune response, impairment of melatonin release, or changes in weight, and these changes in immune response, weight, and other regulatory factors may make specific types of cancer more likely to occur (Figure 2). Yet it is unclear if these causes of sleep disruption may have a causal link or may be a result of confounding factors that also increase the risk of developing cancer. Thus, the role of sleep duration, fragmentation, and other sleep disorders in cancer development and progression needs further delineation to provide a clearer linkage of sleep disorders and cancer development.

3. Sleep Disorders in Cancer

3.1. Sleep Disorders in Individuals with Cancer

Many people suffer from sleep complaints, and this rate increases in cancer patients [46]. Sleep complaints are reported by as high as 75% of cancer patients in a variety of studies [47,48] (Table 2). Sixty-six patients with cancer reported a sleep disturbance in a meta-analysis of 160 studies [49]. Although there is no consensus on the term sleep quality, many investigators use different sleep questionnaires, such as the Pittsburgh Sleep Quality Index, to assess overall sleep issues. Performing a meta-analysis of 59 epidemiological studies with different sleep quality questionnaires, Chen et al. found a global prevalence of poor sleep quality in 57.4% of patients with cancer [50]. Both adult and pediatric patients with cancer can have a wide array of sleep issues, which are including but not limited to excessive sleepiness, difficulty initiating or maintaining sleep, and unusual nocturnal movements, similar to the general population [51,52]. The specific type of cancer, the treatment plan, and the patient's overall course appears to impact the rate of sleep issues [53]. Over three-fourths of non-small cell lung cancer patients complain of poor sleep, most having their sleep symptoms predate the start of therapy [54]. As discussed in the section on the association of sleep disorders and the risk of developing cancer, sleep issues may start prior to the diagnosis and treatment of cancer, and may last years after the individual's cancer is in remission. This is frequently seen in breast cancer patients, many of whom have sleep issues prior to their cancer diagnosis that are frequently aggravated with chemotherapy [55]. The presence of sleep issues may also increase the likelihood of side effects from the cancer treatment, as Jung et al. found with higher incidence of chemotherapy-induced gastrointestinal symptoms in breast cancer patients with sleep issues [56]. Similarly, patients with head and neck cancers and OSA may have exacerbation of their OSA with therapies such as radiation [57]. In a single-center review of over nine thousand patients, Page et al. found that one in five patients with cancer developed insomnia during treatment [58]. Part of the increase in the prevalence of sleep complaints may be from pre-existing conditions or vulnerabilities, the effects of the tumor on sleep, the influence of cancer-directed therapies, and the stress and emotional burden of a cancer diagnosis. Patients may also have changes in weight, diet, and activity levels that influence sleep and waking. Yet, sleep disruption may also be a prognostic factor in cancer. Palesh et al. found that cancer patients with better sleep efficiency and duration, measured by actigraphy, had lower mortality [59].

Table 2. Common sleep complaints in patients with cancer.

Sleep Complaint	Behaviors	Disruptors	Disorders
Insomnia	Review time in bed (association) and timing of sleep (circadian issue), napping, activity Inquire into the daily routine and sleep-associated behaviors	Inquire into sleep environment Medications, supplements, caffeine, ETOH, nicotine	Sleep-related breathing disorders, pain, reflux, other medical, and psychiatric issues
Excessive Sleepiness	Review time in bed dedicated to sleep and timing of sleep (circadian issue) Inquire into daily routine and sleep-associated behaviors	Inquire into sleep environment Medications, supplements, caffeine, ETOH, nicotine	Sleep-related breathing disorders, pain, reflux, other medical, and psychiatric issues
Sleep-Related Breathing Issues	Ask about sleep position, ETOH, nicotine airway irritants	Weight changes, reflux, nasal congestion	Sleep-related breathing disorders, lung, heart, brain, neuromuscular disorders
Restless Legs and Other Nocturnal Movement Disorders	Ask about environment the movement occurs in, timing of movement and relationship to caffeine, ETOH, nicotine and stress	Caffeine, ETOH, diet	Restless legs syndrome, periodic limb movement disorder, other sleep transition movements, and neurological issues
Nocturnal Events—Parasomnias, Nocturnal Seizures		Other sleep disorders, ETOH, short-acting hypnotics	Parasomnia, nocturnal seizures, delirium

3.2. *Sleep Disorders and Cancer Progression*

Interest in sleep and cancer has increased due to increased understanding of how sleep may directly influence cancer, as well as how sleep may regulate mechanisms that may regulate tumor growth and metastasis. As mentioned in the section on sleep disorders in patients with cancer, cancer patients experience high rates of sleep disturbances. These sleep disturbances may, in turn, have profound consequences. In addition to the reduced quality of life, cancer patients with sleep issues have higher rates of mood disorders, shorter time to progression, and reduced survival [60].

In the Wisconsin Sleep Cohort study, with 22 years of follow-up data, subjects with sleep-disordered breathing were found to have a higher mortality rate from cancer than those without sleep-disordered breathing [61]. This group also found that individuals with increased severity of hypoxemia had higher cancer-related mortality rates. Huang et al. also found a higher mortality rate among individuals with advanced lung cancer and sleep apnea [62]. Similarly, an increase in mortality in patients with melanoma and sleep apnea was noted in a five-year follow-up study [63]. The link between sleep issues and cancer-related mortality is likely complex as, contrary to these findings, the Women's Health Initiative population study failed to find a link of insomnia with cancer mortality [64].

In determining the impact of sleep disorders on cancer progression, it is important to look beyond mortality rate. Sleep issues may impact other aspects of cancer progression, as well as recovery. For example, OSA has been associated with an increase in metastasis rates [31]. Untreated OSA results in intermittent hypoxia, which in turn can give rise to more aggressive growth in melanoma. This has been replicated in animal studies with experimentally created intermittent hypoxia [65]. Martina Garcia et al. found a direct relationship between an increase in the severity of sleep apnea and an increase in the aggressiveness of melanoma [66,67]. Despite this, the same group did not find an increase in markers for aggressiveness in breast cancer in patients with concurrent OSA, suggesting that there may be a tumor-specific component to this interplay [68]. Other sleep disorders such as insomnia may also impact cancer survival. Wang et al. found that ovarian cancer patients with insomnia had shorter survival times [69]. Similarly, a meta-analysis of studies of sleep and multiple cancer types conducted by Strom et al. found that disturbed sleep during treatment was associated with shorter time to disease progression and lower survival [70]. In animal studies, mice that had chronically fragmented sleep had accelerated tumor growth [71]. This raises the question of what are the underlying mechanisms that regulate the connection between sleep disruption or intermittent hypoxemia on increasing tumor growth. It is most likely that both may have a subtle effect through multiple pathways. The reason for this increase in tumor growth and aggressiveness in sleep fragmentation may be connected to the hormonal, immune, and cellular metabolic factors noted above; however, other factors may also be involved in accelerating tumor growth. Beyond the effect of hypoxemia, sleep disruption itself impacts carcinogenesis and cancer growth through its impact on angiogenesis, immune response, metabolism, and hormone regulation (Figure 2). Understanding the mechanisms underpinning the relationship between sleep and cancer has allowed researchers to better define questions, and has led to increased interest in the field. For example, there is a growing body of work on sleep, the immune system, and cancer. There is a bidirectional relationship of the immune system and sleep, with both processes regulating the other. This is demonstrated in the increase in sleep complaints with increased levels of inflammation frequently seen in cancer patients [72]. Increased inflammation, such as that seen in cancer, can have a key impact on sleep quality, fatigue, pain, and mood [73]. Cancer progression may be impacted by the inflammation caused by sleep issues [74]. Fragmentation of sleep is associated with increased inflammatory markers and glucocorticoid and catecholamine levels. Elevated glucocorticoid and catecholamine levels may weaken the immune response and promote angiogenesis. Beyond inflammation, sleep disruption has been shown to impact the expression of other growth factors and hormones, as well as their receptors. Through this and other mechanisms, sleep disruption and fragmentation aid tumor progression. Beyond the direct impact on cancer, sleep disruption can negatively impact healing and resilience by limiting cognitive and emotional spheres. This prolongs the negative impacts of cancer, even after there is no evidence of disease.

Sleep disruption and fragmentation in cancer patients result in multiple physiological changes that impact tumor progression and recovery in a tumor-specific manor. Understanding this relationship may help us to better care for cancer patients; therefore, more research on this topic is needed [48].

4. The Impact of Cancer and Cancer Treatments on Sleep

Cancer and cancer-directed therapies may have direct and indirect effects on the brain circuits involved in the regulation of the wake and sleep states. These effects may be altering the molecular signaling pathways of the homeostatic and circadian drives. These signaling pathways may be influenced by changes in cellular metabolic products, hormonal regulation, and inflammatory and immune products. Similarly, the side effects of chemotherapy, radiation therapy, and surgery can include nausea, pain, and fatigue, which frequently result in disturbed sleep. Sleep changes can also occur because of the changes in activity level, diet, and mood that come with cancer and cancer treatment. The understandable emotional toll of the diagnosis of cancer creates substantial stress on the individual, worsening their quality of sleep.

In understanding the influence of cancer on sleep and sleep issues, it is important to understand the impact on each stage. Unfortunately, very few studies have used polysomnography to characterize sleep stages in cancer patients. One study that explored this question was conducted by Parker et al., who used ambulatory polysomnography to characterize sleep stages in 114 cancer patients, and found that people with cancer have reduced total sleep and less slow wave and REM sleep compared to people who did not have cancer. In this study, cancer patients also had increased arousals and more sleep continuity compared to the participants who did not have cancer [75]. This study also found that individuals who slept more during the day had less sleep at night. Reinsel et al. conducted a two-night sleep study protocol of patients with breast cancer, and found a normal average sleep efficiency at 86.7%, with relatively normal distribution of sleep stages. Patients with a higher intensity of sleep disruption had higher periodic limb movements indices in sleep [76]. Unfortunately, the subjects were not asked about symptoms of restless legs syndrome. Although the connection between periodic limb movements in sleep and breast cancer is unclear, studies like these suggest that each cancer type may have a unique effect on sleep regulation.

Physiologically, cancer may also play a direct role in sleep regulation and drive. Frequently, tumor–immune system interactions result in the release of several cytokines that contribute to the homeostatic sleep drive, including TNF-α, I-1β, and IL-6, which can cause daytime fatigue and lead to sleep problems such as insomnia and sleep disruption [77]. These cytokines and molecules can increase after cytolytic therapies. The hypothalamic sleep–wake circuitry may also be impacted by cancer through the impact of cancer on hormones such as leptin and ghrelin [78]. More directly, cancer may directly invade the brain centers that control sleep–wake state. Craniopharyngiomas specifically invade the hypothalamus, potentially disrupting both centers in the control of sleep and circadian rhythm [79]. Patients with damage to the hypothalamic center may show an inability to stabilize their sleep state, including REM sleep, similar to the instability of sleep state that occurs in narcolepsy. The diagnosis of cancer and the implications of cancer can influence the patient's emotional balance. This secondary effect on mood and mood disorders, such as depression and anxiety, can frequently present sleep issues [80]. Lastly, patients with cancer may change their daily routine, causing disruption to their schedule and causing less activity, which subsequently influences sleep. Thus, cancer has numerous pathways to cause disruption of sleep.

In addition to the physiological and psychological burden of cancer, the treatment of cancer may also disrupt sleep. Several studies have demonstrated that both radiation therapy and chemotherapy cause fatigue and insomnia [81]. Medications such as glucocorticoid steroids are commonly used in cancer therapy regimens, yet these frequently cause insomnia, especially when the steroid has a longer half-life or is taken later in the day or requires twice-daily dosing [82]. Other chemotherapies are also associated with insomnia. Kiss, in a meta-analysis, found insomnia was a common side effect for most chemotherapies, hormonal therapies, and immunotherapies [83]. This included finding that checkpoint inhibitor therapies had similar rates of insomnia as other immuno- and non-immuno-targeted therapies, with odds ratios for insomnia ranging from 1.4 to 1.49 [83]. In another study, Ancoli-Israel et al. found that in breast cancer patients, chemotherapy was shown to increase the severity and chronicity of insomnia, especially in those who had a tendency for insomnia prior to the cancer diagnosis [55]. Immunotherapies for cancer may also influence sleep and the indirect pathways that impact sleep [84]. Zarogoulidis et al. studied 49 patients with lung cancer undergoing only immunotherapy directed toward programmed cell death ligand 1 (PD-L1), and found that those with higher PD-L1 expression had a higher likelihood of improvement in sleep latency and sleep duration reduction in fatigue compared to patients with lower PD-L1 expression [85]. They also found that after nine months of therapy, those who had a complete response of their tumor also had near-complete resolution of their sleep issues. This included cancer-related fatigue, as well as fatigue related to confounding factors. Patients who had partial and complete response of their tumor also had an improvement in emotional status, pain status, fatigue, and overall sleep quality. There is a growing interest in modifiable moderating factors of the relationship between cancer and sleep, such as the gut microbiome. Studying fatigue in cancer patients, Hajjar et al. found that the gut microbial species, Eubacterium hallii, was associated with lower fatigue scores, whereas Cosenzaea was associated with high fatigue scores [86]. This demonstrates the inter-relationship of multiple systems that may change with cancer and cancer therapies, and their potential influence on sleep.

Overall, the impact of cancer and cancer treatment on sleep may occur through both tumor-specific and general systemic mechanisms. Additional studies are needed to better define both these direct and indirect pathways, and to determine the best interventions for patients.

5. The Effects of Treating Sleep Disorders in Cancer Patients

In light of the possible impact of sleep disorders on carcinogenesis, as described above, treating a cancer patient's sleep disorders could conceivably influence their outcomes. To date, data are still limited on the impact of treating sleep disorders on cancer outcomes. Most studies show that treatment of the sleep disorder improves sleep-related symptoms. As an example, Ganjei et al. found that treatment of OSA with continuous positive airway pressure improved the daytime sleepiness and fatigue in patients with cancer and OSA, but the study did not include any data on the subsequent cancer status [87]. Similarly, the treatment of insomnia in patients with cancer with pharmacological and nonpharmacological therapies improved the insomnia symptoms, with little information on the effect on cancer progression [88,89].

Although intermittent hypoxia triggered more aggressive growth of melanoma and other tumors in both animal and human studies, clinical evidence of improved cancer-related outcomes in those treated for their sleep issues is sparse [65,66]. In a small study of patients with sleep apnea, Gharib et al. found a reduction in cancer-associated transcriptional signatures with continuous positive airway pressure (CPAP) treatment of OSA, suggesting that an improvement in sleep hindered the environment for tumor growth [90]. Another study found a decrease in inflammatory factors, improved immune response, and reduced vascular endothelial growth factor in patients who were complaint with long-term CPAP [91]. Other treatment paradigms for sleep disorders may add to other improvements in cancer outcomes [92]. Insomnia can be treated with cognitive behavioral therapies for insomnia (CBT-I). For cancer patients with insomnia, CBT-I can improve not only their sleep quality, but also their quality of life, whilst also decreasing comorbidities, and potentially even reducing healthcare costs [93–95]. CBT has been shown to improve insomnia, in fact, Peoples et al. found that CBT resulted in better outcomes than CBT in combination with armodafinil [96]. In addition to CBT-I, other nonpharmacological interventions for insomnia may provide some benefits to cancer patients [97]. These include acupuncture and progressive muscular relaxation [98–100]. Medications appear to have mixed results. Few pharmacological studies examining the treatment of insomnia exist. In one small study of temazepam versus a melatonin group and a placebo group, both melatonin and temazepam showed an improvement in sleep issues, but no improvement in quality of life [101]. Another small study of 30 patients with advanced cancer demonstrated that trazadone as a treatment for insomnia both improved sleep quality and reduced nightmares [102]. However, a meta-analysis of seven randomized studies with trazadone in the general population failed to show significant improvements in sleep latency, duration, or efficiency. Despite this, patients randomized to trazadone did perceive better sleep quality in three of the studies [103]. Melatonin at a nightly dosage of 3 mg was also found to reduce insomnia severity in cancer patients [104]. Exogenous melatonin at low doses (1–3 mg), timed appropriately, can also have an effect on circadian rhythm, but at high doses, it may provide antioxidant properties. In another study of patients with breast cancer and neuropathy, pregabalin improved both insomnia and pain better than duloxetine [105]. The key information lacking for these studies is the impact on the cancer itself. Further research is needed to elucidate the benefits of treating sleep disorders for cancer patients.

6. Clinical Approach to Sleep Issues in Patients with Cancer

The approach to sleep issues in patients with cancer should be holistic, including a review of daily routine, sleep and wake timing, sleep environment, diet, supplements, additional medical issues, recent therapies, and attitudes towards sleep. Sleep issues in cancer patients can fall into three subtypes: sleep issues independent from the cancer, sleep issues related to the cancer or cancer therapy, or sleep issues related to the stress of the diagnosis. Understanding the driver is important for the clinician to best address the sleep issue. Each of these possibilities are not exclusive, and thus deserves clinical introspection as the drivers may offer unique opportunities in approach. In many situations, treating the sleep issue as well as the underlying driver may result in better outcomes.

As many as three-fourths of patients with cancer may have a sleep-related complaint. A methodical approach should be taken when evaluating sleep disturbances in cancer patients (Table 2). Simple screening questions may aid the clinician to identify a sleep issue. The following three questions from the Patient-Reported Outcomes Measurement Information System (PROMIS) questionnaire may provide an entry route: "Are you sleepy during the day", "Do you feel refreshed during the day", and "Are you satisfied with your sleep" [106]. The backbone of the evaluation rests on the patient's history. For clinicians who are not formally trained in sleep medicine, questionnaires such as the Pittsburgh Sleep Questionnaire Index can provide general coverage of sleep issues, with subsections highlighting specific symptoms of sleep apnea, insomnia, or movement issues (Table 3) [107].

Table 3. Sleep questionnaires by category.

Questionnaire Category	Questionnaire	Questionnaire Overview
Introductory Questions	PROMIS Sleep Questions	"Are you sleepy during the day", "Do you feel refreshed during the day", and "Are you satisfied with your sleep"
General Sleep Assessments	Pittsburgh Sleep Quality Index	General questionnaire of 19 items for review of sleep issues
	Sleep Disorder Questionnaire	175-item assessment of sleep habits and disturbance
	Sleep Diary	To track sleep schedule and time
Daytime Sleepiness	Epworth Sleepiness Scale	Able to quantify subjective sleepiness over time
OSA	STOP-BANG Questionnaire	Assesses risk of underlying obstructive sleep apnea
Insomnia	Pittsburgh Sleep Quality Index	Can also be used to track sleep symptoms over time
	Insomnia Severity Index	Assesses severity and impact of insomnia on the patient
	Athens Insomnia Scale	Assesses severity of insomnia
RLS	International Restless Legs Syndrome Scale	Questionnaire to assess the impact of RLS on the patient—can be followed over time

A clinical history should detail the major characteristics relating to possible sleep disturbances, their time of onset, and their course over time in relationship to the patient's cancer. The cancer type may also play a role, as well as the therapies and treatment course. To appropriately support their patient, the clinician should ensure that they have a detailed understanding of the patient's sleep complaints, as well as the factors that may be propagating the sleep issues. Understanding the patient's daily schedule and habits on both work and non-work days necessitates tracking daily therapy routines, sleep location, and environment, habits to prepare for sleep or during middle of the night when awake, use of other substances (caffeine, alcohol, herbs, recreational drugs, etc.), and a description, if possible, from their bed partner of movements, snoring, or witnessed pauses in breathing. Clinicians should gather clues to typical work schedule, wake-up time without an alarm, mealtime, and activity times through the day to assess the timing and strength of the patient's circadian rhythm (Table 4).

Table 4. Evaluation approach for sleep complaints in patients with cancer.

Clinical Approach to Evaluating Sleep Complaints in Patients with Cancer
Sleep History
Bedtime routine and schedule (bedtime and waketime) for work and nonwork days
Sleeping environment (specifically presence of stimulating items, amount of light, noise, temperature, and bed comfort)
Disruptors of sleep
Internal—pain, nausea, reflux, breathing issues
External—light, noise, uncomfortable environment
Personal history of sleep disorders
Personal history of sleep disorder symptoms (daytime fatigue, morning headache)
Personal history of maladaptive behaviors (such as needing to perform specific stimulating routines before bed, worrying or reviewing a mental list in bed, sleeping on couch, or leaving lights or television on at night)
Beliefs about sleep or features that help or impair sleep
History from bed partner (snoring, witnessed apneas, abnormal movements)
Presence of insomnia or hypersomnia (Epworth Sleepiness Scale)
Presence of nocturnal events
Daily activities
Daily routine including meals, activities, social interaction, and sunshine exposure
Work history and job activities and environment
Intake amount and timing of alcohol, caffeine, and/or supplements
Cancer History
Treatment regimen
Therapy dosage, timing, and adverse effects
Relationship of symptoms to the treatment
Additional medical or mental health concerns
Review medication list
Current or personal history of substance use

Approximately one-fifth of workers work a rotating or night shift; thus, shift work may be an important factor for sleep deprivation and circadian rhythm. Furthermore, understanding the patient's perspective on sleep and their daily symptoms is important to assess if the patient views sleep as an important or not-so-important aspect of their health. Additionally, understanding the treatment schedule may also help, as these can also attenuate or induce brief shifts in sleep–wake times. Given the limited availability of some treatments, some patients may need to arrive at the health facility very early, earlier than their normal start of day, or stay late at night to receive their therapy, thus causing added disruption to their schedule. Tools such as a sleep diary or actigraphy can help elucidate the patients sleep–wake pattern, and provide evidence for a circadian rhythm issue.

For many patients with cancer, multiple drivers may play a role in the development and accentuation of sleep disturbances, and conversely, their importance for good sleep (Figure 3, Table 5). Thinking of the homeostatic drive, factors influencing adenosine, cytokines, or other metabolic byproducts may be either enhanced or blocked. Caffeine, which blocks the effects of adenosine, may play a significant role in insomnia and sleep disruption, leading to more daytime fatigue, and thus added caffeine use.

Table 5. Approach to good sleep.

Sleep Environment
Dark, quiet, comfortable bed and pillow; temperature (68–72 F°)
Adequate time for sleep
Dedicating 8 h for sleep
Circadian Rhythm Timing and Reinforcement
Activity, exercise, sunlight, regular meal times, social interaction during the day
Decreased light (especially blue light blocking), activity, large meals, and social interaction in evening close to bedtime
Consider a hot bath or shower in the evening
Promoting the Homeostatic Drive
Activity for brain and body, avoidance of caffeine
Encouraging Good Sleep Associations
Bedroom is only for sleep or intimacy, no television or cell phone, no exercising, working, fighting, worrying in bedroom
Possible use of worry book in a room other than bedroom
Avoidance of Disrupting Agents
Avoid caffeine, alcohol, and nicotine products
Optimizing Medication Regimen
Maximizing alerting agents in the AM
Timing sedating agents in the PM

Other factors such as the total time in bed; the timing of sleep; the possibility of something disturbing sleep(such as OSA, or periodic limb movements), or reflux; or external factors, such as an uncomfortable bed or a noisy or lighted sleep environment, should be considered. Also, mood and conditioned associations, such as worrying in bed, may contribute to poor sleep. The clinician should consider agents that may initiate these factors, as well as additional drivers that may perpetuate sleep issues (Table 5). Patients may start with insomnia as part of chemotherapy, but perpetuate this insomnia with maladaptive behaviors, such as sleeping with the television on. Some patients may require formal sleep testing, such as polysomnography, especially when considering that the patient may have a sleep-related breathing disorder, nocturnal movement disorder, or is at risk for injury from nocturnal events (Table 6).

Table 6. Indications for polysomnography,.

Polysomnography is routinely indicated for:

Evaluation for sleep apnea
Differentiating central vs. obstructive sleep apnea
Evaluation for sleep-related hypoxemia
Evaluation for hypoventilation
Evaluation for narcolepsy/primary hypersomnolence in combination with multiple sleep latency tests the next day
Positive airway pressure titration for patients requiring nocturnal respiratory support
Evaluation prior to upper airway surgery when surgery is being considered for snoring or OSA
Patients with heart failure or cardiovascular disease who have disturbed sleep, nocturnal dyspnea, snoring, or other nocturnal symptoms suggestive of sleep-related breathing disorders
Patients who have symptoms of sleep apnea or hypoventilation when symptoms persist despite appropriate medical management
Evaluation of sleep-related symptoms in patients with neuromuscular disorders
Evaluation of patients with nocturnal movements and daytime sleepiness
Subsequent sleep studies needed for follow up:
    Patients with oral appliance treatment for OSA after clinical titration
    Following appropriate healing from surgical treatment to assess residual OSA
    Re-evaluate return of symptoms in patients with SRBDs after surgical or dental treatment
    Re-evaluate PAP settings in patients with SRBD after significant changes in weight
    Re-evaluate patients who do not respond appropriately after initiation of PAP

Polysomnography should be considered for

Suspicion of sleep apnea in patients with:
    Coronary artery disease
    Previous stroke or TIA
    Tachyarrhythmias or bradyarrhythmias
Evaluation of unusual or atypical parasomnias or those with specific motor patterns
To evaluate if SRBD improved after final fitting of oral appliance

Polysomnography is an option for
Evaluation of patients with sleep-related events, suggestive of parasomnias or nocturnal epilepsy, that are potentially injurious, have forensic implications, or insufficient response to conventional therapy Patients with intractable insomnia that have failed both cognitive behavioral therapy and pharmacological therapy

Further investigations should address specific questions assessing symptoms of OSA, restless legs syndrome (RLS), insomnia, and hypersomnia (i.e., narcolepsy). Additionally, the subjective estimate of daytime sleepiness may provide further clues [108]. The Epworth Sleepiness Scale (ESS) is a reliable measure to assess subjective sleepiness, but it has not been specifically validated for cancer patients [108] (Table 3). Clinically significant daytime sleepiness is demonstrated by a score of greater than or equal to 10. Originally validated in patients with OSA, sleepiness scores from 10 to 15 are typically associated with OSA, whereas lower scores are more likely in those with insomnia or restless legs syndrome, which are typically low; thus, higher scores raise suspicion of primary hypersomnia disorders or additional causes of sleepiness.

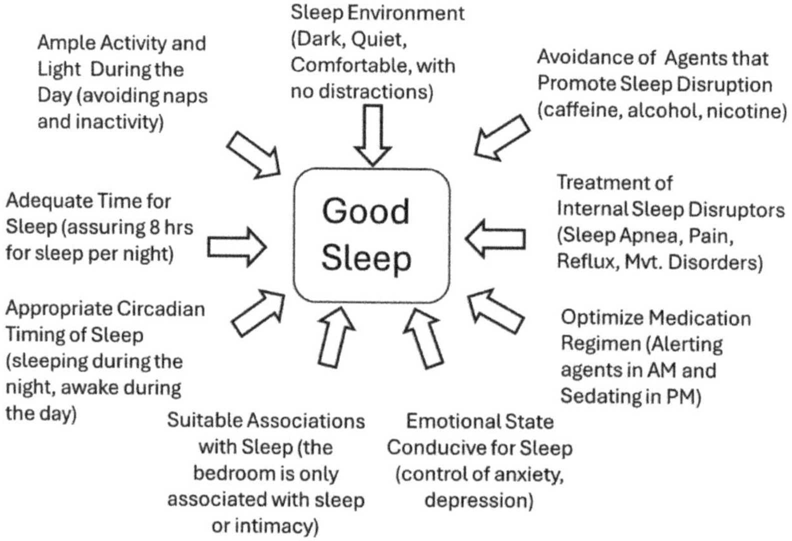

Figure 3. Many factors can influence sleep. This diagram illustrates the variety of components involved in achieving good sleep and the domains by which sleep may be disrupted.

6.1. Clinical Approach to OSA

Obstructive sleep apnea can be prevalent in patients with cancer ranging from 4 to 50%, and some outcome studies suggest that certain cancers progress in relation to the severity of the OSA [62,109]. Consequently, given the prevalence in and potential impacts of OSA on cancer patients, it is important for clinicians to screen for sleep apnea [40]. Symptoms to monitor include daytime sleepiness, snoring, or witnessed apnea events by bedpartner. To best identify patients at risk for sleep apnea, clinicians can use the STOPBANG questionnaire. The tool contains eight items, and a score of three indicates that a patient should be further evaluate for sleep apnea (Table 3) [110]. While the STOPBANG questionnaire was validated in the general population and not specifically for cancer patients, Wong et al. determined that it had a 73% sensitivity and 71% specificity in a group of 249 cancer patients [111]. In the laboratory, polysomnography is the gold standard for determining the type and severity of sleep-related breathing disorders (Table 6). Treatment plans are typically based upon these polysomnographic results and adapted to the severity and patient's acceptance of the therapy. To determine severity, the apnea hypopnea index is typically used to indicate the average number of respiratory events per hour of sleep [112]. For adults, 0–5 is considered normal, while 5–15 is mild, 15–30 is moderate, and >30 events per hour is severe. Patients without daytime symptoms and mild sleep apnea may respond to conservative therapies such as nasal steroids or decongestants, sleeping in the side position, weight loss, and avoiding alcohol and respiratory suppressants. If there is a presence of daytime symptoms or patients have moderately severe sleep apnea, there is a possible benefit to the use of oral appliances, positive airway pressure devices, or surgery. Notably, no matter the degree of sleep apnea, all severity levels may respond to positive airway pressure. Special consideration may be given to challenging issues. Those patients with mucosal ulcers due to chemotherapeutic agents, or radiation therapy or skin breakdown from radiation or surgery, may be physically limited for wearing a CPAP mask or oral appliance. Patients who have developed claustrophobia or significant anxiety may benefit from less intrusive CPAP interfaces such as nasal pillows, and patients may find less leaks from the mask using a variety of "CPAP" fitting pillows. Finding a mask that is comfortable and well-fitting is crucial to success. Nevertheless, the patient must accept and see the therapy as a necessary and key part of the overall strategy to improve their prognosis and health.

6.2. Clinical Approach to RLS

Restless legs syndrome (RLS) can be easily diagnosed by the constellation of having uncomfortable and unpleasant sensations with the urge to move their legs that is worse with rest, totally or partially relieved with movement, and primarily occurring in the evening or night. Although the overall prevalence of RLS in patients with cancer is not known, few case reports suggest RLS can be observed. Moreover, some therapies, such as dopamine antagonists used to treat nausea and aromatase inhibitors used in breast cancer, may increase the frequency of RLS [113]. RLS also may become prevalent in cancer patients as sequelae of cancer treatments, such as anemia, iron deficiency, the use of antipsychotics for sleep, and even environmental issues, such as being still for prolonged periods of time in small spaces, are risk factors for exacerbating RLS. In a small study, Yennurajalingam et al. found that 38% of patients with advanced cancer had symptoms of RLS [114]. Conversely, adjunctive therapies used to treat cancer and cancer treatment-associated pain and nausea, such as gabapentin and narcotics for pain, or pregabalin and benzodiazepines, may improve RLS symptoms [115]. RLS frequently causes sleep disruption and reduces overall total sleep time, triggering difficulty falling asleep and increasing daytime fatigue, consequently adding to the comorbidity of cancer. Gabapentinoid medications can provide significant improvement in RLS symptoms and improve sleep. These medications can be used as first-line therapies for RLS, and are an excellent option for treating RLS symptoms in patients with cancer. Focusing on alleviating the patient's symptoms of feeling an uncontrollable urge to move is key, especially when their therapy requires them to remain still for prolonged periods of time. Similarly, treatment using oral iron or iron infusion or therapy of low iron levels, ferritin levels below 75 mcg/L, or iron saturation below 30% may reduce symptoms and medication requirements [116,117].

6.3. Clinical Approach to Excessive Sleepiness

Frequently, patients with cancer complain of excessive sleepiness. This is frequently confused with fatigue, the sense of loss of energy. The distinguishing feature is the ability to fall asleep, as fatigue is the loss of energy without an increased ability to fall asleep, and sleepiness is an increased ability to sleep or doze. Common drivers of sleepiness include sleep deprivation, sleep disruption such as sleep apnea, or factors adding to the homeostatic pathway, such as adenosines or cytokines, medication effects, or circadian rhythm issues (Table 3). Some of these patients should be considered for polysomnographic evaluation, especially if there is snoring or concerns of hypoventilation (Table 6). Less commonly, if these etiologies are excluded, the clinician should consider the possibility of a primary hypersomnia issue, such as narcolepsy or idiopathic hypersomnia. These conditions require further evaluation and treatment in a sleep center. Narcolepsy is divided into type 1, associated with loss of the wake-stabilizing neurotransmitter orexin (or also defined by presence of cataplexy), and type 2, which is not associated with cataplexy. Patients with narcolepsy may have symptoms related to the dysregulation of REM sleep, including irresistible bouts of excessive daytime sleep, hypnogogic and/or hypnopompic hallucinations, or sleep paralysis. The diagnosis of narcolepsy is confirmed by an overnight monitoring of sleep of least 6 h, followed by a multiple sleep latency test (MSLT) demonstrating a mean sleep latency of less than 8 min and the presence of two of the five naps showing sleep-onset REM periods [112]. Other primary hypersomnias, such as idiopathic hypersomnia, may be possible. Idiopathic hypersomnia is defined as a continuous feeling of dogged sleepiness despite prolonged periods of sleep, similar to that described by some patients undergoing radiation or chemotherapy. Idiopathic hypersomnia is uncommon; however, it is important to consider the differences. The mainstay of therapies for primary hypersomnias is treatment with wake-promoting agents and stimulants during the day and therapies to consolidate and deepen sleep at night. Newer stimulants, such as pitolisant and solriamfetol, add to the existing list of stimulants, such as modafinil and armodafinil. Medications such as sodium oxybate and low-sodium oxybates are proving helpful to improve daytime sleepiness in both narcolepsy and idiopathic hypersomnia [118]. While a mechanistic relationship between narcolepsy, hypersomnia, and cancer is still unclear, the clinician should first address issues such as assuring enough time is dedicated to sleep, optimizing medication timing of sedating medications in the evening and alerting drugs in the morning, addressing sleep disruption from sleep apnea, reflux, pain and environmental disrupters, and optimizing the patient's circadian rhythm by including light exposure and activity during the day.

6.4. Clinical Approach to Insomnia

Insomnia may present at any time in the course of a patient's cancer. Insomnia is defined by difficulty initiating sleep or difficulty maintaining sleep with daytime consequences. In cancer patients, insomnia can be triggered by or worsened by the cancer itself; the medications used to treat the cancer; the anxiety and fear associated with a cancer diagnosis; the use of alcohol, caffeine or herbs; and a lack of activity during the day (Figure 3, Table 4). The clinician should consider the patient's comorbidities, including underlying anxiety and depression, which are frequently associated with insomnia. Insomnia may be triggered by a sudden change in the patient's life or even medication, yet insomnia commonly persists as a result of adopting a maladaptive behavior. These behaviors regularly include sleeping with the television or lights on, sleeping in a recliner chair or away from the bedroom, reading on a computer or getting involved in an engaging activity before bed, or having foods such as alcohol or coffee in the evening. A few studies have attempted to measure the effects of specific nonpharmacological approaches to insomnia. Jung et al. found that cognitive behavioral therapy for insomnia (CBT-i) was effective in cancer patients for reducing sleep complaints and decreasing dependence on hypnotics [98]. CBT-I can be directed at restructuring maladaptive beliefs and breaking these sleep-prohibitive behaviors, and may benefit these patients in other domains [119,120]. Acupuncture was also found to reduce symptoms of insomnia in cancer patients [99]. Additionally, cancer patients may turn to supplements and herbs to improve their prognosis or reduce their symptoms, although these should first be cleared by their oncologist to ensure that the herbs and supplements do not interact with their chemotherapy. In one study, melatonin at 3 mg was found to reduce insomnia symptoms, and in another study, lavender combined with footbaths appeared to provide some benefits [101,121]. The clinician may also wish to identify possible over-the-counter remedies or supplements that do not improve sleep long-term, but may interact with other aspects of the patient's cancer therapy.

Insomnia is best approached with a multi-pronged strategy. Important components of this approach include promoting the correct clues for sleep and waking, bringing an end to maladaptive behaviors, optimizing current medications, and then considering medication (Table 5). Patients should be counseled to set a regular schedule, accentuating activity and light during the day, avoiding napping and caffeine during the day, while making sure the bedroom is dark, comfortable, and quiet at night. These features promote the natural signals for sleep and wake periods. Including CBT-I will also encourage these behaviors, while working to forgo maladaptive behaviors. CBT-I does require trained personnel, and these resources can be limited. Digital CBT-I can provide an accessible effective alternative to in-person CBT-I [122]. CBT-I can be offered as an online or phone application in the form of cost-effective programs that have demonstrated benefits, especially to those patients with limited access [122–124]. While few studies exist on many of these programs, the program Somryst (formerly the SHUTi application) has demonstrated effectiveness in the published studies, and is cleared by the United States Food and Drug Administration (FDA) for digital CBT-I. Given that these patients may be on many medications, many cancer patients are willing to try behavioral therapies, yet those with severe insomnia will still request hypnotic medications [125]. Pharmacotherapy for insomnia is best when directed as a short-term therapy, and most helpful for those sleeping less than 6 h due to this group having a limited response to CBT-I [126]. Although frequently prescribed initially as short-term, many hypnotic medications become chronic in this patient population [127]. Medications such as benzodiazepine receptor agonists (zolpidem, eszopiclone), low-dose doxepin, or orexin receptor antagonists (suvorexants, lemborexants, daridorexants) are approved by the FDA for insomnia. Each provide benefits for the general population, but evidence for cancer patients is minimal [92]. These patients have successfully tapered off medication with continued sleep benefits through the use of directed CBT-I [98]. For patients who have intractable insomnia, it is important to consider additional underlying sleep disorders, such as restless leg syndrome or sleep apnea, or other underlying medical or psychiatric disorders. If these are identified, treatment of the underlying issue, in addition to addressing the insomnia, is important to best care for the patient [128].

6.5. Clinical Approach to Parasomnias

Parasomnias as a result of cancer is an area with little information. While some patients with cancer may develop nocturnal events, many of these are during treatment, and may involve periods of delirium caused by metabolic derangement, medications, or toxins, and can be confused for a parasomnia (Table 3). These nocturnal events can be difficult to differentiate from classical NREM and REM-related parasomnias, even for a highly skilled clinician. As with other sleep disturbances, a clear description of the events is the cornerstone of the evaluation. Clinical details such as time of occurrence, duration, frequency of events, behavior and clarity of speech, retained memory for the event, dream mentation, and specific characteristics observed, such as eyes open or closed, are clues to the underlying etiology. Additional features such as a family history of events, age of onset, and exacerbating factors are also helpful. If these events appear to increase the risk of injury to self or others, or the patient has additional symptoms of other sleep disorders, a video polysomnography with an extended EEG montage should be performed [129] (Table 6). Typically, parasomnias are divided into the stage of sleep from which they arise [112]. Disorders of arousal which arise from NREM and consist of sleepwalking, sleep terrors, and confusional arousals usually occur in the first third of the night, and comprise variable behaviors lasting typically minutes, for which the patient has minimal or partial memory of the event. Although there are other REM parasomnias, REM sleep behavior disorder is associated with patients acting out their dreams, which many times are violent. These events are more common in the latter half of the night, and patients and bedpartners may be seriously injured. A key feature of all these parasomnias is that the behavior described varies between events. When events do not vary and appear to have the same pattern of movements with each episode, these stereotypical events are more concerning for epileptic seizures. Epileptic seizures are classically stereotypic, demonstrating the same behavior each time, and can vary in onset and duration during the night. These events, too, require a more thorough investigation, as the seizures may be a result of metastasis to the brain.

Cancer patients can have a wide array of sleep issues arising from many factors; thus, taking a personalized approach to treatment is essential. As these cases may have multiple domains of medical issues, the same range of domains may exist driving the sleep symptoms in these, requiring a multifaceted diagnostic and therapeutic approach.

7. Future Directions

Sleep influences many physiological and molecular processes. Understanding how these processes impact the development and progression of specific cancer types could help us to better elucidate the pathophysiology of and risk factors for cancer. Further research is needed to understand these mechanisms, as well as the individual impact of each stage of sleep on these processes. These same pathways may present opportunities for therapeutic intervention both directly influencing the cancer, as well as improving the resilience and quality of life of patients with cancer.

8. Conclusions

In summary, the relationship between sleep and cancer is complex and confounded by many variables. Additional research is needed to delineate the mechanisms by which various sleep issues impact the mechanisms that underpin cancer risk and development. While the impact of sleep on various cancer types is still not well defined, it is important for clinicians to evaluate for and treat sleep disturbances in cancer patients, as this may improve overall health, quality of life, and possibly improve the individual's cancer outcomes.

Author Contributions: Conceptualization, C.M.V. and B.V.V.; data curation, C.M.V. and B.V.V.; writing—original draft preparation, C.M.V.; writing—review and editing, B.V.V. All authors have read and agreed to the published version of the manuscript.

Funding: This research received no external funding.

Institutional Review Board Statement: Not applicable.

Informed Consent Statement: Not applicable.

Data Availability Statement: No new data were created for this publication.

Conflicts of Interest: The authors declare no conflicts of interest.

Abbreviations

The following abbreviations are used in this manuscript:

DNA	Deoxyribonucleic acid
CBT-I	Cognitive behavioral therapy for insomnia
CPAP	Continuous positive airway pressure
FDA	United States Food and Drug Administration
NREM	Non-rapid eye movement sleep
OSA	Obstructive sleep apnea
PROMIS	Patient-Reported Outcomes Measurement Information System
REM	Rapid eye movement sleep
RLS	Restless legs syndrome
RNA	Ribonucleic acid
STOPBANG	Snore, tired, observed apnea, pressure (hypertension), body mass index, age, neck, gender

References

1. Tononi, G.; Boly, M.; Cirelli, C. Consciousness and sleep. *Neuron* **2024**, *112*, 1568–1594. [CrossRef] [PubMed]
2. Borbély, A. The two-process model of sleep regulation: Beginnings and outlook. *J. Sleep Res.* **2022**, *31*, e13598. [CrossRef] [PubMed]
3. Feinberg, I.; Floyd, T.C. Systematic trends across the night in human sleep cycles. *Psychophysiology* **1979**, *16*, 283–291. [CrossRef]
4. Frank, M.G.; Heller, H.C. The Function(s) of Sleep. *Handb. Exp. Pharmacol.* **2019**, *253*, 3–34. [CrossRef] [PubMed]
5. Global Cancer Burden Growing, Amidst Mounting Need for Services. Available online: https://www.who.int/news/item/01-02-2024-global-cancer-burden-growing--amidst-mounting-need-for-services (accessed on 15 December 2024).
6. Cancer Facts & Figures. Available online: https://www.cancer.org/research/cancer-facts-statistics/all-cancer-facts-figures/2024-cancer-facts-figures.html (accessed on 15 December 2024).
7. Pariollaud, M.; Lamia, K.A. Cancer in the Fourth Dimension: What Is the Impact of Circadian Disruption? *Cancer Discov.* **2020**, *10*, 1455–1464. [CrossRef]
8. Sancar, A.; Van Gelder, R.N. Clocks, cancer, and chronochemotherapy. *Science* **2021**, *371*, eabb0738. [CrossRef]
9. Richmond, R.C.; Anderson, E.L.; Dashti, H.S.; Jones, S.E.; Lane, J.M.; Strand, L.B.; Brumpton, B.; Rutter, M.K.; Wood, A.R.; Straif, K.; et al. Investigating causal relations between sleep traits and risk of breast cancer in women: Mendelian randomisation study. *BMJ* **2019**, *365*, l2327. [CrossRef] [PubMed]
10. Zhang, X.; Giovannucci, E.L.; Wu, K.; Gao, X.; Hu, F.; Ogino, S.; Schernhammer, E.S.; Fuchs, C.S.; Redline, S.; Willett, W.C.; et al. Associations of self-reported sleep duration and snoring with colorectal cancer risk in men and women. *Sleep* **2013**, *36*, 681–688. [CrossRef]
11. Royse, K.E.; El-Serag, H.B.; Chen, L.; White, D.L.; Hale, L.; Sangi-Haghpeykar, H.; Jiao, L. Sleep Duration and Risk of Liver Cancer in Postmenopausal Women: The Women's Health Initiative Study. *J. Womens Health* **2017**, *26*, 1270–1277. [CrossRef]
12. Wong, J.Y.; Bassig, B.A.; Vermeulen, R.; Hu, W.; Ning, B.; Seow, W.J.; Ji, B.T.; Downward, G.S.; Katki, H.A.; Barone-Adesi, F.; et al. Sleep Duration across the Adult Lifecourse and Risk of Lung Cancer Mortality: A Cohort Study in Xuanwei, China. *Cancer Prev. Res.* **2017**, *10*, 327–336. [CrossRef]
13. Verkasalo, P.K.; Lillberg, K.; Stevens, R.G.; Hublin, C.; Partinen, M.; Koskenvuo, M.; Kaprio, J. Sleep duration and breast cancer: A prospective cohort study. *Cancer Res.* **2005**, *65*, 9595–9600. [CrossRef] [PubMed]
14. Kakizaki, M.; Kuriyama, S.; Sone, T.; Ohmori-Matsuda, K.; Hozawa, A.; Nakaya, N.; Fukudo, S.; Tsuji, I. Sleep duration and the risk of breast cancer: The Ohsaki Cohort Study. *Br. J. Cancer* **2008**, *99*, 1502–1505. [CrossRef] [PubMed]
15. Pinheiro, S.P.; Schernhammer, E.S.; Tworoger, S.S.; Michels, K.B. A prospective study on habitual duration of sleep and incidence of breast cancer in a large cohort of women. *Cancer Res.* **2006**, *66*, 5521–5525. [CrossRef] [PubMed]
16. McElroy, J.A.; Newcomb, P.A.; Titus-Ernstoff, L.; Trentham-Dietz, A.; Hampton, J.M.; Egan, K.M. Duration of sleep and breast cancer risk in a large population-based case-control study. *J. Sleep Res.* **2006**, *15*, 241–249. [CrossRef]
17. Zhou, T.; Wang, Z.; Qiao, C.; Wang, S.; Hu, S.; Wang, X.; Ma, X.; Wang, D.; Li, J.; Li, Z.; et al. Sleep disturbances and the risk of lung cancer: A meta-epidemiological study. *BMC Cancer* **2023**, *23*, 884. [CrossRef]
18. Thompson, C.L.; Larkin, E.K.; Patel, S.; Berger, N.A.; Redline, S.; Li, L. Short duration of sleep increases risk of colorectal adenoma. *Cancer* **2011**, *117*, 841–847. [CrossRef]
19. Gapstur, S.M.; Diver, W.R.; Stevens, V.L.; Carter, B.D.; Teras, L.R.; Jacobs, E.J. Work schedule, sleep duration, insomnia, and risk of fatal prostate cancer. *Am. J. Prev. Med.* **2014**, *46*, S26–S33. [CrossRef]
20. Sigurdardottir, L.G.; Valdimarsdottir, U.A.; Mucci, L.A.; Fall, K.; Rider, J.R.; Schernhammer, E.; Czeisler, C.A.; Launer, L.; Harris, T.; Stampfer, M.J.; et al. Sleep disruption among older men and risk of prostate cancer. *Cancer Epidemiol. Biomark. Prev.* **2013**, *22*, 872–879. [CrossRef]
21. Lu, Y.; Tian, N.; Yin, J.; Shi, Y.; Huang, Z. Association between sleep duration and cancer risk: A meta-analysis of prospective cohort studies. *PLoS ONE* **2013**, *8*, e74723. [CrossRef]
22. Titova, O.E.; Michaelsson, K.; Vithayathil, M.; Mason, A.M.; Kar, S.; Burgess, S.; Larsson, S.C. Sleep duration and risk of overall and 22 site-specific cancers: A Mendelian randomization study. *Int. J. Cancer* **2021**, *148*, 914–920. [CrossRef]
23. Lanza, G.; Mogavero, M.P.; Salemi, M.; Ferri, R. The Triad of Sleep, Immunity, and Cancer: A Mediating Perspective. *Cells* **2024**, *13*, 1246. [CrossRef] [PubMed]
24. Zielinski, M.R.; Davis, J.M.; Fadel, J.R.; Youngstedt, S.D. Influence of chronic moderate sleep restriction and exercise on inflammation and carcinogenesis in mice. *Brain Behav. Immun.* **2012**, *26*, 672–679. [CrossRef]
25. Sen, A.; Opdahl, S.; Strand, L.B.; Vatten, L.J.; Laugsand, L.E.; Janszky, I. Insomnia and the Risk of Breast Cancer: The HUNT Study. *Psychosom. Med.* **2017**, *79*, 461–468. [CrossRef]
26. Shi, T.; Min, M.; Sun, C.; Zhang, Y.; Liang, M.; Sun, Y. Does insomnia predict a high risk of cancer? A systematic review and meta-analysis of cohort studies. *J. Sleep Res.* **2020**, *29*, e12876. [CrossRef]
27. Chiu, H.Y.; Huang, C.J.; Fan, Y.C.; Tsai, P.S. Insomnia but Not Hypnotics Use Associates with the Risk of Breast Cancer: A Population-Based Matched Cohort Study. *J. Womens Health* **2018**, *27*, 1250–1256. [CrossRef] [PubMed]

28. Fang, Y.Y.; Hung, C.T.; Chan, J.C.; Huang, S.M.; Lee, Y.H. Meta-analysis: Exercise intervention for sleep problems in cancer patients. *Eur. J. Cancer Care* **2019**, *28*, e13131. [CrossRef]
29. Yap, D.W.T.; Tan, N.K.W.; Tan, B.K.J.; Teo, Y.H.; Tan, V.K.M.; See, A.; Toh, S.T. The Association of Obstructive Sleep Apnea with Breast Cancer Incidence and Mortality: A Systematic Review and Meta-analysis. *J. Breast Cancer* **2022**, *25*, 149–163. [CrossRef] [PubMed]
30. Fang, H.F.; Miao, N.F.; Chen, C.D.; Sithole, T.; Chung, M.H. Risk of Cancer in Patients with Insomnia, Parasomnia, and Obstructive Sleep Apnea: A Nationwide Nested Case-Control Study. *J. Cancer* **2015**, *6*, 1140–1147. [CrossRef]
31. Gozal, D.; Ham, S.A.; Mokhlesi, B. Sleep Apnea and Cancer: Analysis of a Nationwide Population Sample. *Sleep* **2016**, *39*, 1493–1500. [CrossRef]
32. Sillah, A.; Watson, N.F.; Schwartz, S.M.; Gozal, D.; Phipps, A.I. Sleep apnea and subsequent cancer incidence. *Cancer Causes Control* **2018**, *29*, 987–994. [CrossRef]
33. Lee, S.; Kim, B.G.; Kim, J.W.; Lee, K.L.; Koo, D.L.; Nam, H.; Im, J.P.; Kim, J.S.; Koh, S.J. Obstructive sleep apnea is associated with an increased risk of colorectal neoplasia. *Gastrointest. Endosc.* **2017**, *85*, 568–573.e1. [CrossRef]
34. Tseng, C.M.; Chen, Y.T.; Tao, C.W.; Ou, S.M.; Hsiao, Y.H.; Li, S.Y.; Chen, T.J.; Perng, D.W.; Chou, K.T. Adult narcoleptic patients have increased risk of cancer: A nationwide population-based study. *Cancer Epidemiol.* **2015**, *39*, 793–797. [CrossRef] [PubMed]
35. Vogtmann, E.; Levitan, E.B.; Hale, L.; Shikany, J.M.; Shah, N.A.; Endeshaw, Y.; Lewis, C.E.; Manson, J.E.; Chlebowski, R.T. Association between sleep and breast cancer incidence among postmenopausal women in the Women's Health Initiative. *Sleep* **2013**, *36*, 1437–1444. [CrossRef] [PubMed]
36. Xia, L.; Chen, G.H.; Li, Z.H.; Jiang, S.; Shen, J. Alterations in hypothalamus-pituitary-adrenal/thyroid axes and gonadotropin-releasing hormone in the patients with primary insomnia: A clinical research. *PLoS ONE* **2013**, *8*, e71065. [CrossRef]
37. Veler, H. Sleep and Inflammation: Bidirectional Relationship. *Sleep Med. Clin.* **2023**, *18*, 213–218. [CrossRef] [PubMed]
38. Marriott, R.J.; Singh, B.; McArdle, N.; Darcey, E.; King, S.; Bond-Smith, D.; Reynor, A.; Noffsinger, W.; Ward, K.; Mukherjee, S.; et al. Does OSA Increase Risk for Cancer?: A Large Historical Sleep Clinic Cohort Study. *Chest* **2023**, *164*, 1042–1056. [CrossRef]
39. Prabhakar, N.R.; Peng, Y.J.; Nanduri, J. Hypoxia-inducible factors and obstructive sleep apnea. *J. Clin. Invest.* **2020**, *130*, 5042–5051. [CrossRef]
40. Marrone, O.; Bonsignore, M.R. Obstructive sleep apnea and cancer: A complex relationship. *Curr. Opin. Pulm. Med.* **2020**, *26*, 657–667. [CrossRef]
41. Jordan, W.; Cohrs, S.; Degner, D.; Meier, A.; Rodenbeck, A.; Mayer, G.; Pilz, J.; Rüther, E.; Kornhuber, J.; Bleich, S. Evaluation of oxidative stress measurements in obstructive sleep apnea syndrome. *J. Neural. Transm.* **2006**, *113*, 239–254. [CrossRef]
42. Gozal, D.; Almendros, I.; Phipps, A.I.; Campos-Rodriguez, F.; Martinez-Garcia, M.A.; Farre, R. Sleep Apnoea Adverse Effects on Cancer: True, False, or Too Many Confounders? *Int. J. Mol. Sci.* **2020**, *21*, 8779. [CrossRef]
43. Couvineau, A.; Dayot, S.; Nicole, P.; Gratio, V.; Rebours, V.; Couvelard, A.; Voisin, T. The Anti-tumoral Properties of Orexin/Hypocretin Hypothalamic Neuropeptides: An Unexpected Therapeutic Role. *Front. Endocrinol.* **2018**, *9*, 573. [CrossRef] [PubMed]
44. Graybill, N.L.; Weissig, V. A review of orexin's unprecedented potential as a novel, highly-specific treatment for various localized and metastatic cancers. *SAGE Open Med.* **2017**, *5*, 2050312117735774. [CrossRef]
45. Dayot, S.; Speisky, D.; Couvelard, A.; Bourgoin, P.; Gratio, V.; Cros, J.; Rebours, V.; Sauvanet, A.; Bedossa, P.; Paradis, V.; et al. In vitro, in vivo and ex vivo demonstration of the antitumoral role of hypocretin-1/orexin-A and almorexant in pancreatic ductal adenocarcinoma. *Oncotarget* **2018**, *9*, 6952–6967. [CrossRef] [PubMed]
46. Roscoe, J.A.; Kaufman, M.E.; Matteson-Rusby, S.E.; Palesh, O.G.; Ryan, J.L.; Kohli, S.; Perlis, M.L.; Morrow, G.R. Cancer-related fatigue and sleep disorders. *Oncologist* **2007**, *12* (Suppl. S1), 35–42. [CrossRef] [PubMed]
47. Davidson, J.R.; MacLean, A.W.; Brundage, M.D.; Schulze, K. Sleep disturbance in cancer patients. *Soc. Sci. Med.* **2002**, *54*, 1309–1321. [CrossRef]
48. Otte, J.L.; Carpenter, J.S.; Manchanda, S.; Rand, K.L.; Skaar, T.C.; Weaver, M.; Chernyak, Y.; Zhong, X.; Igega, C.; Landis, C. Systematic review of sleep disorders in cancer patients: Can the prevalence of sleep disorders be ascertained? *Cancer Med.* **2015**, *4*, 183–200. [CrossRef]
49. Al Maqbali, M.; Al Sinani, M.; Alsayed, A.; Gleason, A.M. Prevalence of Sleep Disturbance in Patients with Cancer: A Systematic Review and Meta-Analysis. *Clin. Nurs. Res.* **2022**, *31*, 1107–1123. [CrossRef]
50. Chen, M.Y.; Zheng, W.Y.; Liu, Y.F.; Li, X.H.; Lam, M.I.; Su, Z.; Cheung, T.; Ungvari, G.S.; Tang, L.; Ng, C.H.; et al. Global prevalence of poor sleep quality in cancer patients: A systematic review and meta-analysis. *Gen. Hosp. Psychiatry* **2024**, *87*, 92–102. [CrossRef]
51. Berger, A.M.; Parker, K.P.; Young-McCaughan, S.; Mallory, G.A.; Barsevick, A.M.; Beck, S.L.; Carpenter, J.S.; Carter, P.A.; Farr, L.A.; Hinds, P.S.; et al. Sleep wake disturbances in people with cancer and their caregivers: State of the science. *Oncol. Nurs. Forum* **2005**, *32*, E98–E126. [CrossRef]
52. Kaleyias, J.; Manley, P.; Kothare, S.V. Sleep disorders in children with cancer. *Semin. Pediatr. Neurol.* **2012**, *19*, 25–34. [CrossRef]

53. Mogavero, M.P.; DelRosso, L.M.; Fanfulla, F.; Bruni, O.; Ferri, R. Sleep disorders and cancer: State of the art and future perspectives. *Sleep Med. Rev.* **2020**, *56*, 101409. [CrossRef] [PubMed]
54. Dean, G.E.; Abu Sabbah, E.; Yingrengreung, S.; Ziegler, P.; Chen, H.; Steinbrenner, L.M.; Dickerson, S.S. Sleeping with the enemy: Sleep and quality of life in patients with lung cancer. *Cancer Nurs.* **2015**, *38*, 60–70. [CrossRef] [PubMed]
55. Ancoli-Israel, S.; Liu, L.; Rissling, M.; Natarajan, L.; Neikrug, A.B.; Palmer, B.W.; Mills, P.J.; Parker, B.A.; Sadler, G.R.; Maglione, J. Sleep, fatigue, depression, and circadian activity rhythms in women with breast cancer before and after treatment: A 1-year longitudinal study. *Support. Care Cancer* **2014**, *22*, 2535–2545. [CrossRef] [PubMed]
56. Jung, D.; Lee, K.M.; Kim, W.H.; Lee, J.Y.; Kim, T.Y.; Im, S.A.; Lee, K.H.; Spiegel, D.; Hahm, B.J. Longitudinal Association of Poor Sleep Quality with Chemotherapy-Induced Nausea and Vomiting in Patients with Breast Cancer. *Psychosom. Med.* **2016**, *78*, 959–965. [CrossRef]
57. Zhou, J.; Jolly, S. Obstructive sleep apnea and fatigue in head and neck cancer patients. *Am. J. Clin. Oncol.* **2015**, *38*, 411–414. [CrossRef]
58. Page, J.M.; Morgans, A.K.; Hassett, M.J.; Haakenstad, E.; Manni, M.; McCleary, N.J.; Zhou, E.S. Insomnia Prevalence and Correlates in Cancer Patients Undergoing Treatment. *Psychooncology* **2025**, *34*, e70079. [CrossRef]
59. Palesh, O.; Aldridge-Gerry, A.; Zeitzer, J.M.; Koopman, C.; Neri, E.; Giese-Davis, J.; Jo, B.; Kraemer, H.; Nouriani, B.; Spiegel, D. Actigraphy-measured sleep disruption as a predictor of survival among women with advanced breast cancer. *Sleep* **2014**, *37*, 837–842. [CrossRef]
60. Gottfried, T.; Kamer, I.; Salant, I.; Urban, D.; Lawrence, Y.R.; Onn, A.; Bar, J. Self-reported sleep quality as prognostic for survival in lung cancer patients. *Cancer Manag. Res.* **2020**, *12*, 313–321. [CrossRef]
61. Nieto, F.J.; Peppard, P.E.; Young, T.; Finn, L.; Hla, K.M.; Farré, R. Sleep-disordered breathing and cancer mortality: Results from the Wisconsin Sleep Cohort Study. *Am. J. Respir. Crit. Care Med.* **2012**, *186*, 190–194. [CrossRef]
62. Huang, H.Y.; Lin, S.W.; Chuang, L.P.; Wang, C.L.; Sun, M.H.; Li, H.Y.; Chang, C.J.; Chang, S.C.; Yang, C.T.; Chen, N.H. Severe OSA associated with higher risk of mortality in stage III and IV lung cancer. *J. Clin. Sleep Med.* **2020**, *16*, 1091–1098. [CrossRef]
63. Sillah, A.; Faria, F.; Watson, N.F.; Gozal, D.; Phipps, A.I. Five-year relative survival in sleep apnea patients with a subsequent cancer diagnosis. *J. Clin. Sleep Med.* **2020**, *16*, 667–673. [CrossRef] [PubMed]
64. Kabat, G.C.; Xue, X.; Kamensky, V.; Zaslavsky, O.; Stone, K.L.; Johnson, K.C.; Wassertheil-Smoller, S.; Shadyab, A.H.; Luo, J.; Hale, L.; et al. The association of sleep duration and quality with all-cause and cause-specific mortality in the Women's Health Initiative. *Sleep Med.* **2018**, *50*, 48–54. [CrossRef] [PubMed]
65. Martinez-Garcia, M.A.; Campos-Rodriguez, F.; Almendros, I.; Garcia-Rio, F.; Sanchez-de-la-Torre, M.; Farre, R.; Gozal, D. Cancer and Sleep Apnea: Cutaneous Melanoma as a Case Study. *Am. J. Respir. Crit. Care Med.* **2019**, *200*, 1345–1353. [CrossRef]
66. Martínez-García, M.; Martorell-Calatayud, A.; Nagore, E.; Valero, I.; Selma, M.J.; Chiner, E.; Landete, P.; Montserrat, J.M.; Carrera, C.; Pérez-Gil, A.; et al. Association between sleep disordered breathing and aggressiveness markers of malignant cutaneous melanoma. *Eur. Respir. J.* **2014**, *43*, 1661–1668. [CrossRef]
67. Martinez-Garcia, M.A.; Campos-Rodriguez, F.; Nagore, E.; Martorell, A.; Rodriguez-Peralto, J.L.; Riveiro-Falkenbach, E.; Hernandez, L.; Bañuls, J.; Arias, E.; Ortiz, P.; et al. Sleep-Disordered Breathing Is Independently Associated with Increased Aggressiveness of Cutaneous Melanoma: A Multicenter Observational Study in 443 Patients. *Chest* **2018**, *154*, 1348–1358. [CrossRef]
68. Campos-Rodriguez, F.; Cruz-Medina, A.; Selma, M.J.; Rodriguez-de-la-Borbolla-Artacho, M.; Sanchez-Vega, A.; Ripoll-Orts, F.; Almeida-Gonzalez, C.V.; Martinez-Garcia, M.A. Association between sleep-disordered breathing and breast cancer aggressiveness. *PLoS ONE* **2018**, *13*, e0207591. [CrossRef]
69. Wang, H.; Reid, B.M.; Richmond, R.C.; Lane, J.M.; Saxena, R.; Gonzalez, B.D.; Fridley, B.L.; Redline, S.; Tworoger, S.S.; Wang, X. Impact of insomnia on ovarian cancer risk and survival: A Mendelian randomization study. *EBioMedicine* **2024**, *104*, 105175. [CrossRef] [PubMed]
70. Strøm, L.; Danielsen, J.T.; Amidi, A.; Cardenas Egusquiza, A.L.; Wu, L.M.; Zachariae, R. Sleep During Oncological Treatment—A Systematic Review and Meta-Analysis of Associations with Treatment Response, Time to Progression and Survival. *Front. Neurosci.* **2022**, *16*, 817837. [CrossRef]
71. Hakim, F.; Wang, Y.; Zhang, S.X.; Zheng, J.; Yolcu, E.S.; Carreras, A.; Khalyfa, A.; Shirwan, H.; Almendros, I.; Gozal, D. Fragmented sleep accelerates tumor growth and progression through recruitment of tumor-associated macrophages and TLR4 signaling. *Cancer Res.* **2014**, *74*, 1329–1337. [CrossRef]
72. Tong, H.H.; Li, J.R.; Feng, Y.; Li, S.W.; Qiu, H.; Hong, J.F. The Association Between Sleep Disturbance and Proinflammatory Markers in Patients with Cancer: A Meta-analysis. *Cancer Nurs.* **2023**, *46*, E91–E98. [CrossRef]
73. Kwekkeboom, K.L.; Tostrud, L.; Costanzo, E.; Coe, C.L.; Serlin, R.C.; Ward, S.E.; Zhang, Y. The Role of Inflammation in the Pain, Fatigue, and Sleep Disturbance Symptom Cluster in Advanced Cancer. *J. Pain Symptom Manag.* **2018**, *55*, 1286–1295. [CrossRef] [PubMed]

74. Greten, F.R.; Grivennikov, S.I. Inflammation and Cancer: Triggers, Mechanisms, and Consequences. *Immunity* **2019**, *51*, 27–41. [CrossRef] [PubMed]
75. Parker, K.P.; Bliwise, D.L.; Ribeiro, M.; Jain, S.R.; Vena, C.I.; Kohles-Baker, M.K.; Rogatko, A.; Xu, Z.; Harris, W.B. Sleep/Wake patterns of individuals with advanced cancer measured by ambulatory polysomnography. *J. Clin. Oncol.* **2008**, *26*, 2464–2472. [CrossRef] [PubMed]
76. Reinsel, R.A.; Starr, T.D.; O'Sullivan, B.; Passik, S.D.; Kavey, N.B. Polysomnographic Study of Sleep in Survivors of Breast Cancer. *J. Clin. Sleep Med.* **2015**, *11*, 1361–1370. [CrossRef]
77. Shi, W.; Misra, S.; Li, M.; Su, J.; Chong, L.P.; McCuske, M.; Williams, J.; Xu, W.; Ghoraie, L.S.; Sutherland, D.R.; et al. Inflammatory Biomarkers, Hematopoietic Stem Cells, and Symptoms in Breast Cancer Patients Undergoing Adjuvant Radiation Therapy. *JNCI Cancer Spectr.* **2020**, *4*, pkaa037. [CrossRef]
78. Wolf, I.; Sadetzki, S.; Kanety, H.; Kundel, Y.; Pariente, C.; Epstein, N.; Oberman, B.; Catane, R.; Kaufman, B.; Shimon, I. Adiponectin, ghrelin, and leptin in cancer cachexia in breast and colon cancer patients. *Cancer* **2006**, *106*, 966–973. [CrossRef]
79. Mandrell, B.N.; LaRosa, K.; Hancock, D.; Caples, M.; Sykes, A.; Lu, Z.; Wise, M.S.; Khan, R.B.; Merchant, T.E.; McLaughlin-Crabtree, V. Predictors of narcolepsy and hypersomnia due to medical disorder in pediatric craniopharyngioma. *J. Neurooncol.* **2020**, *148*, 307–316. [CrossRef]
80. El Kherchi, O.; Aquil, A.; El Khoudri, N.; Mouallif, M.; Daghi, M.; Guerroumi, M.; Saad, E.M.; Benider, A.; Jayakumar, A.R.; Elgot, A. Anxiety and Depression Comorbidities in Moroccan Patients with Breast Cancer. *Front. Psychiatry* **2020**, *11*, 584907. [CrossRef]
81. Tag Eldin, E.S.; Younis, S.G.; Aziz, L.; Eldin, A.T.; Erfan, S.T. Evaluation of sleep pattern disorders in breast cancer patients receiving adjuvant treatment (chemotherapy and/or radiotherapy) using polysomnography. *J. BUON* **2019**, *24*, 529–534.
82. Pound, C.M.; Clark, C.; Ni, A.; Athale, U.; Lewis, V.; Halton, J.M. Corticosteroids, behavior, and quality of life in children treated for acute lymphoblastic leukemia; a multicentered trial. *J. Pediatr. Hematol. Oncol.* **2012**, *34*, 517–523. [CrossRef]
83. Kiss, I.; Kuhn, M.; Hrusak, K.; Buchler, B.; Boublikova, L.; Buchler, T. Insomnia in patients treated with checkpoint inhibitors for cancer: A meta-analysis. *Front. Oncol.* **2022**, *12*, 946307. [CrossRef]
84. Balachandran, D.D.; Bashoura, L.; Sheshadri, A.; Manzullo, E.; Faiz, S.A. The Impact of Immunotherapy on Sleep and Circadian Rhythms in Patients with Cancer. *Front. Oncol.* **2023**, *13*, 1295267. [CrossRef] [PubMed]
85. Zarogoulidis, P.; Petridis, D.; Kosmidis, C.; Sapalidis, K.; Nena, L.; Matthaios, D.; Papadopoulos, V.; Perdikouri, E.I.; Porpodis, K.; Kakavelas, P.; et al. Non-Small-Cell Lung Cancer Immunotherapy and Sleep Characteristics: The Crossroad for Optimal Survival. *Diseases* **2023**, *11*, 26. [CrossRef]
86. Hajjar, J.; Mendoza, T.; Zhang, L.; Fu, S.; Piha-Paul, S.A.; Hong, D.S.; Janku, F.; Karp, D.D.; Ballhausen, A.; Gong, J.; et al. Associations between the gut microbiome and fatigue in cancer patients. *Sci. Rep.* **2021**, *11*, 5847. [CrossRef] [PubMed]
87. Ganjaei, K.G.; Wong, K.A.; Strauss, S.M.; Carlsson, S.V.; Barton-Burke, M.; Tan, M. Treatment of obstructive sleep apnea with CPAP improves daytime sleepiness and fatigue in cancer patients. *Cancer Med.* **2024**, *13*, e7198. [CrossRef]
88. Nissen, E.R.; Neumann, H.; Knutzen, S.M.; Henriksen, E.N.; Amidi, A.; Johansen, C.; von Heymann, A.; Christiansen, P.; Zachariae, R. Interventions for insomnia in cancer patients and survivors—A comprehensive systematic review and meta-analysis. *JNCI Cancer Spectr.* **2024**, *8*, pkae041. [CrossRef]
89. Grassi, L.; Zachariae, R.; Caruso, R.; Palagini, L.; Campos-Ródenas, R.; Riba, M.B.; Lloyd-Williams, M.; Kissane, D.; Rodin, G.; McFarland, D.; et al. Insomnia in adult patients with cancer: ESMO Clinical Practice Guideline. *ESMO Open* **2023**, *8*, 102047. [CrossRef] [PubMed]
90. Gharib, S.A.; Seiger, A.N.; Hayes, A.L.; Mehra, R.; Patel, S.R. Treatment of obstructive sleep apnea alters cancer-associated transcriptional signatures in circulating leukocytes. *Sleep* **2014**, *37*, 709–714. [CrossRef]
91. Perrini, S.; Cignarelli, A.; Quaranta, V.N.; Falcone, V.A.; Kounaki, S.; Porro, S.; Ciavarella, A.; Ficarella, R.; Barbaro, M.; Genchi, V.A.; et al. Correction of intermittent hypoxia reduces inflammation in obese subjects with obstructive sleep apnea. *JCI Insight* **2017**, *2*, e94379. [CrossRef]
92. Saeki, Y.; Sumi, Y.; Ozaki, Y.; Hosonaga, M.; Kenmotsu, Y.; Onoe, T.; Yamaguchi, K.; Matsumoto, Y. Proposal for Managing Cancer-Related Insomnia: A Systematic Literature Review of Associated Factors and a Narrative Review of Treatment. *Cancer Med.* **2024**, *13*, e70365. [CrossRef]
93. Woodward, S.C. Cognitive-behavioral therapy for insomnia in patients with cancer. *Clin. J. Oncol. Nurs.* **2011**, *15*, E42–E52. [CrossRef] [PubMed]
94. Arico, D.; Raggi, A.; Ferri, R. Cognitive Behavioral Therapy for Insomnia in Breast Cancer Survivors: A Review of the Literature. *Front. Psychol.* **2016**, *7*, 1162. [CrossRef]
95. Irwin, M.R. Innovation in the Treatment of Insomnia in Breast Cancer Survivors. *J. Natl. Cancer Inst.* **2018**, *110*, 799–800. [CrossRef]
96. Peoples, A.R.; Garland, S.N.; Perlis, M.L.; Savard, J.; Heckler, C.E.; Kamen, C.S.; Ryan, J.L.; Mustian, K.M.; Janelsins, M.C.; Peppone, L.J.; et al. Effects of cognitive behavioral therapy for insomnia and armodafinil on quality of life in cancer survivors: A randomized placebo-controlled trial. *J. Cancer Surviv.* **2017**, *11*, 401–409. [CrossRef] [PubMed]

97. Papadopoulos, D.; Papadoudis, A.; Kiagia, M.; Syrigos, K. Nonpharmacologic Interventions for Improving Sleep Disturbances in Patients with Lung Cancer: A Systematic Review and Meta-analysis. *J. Pain Symptom Manag.* **2018**, *55*, 1364–1381.e5. [CrossRef] [PubMed]
98. Jung, H.J.; Yu, E.S.; Kim, J.H. Combined Program of Cognitive-Behavioral Therapy for Insomnia and Medication Tapering in Cancer Patients: A Clinic-Based Pilot Study. *Behav. Sleep Med.* **2020**, *18*, 386–395. [CrossRef]
99. Zhang, J.; Zhang, Z.; Huang, S.; Qiu, X.; Lao, L.; Huang, Y.; Zhang, Z.J. Acupuncture for cancer-related insomnia: A systematic review and meta-analysis. *Phytomedicine* **2022**, *102*, 154160. [CrossRef]
100. Wang, Y.; Yang, L.; Lin, G.; Huang, B.; Sheng, X.; Wang, L.; Chen, L.; Qiu, X.; Wu, X.; Lin, R. The efficacy of progressive muscle relaxation training on cancer-related fatigue and quality of life in patients with cancer: A systematic review and meta-analysis of randomized controlled studies. *Int. J. Nurs. Stud.* **2024**, *152*, 104694. [CrossRef]
101. Mendis, R.; Wong, A.; Frenkel, S.; Southcott, A.M.; Selman, C.J.; Martin, J.; Grobler, A.; Currow, D.; Agar, M.; Le, B.; et al. Temazepam or Melatonin Versus Placebo for the Treatment of Insomnia in Advanced Cancer: A Three-Arm, Double-Blind, Phase III, Multicenter, Randomized Clinical Trial. *J. Palliat. Med.* **2024**, *27*, 1368–1373. [CrossRef]
102. Tanimukai, H.; Murai, T.; Okazaki, N.; Matsuda, Y.; Okamoto, Y.; Kabeshita, Y.; Ohno, Y.; Tsuneto, S. An observational study of insomnia and nightmare treated with trazodone in patients with advanced cancer. *Am. J. Hosp. Palliat. Care* **2013**, *30*, 359–362. [CrossRef]
103. Yi, X.Y.; Ni, S.F.; Ghadami, M.R.; Meng, H.Q.; Chen, M.Y.; Kuang, L.; Zhang, Y.Q.; Zhang, L.; Zhou, X.Y. Trazodone for the treatment of insomnia: A meta-analysis of randomized placebo-controlled trials. *Sleep Med.* **2018**, *45*, 25–32. [CrossRef]
104. Kurdi, M.S.; As, A.; Ladhad, D.A.; Mitragotri, M.V.; Baiju, A. Comparison Between Efficacy of Oral Melatonin and Oral L-theanine in Improving Sleep in Cancer Patients Suffering From Insomnia: A Randomised Double-blinded Placebo-controlled Study. *Indian. J. Palliat. Care* **2024**, *30*, 176–181. [CrossRef]
105. Avan, R.; Janbabaei, G.; Hendouei, N.; Alipour, A.; Borhani, S.; Tabrizi, N.; Salehifar, E. The effect of pregabalin and duloxetine treatment on quality of life of breast cancer patients with taxane-induced sensory neuropathy: A randomized clinical trial. *J. Res. Med. Sci.* **2018**, *23*, 52. [CrossRef] [PubMed]
106. Buysse, D.J.; Yu, L.; Moul, D.E.; Germain, A.; Stover, A.; Dodds, N.E.; Johnston, K.L.; Shablesky-Cade, M.A.; Pilkonis, P.A. Development and validation of patient-reported outcome measures for sleep disturbance and sleep-related impairments. *Sleep* **2010**, *33*, 781–792. [CrossRef]
107. Buysse, D.J.; Reynolds, C.F., 3rd; Monk, T.H.; Berman, S.R.; Kupfer, D.J. The Pittsburgh Sleep Quality Index: A new instrument for psychiatric practice and research. *Psychiatry Res.* **1989**, *28*, 193–213. [CrossRef]
108. Kendzerska, T.B.; Smith, P.M.; Brignardello-Petersen, R.; Leung, R.S.; Tomlinson, G.A. Evaluation of the measurement properties of the Epworth sleepiness scale: A systematic review. *Sleep Med. Rev.* **2014**, *18*, 321–331. [CrossRef]
109. Huppertz, T.; Horstmann, V.; Scharnow, C.; Ruckes, C.; Bahr, K.; Matthias, C.; Gouveris, H. OSA in patients with head and neck cancer is associated with cancer size and oncologic outcome. *Eur. Arch. Otorhinolaryngol.* **2020**, *278*, 2485–2491. [CrossRef]
110. Chung, F.; Subramanyam, R.; Liao, P.; Sasaki, E.; Shapiro, C.; Sun, Y. High STOP-Bang score indicates a high probability of obstructive sleep apnoea. *Br. J. Anaesth.* **2012**, *108*, 768–775. [CrossRef] [PubMed]
111. Wong, K.A.; Paul, A.; Fuentes, P.; Lim, D.C.; Das, A.; Tan, M. Screening for obstructive sleep apnea in patients with cancer—A machine learning approach. *Sleep Adv.* **2023**, *4*, zpad042. [CrossRef] [PubMed]
112. The AASM International Classification of Sleep Disorders—Third Edition, Text Revision (ICSD-3-TR). Available online: https://aasm.org/clinical-resources/international-classification-sleep-disorders/ (accessed on 5 January 2025).
113. Pedersini, R.; di Mauro, P.; Amoroso, V.; Castronovo, V.; Zamparini, M.; Monteverdi, S.; Laini, L.; Schivardi, G.; Cosentini, D.; Grisanti, S.; et al. Sleep disturbances and restless legs syndrome in postmenopausal women with early breast cancer given adjuvant aromatase inhibitor therapy. *Breast* **2022**, *66*, 162–168. [CrossRef]
114. Yennurajalingam, S.; Balachandran, D.; Pedraza Cardozo, S.L.; Berg, E.A.; Chisholm, G.B.; Reddy, A.; DeLa Cruz, V.; Williams, J.L.; Bruera, E. Patient-reported sleep disturbance in advanced cancer: Frequency, predictors and screening performance of the Edmonton Symptom Assessment System sleep item. *BMJ Support. Palliat. Care* **2017**, *7*, 274–280. [CrossRef]
115. Gartner, J.; Jaroslawski, K.; Becker, G.; Boehlke, C. Improvement of Restless Legs Syndrome Under Treatment of Cancer Pain with Morphine and Fentanyl. *Front. Neurol.* **2019**, *10*, 457. [CrossRef] [PubMed]
116. Allen, R.P.; Picchietti, D.L.; Auerbach, M.; Cho, Y.W.; Connor, J.R.; Earley, C.J.; Garcia-Borreguero, D.; Kotagal, S.; Manconi, M.; Ondo, W.; et al. Evidence-based and consensus clinical practice guidelines for the iron treatment of restless legs syndrome/Willis-Ekbom disease in adults and children: An IRLSSG task force report. *Sleep Med.* **2018**, *41*, 27–44. [CrossRef]
117. Winkelman, J.W.; Berkowski, J.A.; DelRosso, L.M.; Koo, B.B.; Scharf, M.T.; Sharon, D.; Zak, R.S.; Kazmi, U.; Falck-Ytter, Y.; Shelgikar, A.V.; et al. Treatment of restless legs syndrome and periodic limb movement disorder: An American Academy of Sleep Medicine clinical practice guideline. *J. Clin. Sleep Med.* **2025**, *21*, 137–152. [CrossRef] [PubMed]
118. Morse, A.M.; Bogan, R.K.; Roy, A.; Thorpy, M.J. Dosing Optimization of Low-Sodium Oxybate in Narcolepsy and Idiopathic Hypersomnia in Adults: Consensus Recommendations. *Neurol. Ther.* **2024**, *13*, 785–807. [CrossRef]

119. Ma, Y.; Hall, D.L.; Ngo, L.H.; Liu, Q.; Bain, P.A.; Yeh, G.Y. Efficacy of cognitive behavioral therapy for insomnia in breast cancer: A meta-analysis. *Sleep Med. Rev.* **2021**, *55*, 101376. [CrossRef] [PubMed]
120. Liou, K.T.; Root, J.C.; Garland, S.N.; Green, J.; Li, Y.; Li, Q.S.; Kantoff, P.W.; Ahles, T.A.; Mao, J.J. Effects of acupuncture versus cognitive behavioral therapy on cognitive function in cancer survivors with insomnia: A secondary analysis of a randomized clinical trial. *Cancer* **2020**, *126*, 3042–3052. [CrossRef]
121. Şahin, F.; Özkaraman, A.; Irmak Kaya, Z. The effect of a combined treatment of foot soak and lavender oil inhalation therapy on the severity of insomnia of patients with cancer: Randomized interventional study. *Explore* **2023**, *19*, 426–433. [CrossRef]
122. Zachariae, R.; Lyby, M.S.; Ritterband, L.M.; O'Toole, M.S. Efficacy of internet-delivered cognitive-behavioral therapy for insomnia—A systematic review and meta-analysis of randomized controlled trials. *Sleep Med. Rev.* **2016**, *30*, 1–10. [CrossRef]
123. Savard, J.; Ivers, H.; Morin, C.M.; Lacroix, G. Video cognitive-behavioral therapy for insomnia in cancer patients: A cost-effective alternative. *Psychooncology* **2021**, *30*, 44–51. [CrossRef]
124. Felder, J.N.; Epel, E.S.; Neuhaus, J.; Krystal, A.D.; Prather, A.A. Efficacy of Digital Cognitive Behavioral Therapy for the Treatment of Insomnia Symptoms Among Pregnant Women: A Randomized Clinical Trial. *JAMA Psychiatry* **2020**, *77*, 484–492. [CrossRef] [PubMed]
125. Delpachitra, S.; Campbell, A.; Wibowo, E. Preference for sleep management strategies among prostate cancer patients: An Aotearoa/New Zealand perspective. *Cancer Treat. Res. Commun.* **2020**, *25*, 100219. [CrossRef] [PubMed]
126. Bathgate, C.J.; Edinger, J.D.; Krystal, A.D. Insomnia Patients with Objective Short Sleep Duration Have a Blunted Response to Cognitive Behavioral Therapy for Insomnia. *Sleep* **2017**, *40*, zsw012. [CrossRef] [PubMed]
127. Slade, A.N.; Waters, M.R.; Serrano, N.A. Long-term sleep disturbance and prescription sleep aid use among cancer survivors in the United States. *Support. Care Cancer* **2020**, *28*, 551–560. [CrossRef]
128. Carney, C.E.; Edinger, J.D.; Kuchibhatla, M.; Lachowski, A.M.; Bogouslavsky, O.; Krystal, A.D.; Shapiro, C.M. Cognitive Behavioral Insomnia Therapy for Those with Insomnia and Depression: A Randomized Controlled Clinical Trial. *Sleep* **2017**, *40*, zsx019. [CrossRef]
129. Foldvary, N.; Caruso, A.C.; Mascha, E.; Perry, M.; Klem, G.; McCarthy, V.; Qureshi, F.; Dinner, D. Identifying montages that best detect electrographic seizure activity during polysomnography. *Sleep* **2000**, *23*, 221–229.

cancers

MDPI

Review

Technological Resources for Physical Rehabilitation in Cancer Patients Undergoing Chemotherapy: A Scoping Review

Anabela Amarelo [1,2], Marisa Mota [1], Bruno Amarelo [1], Marta Campos Ferreira [3] and Carla Sílvia Fernandes [4,5,6,*]

1 Gaia-Espinho Local Health Unit, 4434-502 Vila Nova de Gaia, Portugal; anabela.amarelo@ulsge.min-saude.pt (A.A.); marisa.mota@ulsge.min-saude.pt (M.M.); bruno.amarelo@ulsge.min-saude.pt (B.A.)
2 Association for Research and Supportive Care in Oncology (AICSO), 4410-406 Arcozelo, Portugal
3 INESC TEC—Institute for Systems and Computer Engineering, Technology and Science, Faculty of Engineering, University of Porto (FEUP), 4200-465 Porto, Portugal; mferreira@fe.up.pt
4 Nursing School of Porto, 4200-072 Porto, Portugal
5 Research Center RISEHealth, 4200-319 Porto, Portugal
6 Association ADITGames, 4490-582 Póvoa de Varzim, Portugal
* Correspondence: carlafernandes@esenf.pt

Simple Summary: This scoping review explores how technological tools can support cancer rehabilitation for cancer patients undergoing chemotherapy. Technologies such as wearable devices, mobile health (mHealth) applications, telerehabilitation platforms, and virtual reality have emerged as valuable aids for maintaining or improving patients' physical activity levels. By mapping these tools, we highlight their benefits in managing cancer- and treatment-related side effects, such as fatigue and reduced mobility, ultimately enhancing quality of life. This review also identifies areas for integrating these resources into care practices and outlines directions for future research to maximize clinical effectiveness and accessibility.

Abstract: Background/Objectives: Cancer patients undergoing chemotherapy often face challenges that reduce their physical function and quality of life. Technological resources offer innovative solutions for physical rehabilitation, but the extent of their application in this context remains unclear. This scoping review aims to explore and map the various technological tools used to support physical rehabilitation in cancer patients during chemotherapy, focusing on their potential to improve outcomes and enhance patient care. **Methods**: A scoping review was conducted following the Joanna Briggs Institute (JBI) guidelines and the PRISMA-ScR framework. Comprehensive searches were performed in the MEDLINE, CINAHL, Scopus, SPORTDiscus, and COCHRANE databases. The included studies focused on the technological resources used in physical rehabilitation for cancer patients undergoing chemotherapy. Data extraction followed the World Health Organization's "Classification of Digital Health Interventions v1.0" to categorize the technologies. **Results**: A total of 32 studies met the inclusion criteria. The most commonly used technologies included wearable devices (16 studies), web-based platforms and telerehabilitation systems (7 studies), mHealth applications (6 studies), virtual reality (2 studies), and exergaming (3 studies). These tools were designed to enhance physical function, manage treatment-related symptoms, and improve overall quality of life. Wearable devices were particularly effective for monitoring physical activity, while web-based platforms and mHealth applications supported remote rehabilitation and patient engagement. **Conclusions**: Technological resources offer significant opportunities for personalized rehabilitation interventions in cancer patients undergoing chemotherapy. However, further research is needed to evaluate the long-term effectiveness, cost-efficiency, and clinical integration of these tools to ensure broader accessibility and sustainable impact.

Keywords: oncology rehabilitation; digital health tools; supportive care in cancer; mHealth applications

1. Introduction

Cancer continues to be a leading public health challenge worldwide, with an estimated 20 million new cases and 10 million deaths reported in 2022 alone, according to GLOBOCAN [1–3]. By 2040, global cancer incidence is expected to rise to 29.9 million cases annually, with over 70 million people living after cancer, which will place an increasing burden on healthcare systems and affect the long-term well-being of survivors [3–5]. As the number of cancer survivors grows, the long-term effects of both the disease and its treatments become more critical to address.

Chemotherapy, despite advances in cancer treatment, remains a common therapeutic approach, either used alone or in combination with targeted and immunotherapeutic agents [6,7]. Unfortunately, chemotherapy exposes patients to a range of adverse effects, increasing morbidity and treatment costs while negatively impacting health-related quality of life (HR-QOL), and may limit the administration of future treatments, potentially affecting long-term outcomes [6–8].

Comprehensive care is critical for cancer patients during treatment, as prolonged periods of inactivity and the disease itself can result in fatigue, peripheral neuropathy, nausea, cardiotoxicity, cognitive impairments, and overall functional decline [7,9]. These effects often persist long after treatment, causing long-term functional challenges in returning to normal life, work, or independent living [10]. Although supportive care interventions address some of these effects, many remain difficult to manage, emphasizing the need for continuous improvements in mitigating chemotherapy-related side effects [7,8].

In these context, physical rehabilitation plays a crucial role in helping patients maintain or regain functionality during cancer treatment [10,11]. Exercise has shown substantial benefits, including improved mental health, reduced fatigue, and enhanced well-being, with guidelines recommending at least 150 min of aerobic activity and 2–3 resistance sessions per week during and after treatment [12].

Despite these benefits, several factors have been identified as barriers to exercise, including cancer therapy-related side effects, kinesiophobia, lack of access to tailored facilities, and individual health beliefs and preferences [13]. In recent years, digital technological advancements have introduced new possibilities for health [14–16]. As digital technologies advance, becoming smarter and interconnected through wireless communication, unimaginable possibilities open for the advancement of science, health, and rehabilitation [15].

In this setting, technologies such as mobile health applications, wearable devices, telerehabilitation platforms, and virtual reality systems are designed to remotely monitor, guide, and support physical activity and symptom management [17–19]. These tools enable patients and healthcare providers to engage in rehabilitation programs more efficiently, offering personalized feedback, progress tracking, and symptom management, often in real time [15,16]. However, despite the growing interest in digital health interventions within oncology, the scope of available technological resources for physical rehabilitation in cancer patients undergoing chemotherapy remains unexplored [18,20].

While existing studies suggest that mobile health applications and tele-rehabilitation tools can enhance self-management and symptom control in cancer patients, a comprehensive map of these technologies is necessary to identify trends and gaps in the literature [18,21]. This scoping review aims to map the available technological resources for physical rehabilitation in cancer patients undergoing chemotherapy, highlighting areas where further research is needed to optimize the use of technology in cancer care.

2. Materials and Methods

A scoping review was carried out to explore the current body of scientific literature, following the guidelines established by the Joanna Briggs Institute (JBI) [22,23]. The PRISMA-ScR framework (Preferred Reporting Items for Systematic Reviews and Meta-Analyses for Scoping Reviews) was utilized to ensure systematic organization and transparency throughout the research process, as outlined in the PRISMA-ScR guidelines [22,24,25]. The review protocol was also registered on the Open Science Framework® platform, with the following https://doi.org/10.17605/OSF.IO/RV795.

2.1. Research Method

The research question was developed using the Population, Concept, and Context (PCC) framework, as outlined by the Joanna Briggs Institute [23,25]. The study focused on adults over the age of 18 who were cancer patients undergoing chemotherapy (Population), participating in physical rehabilitation programs (Context), and using technological resources (Concept). These criteria guided the selection of studies for the bibliographic sample, with search terms derived from this framework. To ensure broad coverage, the search included both free terms and database-specific descriptors. The search strategy was tailored for each database using English-language descriptors and syntax customized to the following platforms: MEDLINE®, CINAHL®, Scopus, SPORTDiscuss, and COCHRANE. A combination of medical subject headings (MeSHs), subject headings, and free-text terms was employed, enhancing the search's comprehensiveness (Appendix A Table A1). Additional articles were manually added by examining the reference lists of all publications included in the review, a method referred to as "backward citation searching". The literature search was carried out to include studies published up to 31 March 2024, with no time restrictions.

2.2. Eligibility Criteria

The inclusion and exclusion criteria were established based on the PCC framework, focusing on the guiding question: What technological resources are available for physical rehabilitation in cancer patients undergoing chemotherapy? Sub-questions were posed to refine the focus, exploring which types of technologies are used, what functionalities they provide, and their feasibility or acceptability.

Studies were excluded if they focused on: individuals under the age of 18; patients receiving treatments other than chemotherapy; or programs focused solely on well-being, psychological support, behavior change, or symptom management instead of physical rehabilitation. Additionally, studies focused on the prehabilitation phase or cancer survivors post-treatment were excluded, as well as non-primary research (editorials, letters, reviews, gray literature, dissertations, and book chapters). Only primary research published in English, French, Spanish, or Portuguese was considered. Qualitative, quantitative, and mixed-methods studies were included.

2.3. Data Extraction

The search results from each database were imported into Rayyan® software (https://www.rayyan.ai, accessed on 14 August 2024), a web-based tool designed to assist in the systematic review process, to streamline the review process [26]. After removing duplicate references, two researchers (A.A. and C.S.F.) independently carried out the initial screening of titles and abstracts, applying the previously established inclusion and exclusion criteria. The full texts of the selected references were then obtained to finalize decisions on their inclusion [27]. Any disagreements regarding inclusion or exclusion were resolved by consulting a third researcher (B.A.) to reach a consensus.

Each selected article was assigned an identifier (S) based on the order of review. The PRISMA 2020 framework was used to organize the data and to ensure transparency and consistency throughout the screening and selection process [28].

2.4. Data Analysis

Data were collected using a customized extraction form, capturing the following details for each study: author, year of publication, and country; study design; study objective; participant characteristics; type of technology used; purpose; type of intervention; main instruments; and outcomes (Table 1). Data extraction and synthesis were performed independently by two researchers (A.A. and C.S.F.), with a third researcher (B.A.) available to resolve any disagreements.

To provide a structured categorization of technological resources in healthcare, data were analyzed based on the "Classification of Digital Health Interventions v1.0" from the World Health Organization [29]. This framework provides a structured approach for describing digital technologies in healthcare, categorizing them into four key target groups: clients, healthcare providers, health system managers, and data services. For this analysis, we extracted information regarding the target group and type of technological resource used in each study, aligning it with the WHO classification.

A multi-input table was created to present the relationships between the types of technologies and their targets, functionalities, and primary objectives. Table 2 offers a comprehensive overview of technological interventions.

Table 1. Characteristics of studies included in the scoping review.

ID	Athor/Year/ Country	Study Design	Objective	Population	Technology	Purpose of Technological Resource	Intervention	Instruments	Outcomes
S01 [30]	Albrecht T 2024 (USA)	Single-arm pre–post-interventional study	Evaluate a web-based exercise tool for cancer patients undergoing chemotherapy	12 breast and prostate cancer patients	Web-based app	To promote exercise and monitor anxiety, depression, fatigue	12-week physical activity program	PROMIS, 6MWT	Improved anxiety, depression, walking distance
S02 [31]	Cheong I 2018 (Republic of Korea)	Prospective interventional study	Evaluate the effect of a mobile healthcare program on fatigue and strength	102 colorectal cancer patients	mHealth app + Wearable	To enhance strength and cardiorespiratory endurance	12-week rehabilitation	2MWT, IPAQ, PG-SGA, QLQ-C30	Improved strength, fatigue, endurance
S03 [32]	Qi Y 2024 (China)	Single-center, single-arm, prospective phase I study	Assess feasibility of VR and mHealth rehabilitation	123 lung, gastric, colorectal cancer patients	mHealth + VR	To improve physical and psychological health	8-week mHealth and VR rehabilitation	6MWT, PG-SGA, HADS, QLQ-C30	Improved BMI, anxiety, depression, muscle mass
S04 [33]	Wolff J 2023 (Germany)	Randomized controlled trial (RCT), with a waiting-list control	Evaluate the impact of a cancer exercise program using the PINK! app	60 breast cancer patients	PINK! app	To reduce fatigue and support mental well-being	12-week app-based coaching program	PHQ-9, QLQ-C30, IPAQ	Reduced fatigue, psychological distress
S05 [34]	Feyzioğlu Ö 2022 (Turkey)	Pilot study with a pre-test and post-test design	Evaluate the effectiveness of video game-based exercises for upper extremity function	30 breast cancer patients	Video game-based exercises	To improve upper extremity functionality through interactive gaming	Kinect-based exergaming	DASH, SPADI, ROM	Improved upper extremity functionality
S06 [35]	Ariza-Garcia A 2019 (Spain)	Two-arm, assessor-blinded, parallel, randomized controlled trial	Evaluate the impact of web-based exercise program on functional capacity and strength	78 breast cancer patients (stages I-IIIA)	Web-based system	To enhance functional capacity and muscle strength	Web-based exercise program	SF-36, 6MWT	Improved functional capacity, muscle strength

Table 1. *Cont.*

ID	Athor/Year/ Country	Study Design	Objective	Population	Technology	Purpose of Technological Resource	Intervention	Instruments	Outcomes
S07 [36]	Troschel F 2019 (Germany)	Case report	Track physical fitness and exercise adherence in a glioblastoma patient using a sports watch	1 glioblastoma patient	Sports watch	To track fitness levels and motivate exercise	Personalized fitness program	Garmin Fitness Metrics	Improved fitness, completed marathon
S08 [37]	Coats V 2019 (Canada)	Pilot study, feasibility study	Assess feasibility and effectiveness of telerehabilitation in lung cancer patients	35 lung cancer patients	Telerehabilitation	To deliver remote rehabilitation and improve functional capacity	Supervised home-based rehabilitation	6MWT, IPAQ, FFI	Improved functional capacity, high satisfaction
S09 [38]	Van Blarigan E 2022 (USA)	Pilot RCT	Evaluate physical activity improvement through personalized walking program	45 colorectal cancer patients	Fitbit + SMS	To monitor physical activity and improve adherence	Personalized walking program	Fitbit, IPAQ	Improved physical activity, high adherence
S10 [39]	Moffet H 2015 (Canada)	Longitudinal pilot study	Evaluate telerehabilitation program for lung cancer patients	12 lung cancer patients	Telerehabilitation	To provide home-based rehabilitation with professional supervision	Home-based telerehabilitation	6MWT, CRF, IPAQ	High adherence, reliable platform
S11 [40]	Purdy G M 2022 (Canada)	Feasibility study	Evaluate the use of eHealth apps for physical fitness in multiple myeloma patients	15 multiple myeloma patients	eHealth app	To enhance physical fitness and quality of life	eHealth-based exercise program	QLQ-C30, SF-36, BFI	Improved fitness, quality of life
S12 [41]	Wolff J 2024 (Germany)	Retrospective observational study (real-world data)	Assess the impact of a weight loss program using the PINK! Coach app in breast cancer survivors	100 breast cancer survivors	PINK! Coach app	To support weight loss and physical activity remotely	App-based weight loss program	BMI, 6MWT, IPAQ	Reduced BMI, increased physical activity

Table 1. *Cont.*

ID	Athor/Year/ Country	Study Design	Objective	Population	Technology	Purpose of Technological Resource	Intervention	Instruments	Outcomes
S13 [42]	Poh Loh K 2021 (USA)	Qualitative study	Evaluate the feasibility of a walking and resistance exercise program in myeloid neoplasm patients	20 myeloid neoplasm patients	GO-EXCAP mobile app	To facilitate walking and resistance exercise programs remotely	Walking + resistance exercise	IPAQ, SF-36	Feasible exercise program
S14 [43]	Romero-Elías M 2024 (Spain)	Qualitative study, quasi-experimental research	Evaluate psychological support and physical activity engagement through video conferencing in colorectal cancer patients	22 colorectal cancer patients	Video conferencing	To offer remote psychological support and engage in physical activity	Remote exercise program + mental health	IPAQ, SF-36	Improved psychological well-being, PA
S15 [44]	Nyrop 2017 (USA)	Longitudinal, observational study	Evaluate the impact of Fitbit monitoring on walking adherence in breast cancer patients	56 breast cancer patients	Fitbit Zip	To monitor steps and adherence to exercise	Walking program with step monitoring	Fitbit, IPAQ	Improved walking adherence, reduced fatigue
S16 [45]	Park 2019 (Republic of Korea)	Prospective, single-arm intervention study (pilot study)	Evaluate exercise capacity and distress management through smartphone app	43 NSCLC patients	Smartphone app	To track exercise capacity and provide distress management	Exercise program with remote monitoring	6MWT, PG-SGA, HADS	Improved exercise capacity, reduced distress
S17 [46]	Villaron 2018 (France)	Randomized pilot study	Assess step-tracking and telehealth for fatigue reduction and physical activity promotion	75 cancer patients (various types)	Pedometer, Telehealth	To promote physical activity and reduce fatigue through step tracking	Walking-based physical activity	IPAQ, SF-36	Improved physical activity, reduced fatigue
S18 [47]	Backman 2014 (Sweden)	Randomized controlled trial (RCT)	Evaluate pedometer-based physical activity interventions for cancer patients	97 breast and colorectal cancer patients	Pedometer	To encourage physical activity and track steps	Walking program with pedometer	IPAQ, QLQ-C30	Improved physical activity, breast cancer symptoms

Table 1. *Cont.*

ID	Athor/Year/ Country	Study Design	Objective	Population	Technology	Purpose of Technological Resource	Intervention	Instruments	Outcomes
S19 [48]	Gokal 2015 (UK)	Randomized controlled trial (RCT)	Evaluate the impact of a walking program on fatigue and physical activity in breast cancer patients	60 breast cancer patients	Pedometer	To promote walking and reduce fatigue	Walking program with step goals	PFS, FACIT-F, IPAQ	Improved physical activity, fatigue, self-esteem
S20 [49]	Jarden 2016 (Denmark)	Randomized controlled trial (RCT)	Evaluate the effect of multimodal rehabilitation on quality of life in acute leukemia patients	102 acute leukemia patients	Pedometer, Multi-modal intervention	To track physical activity and improve quality of life	Multimodal rehab with walking program	SF-36, QLQ-C30, IPAQ	Improved physical function, quality of life
S21 [50]	Delrieu 2020 (France)	Single-arm intervention study (feasibility study)	Assess the feasibility of activity trackers in metastatic breast cancer patients	40 metastatic breast cancer patients	Activity tracker	To monitor and increase physical activity	Activity tracker-based PA program	6MWT, IPAQ	Increased physical activity, reduced sitting time
S22 [51]	Edbrooke 2019 (Australia)	Randomized controlled trial (RCT)	Evaluate SenseWear accelerometer for tracking physical activity and intensity in lung cancer patients	56 lung cancer patients	SenseWear accelerometer	To track physical activity and provide feedback on intensity	SenseWear-based activity program	6MWT, SF-36, IPAQ	Improved physical activity, HRQoL
S23 [52]	Gandhi 2020 (India)	Non-randomized controlled trial	Assess the impact of a walking program with pedometer for fatigue and QoL in breast cancer patients	85 breast cancer patients	Pedometer	To track steps and monitor fatigue	Walking program with pedometer	FACIT-F, SF-36, IPAQ	Reduced fatigue, improved quality of life
S24 [53]	Lowe 2013 (Canada)	Quasi-experimental pilot study (case series)	Evaluate the impact of an accelerometer for tracking sedentary behavior in advanced cancer patients	30 advanced cancer patients	activPAL accelerometer	To track sedentary behavior and physical activity	Sedentary behavior intervention	activPAL metrics	Improved quality of life, mixed physical function

Table 1. *Cont.*

ID	Athor/Year/ Country	Study Design	Objective	Population	Technology	Purpose of Technological Resource	Intervention	Instruments	Outcomes
S25 [54]	Marthick 2018 (Australia)	Prospective cohort study	Assess daily physical activity tracking in various cancer patients using Misfit Shine	112 cancer patients	Misfit Shine	To monitor daily physical activity levels	Physical activity intervention	Misfit Shine metrics	Improved physical activity, quality of life
S26 [55]	Nilsson 2020 (Norway)	Prospective cohort study	Evaluate SenseWear Armband for moderate-to-vigorous physical activity tracking in cancer patients	90 cancer patients	SenseWear Armband	To track moderate-to-vigorous physical activity	SenseWear-based PA program	MVPA metrics, SF-36	Reduced fatigue, increased MVPA
S27 [56]	Vallance 2016 (Canada)	Randomized controlled trial (RCT)	Evaluate pedometer-based walking program for physical activity promotion in breast cancer patients	81 breast cancer patients	Pedometer, print materials	To encourage adherence to a physical activity program	Walking program with pedometer	SF-36, IPAQ	High adherence, no significant difference in PA
S28 [57]	Mouri 2018 (Japan)	Prospective, multicenter, single-arm study	Evaluate walking-based outdoor activity program for physical activity in NSCLC and pancreatic cancer patients	59 NSCLC and pancreatic cancer patients	Pedometer	To promote outdoor activity and improve quality of life	Walking-based PA program	6MWT, IPAQ	Increased outdoor activity, improved QoL
S29 [58]	Parker 2019 (USA)	Prospective single-arm study	Evaluate ActiGraph accelerometer for monitoring activity in pancreatic cancer patients	47 pancreatic cancer patients	ActiGraph accelerometer	To monitor activity levels and increase moderate-to-vigorous physical activity	Personalized physical activity intervention	ActiGraph, MVPA metrics	High adherence, increased MVPA
S30 [59]	de Oliveira 2018 (Brazil)	Controlled trial	Evaluate Kinect-based rehabilitation for fatigue reduction in cancer patients	60 cancer patients	Xbox Kinect	To promote interactive rehabilitation and reduce fatigue	Kinect-based rehabilitation program	FACIT-F, SF-36	Reduced fatigue, improved quality of life

Table 1. *Cont.*

ID	Athor/Year/ Country	Study Design	Objective	Population	Technology	Purpose of Technological Resource	Intervention	Instruments	Outcomes
S31 [60]	de Oliveira 2020 (Brazil)	Randomized controlled clinical trial	Assess the impact of Kinect-based exercises on shoulder mobility and disability	50 cancer patients	Xbox Kinect	To improve shoulder mobility and reduce disability	Kinect-based exercise program	DASH, ROM	Reduced shoulder disability, no change in muscle strength
S32 [61]	Tsuda 2016 (Japan)	Prospective single-arm feasibility study	Evaluate the use of Nintendo Wii Fit for maintaining physical performance in hematologic malignancy patients	22 hematologic malignancy patients	Nintendo Wii Fit	To maintain physical performance and improve psychological health	Wii Fit-based exercise program	HADS, PG-SGA, 6MWT	Maintained physical performance, improved anxiety and depression

6MWT: 6-Minute Walk Test; 2MWT: 2-Minute Walk Test; BFI: Brief Fatigue Inventory; BMI: Body Mass Index; CRF: cancer-related fatigue; DASH: disabilities of the arm, shoulder, and hand; FACIT-F: Functional Assessment of Chronic Illness Therapy—Fatigue; FFI: Foot Function Index; HADS: Hospital Anxiety and Depression Scale; IPAQ: International Physical Activity Questionnaire; MVPA: moderate-to-vigorous physical activity; PG-SGA: Patient-Generated Subjective Global Assessment; PHQ-9: Patient Health Questionnaire-9; PROMIS: Patient-Reported Outcomes Measurement Information System; PFS: Piper Fatigue Scale; QLQ-C30: Quality of Life Questionnaire—Core 30; ROM: range of motion; SF-36: Short-Form (36) Health Survey; SPADI: Shoulder Pain and Disability Index.

Table 2. Technological resource types and categorization.

ID.	Technology Type	WHO DHI Classification	Functionality	Feasibility	Usability	Appropriateness/ Suitability	Objective	Key Findings
S01 [30]	Web-based application (EPT tool)	DHI 1.1—Client-targeted (therapy)	Exercise planning, mental health monitoring	High adherence, easy to use for home-based monitoring, no significant cost barriers.	Highly usable for remote use and adaptable for patients undergoing chemotherapy.	Well-suited for promoting physical activity and managing mental health in cancer patients.	Improved physical activity, mental health	Improved anxiety, depression, and walking distance.
S02 [31]	mHealth + Wearable device	DHI 1.2—Client-targeted (self-monitoring)	Exercise guidance, physical activity tracking	Good feasibility: mobile app and wearable devices are practical; adherence was 75%.	Mobile app and wearable are good self-monitoring tools suited for tracking fatigue and performance.	Appropriate for addressing fatigue and endurance, well-targeted for rehabilitation.	Improved strength, endurance, fatigue	Improved strength, endurance, and reduced fatigue.
S03 [32]	mHealth + VR	DHI 1.1—Client-targeted (therapy)	Group exercise, VR therapy	Requires technological familiarity, but feasible for patients comfortable with tech. Adherence varies.	Engaging, but requires more technological knowledge for use.	Suitable for comprehensive physical and psychological rehabilitation, including anxiety reduction.	Improved physical, psychological status	Improved BMI, anxiety, depression, and muscle mass.

Table 2. *Cont.*

ID.	Technology Type	WHO DHI Classification	Functionality	Feasibility	Usability	Appropriateness/ Suitability	Objective	Key Findings
S04 [33]	App-based coaching (PINK!)	DHI 1.4—Client-targeted (coaching)	Exercise, nutrition, mental health coaching	High adherence, practical for patients needing daily support.	Easy to use and provides regular support for psychological and physical health.	Highly suitable for fatigue reduction and mental health management.	Reduced distress, increase PA	Reduced fatigue, distress, and increased physical activity.
S05 [34]	Exergaming (Xbox Kinect)	DHI 1.1—Client-targeted (therapy)	Interactive gaming for physical activity	Feasible for younger patients or those familiar with gaming systems; cost may vary.	Interactive and engaging, but access to technology may limit use.	Well-suited for upper extremity rehabilitation.	Improve upper extremity functionality	Improved range of motion; no significant change in strength.
S06 [35]	Web-based exercise system (e-Cuidate-Chemo)	DHI 1.1—Client-targeted (therapy)	Web-based exercise therapy	High adherence, feasible for remote intervention, accessible to patients with Internet access.	Easy to use for breast cancer patients at home; remote access ensures usability during chemotherapy.	Well-suited for mitigating chemotherapy-related physical deterioration.	Counters physical deterioration	Improved functional capacity and strength, no significant changes in body composition.
S07 [36]	Wearable (Polar V800 sports watch)	DHI 1.2—Client-targeted (self-monitoring)	High-intensity physical training tracking	Feasible for highly active patients but may not be suitable for all cancer patients due to high intensity.	Convenient for tracking fitness levels, but limited to patients capable of engaging in high-intensity activities.	Suitable for motivated, physically fit patients.	Tracks physical activity and fitness	Maintained fitness, completed marathons, improved physical fitness during cancer treatment.
S08 [37]	Telerehabilitation platform (eChez-Soi)	DHI 1.1—Client-targeted (remote care)	Remote exercise monitoring	High adherence, feasible for remote care with sensors, accessible for patients with internet access.	Highly usable for supervised remote rehabilitation, good adherence.	Very suitable for patients needing remote rehabilitation.	Improves functional capacity through remote exercise	High satisfaction, improved 6MWT, significant improvements in functional capacity, no adverse events.
S09 [38]	Wearable (Fitbit) + SMS	DHI 1.2—Client-targeted (self-monitoring)	Physical activity tracking, reminders	High adherence to Fitbit, practical due to automated SMS, though engagement with SMS was moderate.	Easy to use for tracking physical activity and providing reminders through SMS, though SMS engagement may vary.	Suitable for promoting physical activity during chemotherapy.	Promotes physical activity	Improved adherence to daily activity tracking, slight improvements in physical activity.
S10 [39]	Telerehabilitation platform	DHI 1.1—Client-targeted (remote care)	Remote exercise monitoring	Feasible for patients undergoing chemotherapy, high adherence, some technical issues reported but resolved.	Easy to use and practical for telerehabilitation programs with few technical problems.	Suitable for home-based rehabilitation for lung cancer patients.	Evaluates telerehabilitation for lung cancer patients	High adherence, reliable platform, minor technical issues, high patient satisfaction.

Table 2. *Cont.*

ID.	Technology Type	WHO DHI Classification	Functionality	Feasibility	Usability	Appropriateness/ Suitability	Objective	Key Findings
S11 [40]	eHealth app	DHI 1.1—Client-targeted (remote care)	Home-based exercise	High adherence (90%), feasible for multiple myeloma patients across various treatment stages.	Suitable for home-based virtual exercise, highly usable and adaptable for patient needs.	Well-suited for improving fitness and quality of life in multiple myeloma patients.	Improves fitness and quality of life	High adherence, improved physical fitness and quality of life, no adverse events.
S12 [41]	App-based coaching (PINK! Coach)	DHI 1.4—Client-targeted (coaching)	Coaching for PA, nutrition, stress management	Feasible for breast cancer patients undergoing chemotherapy, cost-effective for remote support, high adherence.	Practical and easy to use for maintaining physical activity and lifestyle changes.	Suitable for supporting weight management and physical activity in breast cancer patients.	Supports weight management during chemotherapy	Maintained or reduced BMI, increased physical activity, especially in antihormone therapy patients.
S13 [42]	mHealth (Go-EXCAP mobile app)	DHI 1.1—Client-targeted (remote care)	Remote-supervised exercise, monitoring	High adherence to wearables and remote monitoring, practical for improving fitness during chemotherapy.	Usable for patients requiring close monitoring during rehabilitation, accessible for home use.	Suitable for improving fitness and strength, well-targeted for remote interventions.	Improves fitness and strength	High adherence, improved fitness and strength through remote monitoring.
S14 [43]	Video conferencing (Meet app)	DHI 1.1—Client-targeted (remote care)	Supervised exercise, motivational strategies	Feasible for remote exercise programs, high engagement reported, accessible through standard video conferencing tools.	Highly usable for remote supervision, provides motivational support during exercise programs.	Suitable for colorectal cancer patients needing both physical and psychological support during chemotherapy.	Improves physical activity and psychological well-being	Improved physical activity and psychological well-being, high engagement, effective motivational strategies.
S15 [44]	Pedometer-based walking program	DHI 1.2—Client-targeted (self-monitoring)	Physical activity tracking	Feasible with high adherence, accessible for patients with limited physical activity experience, low-cost.	Easy to use pedometer-based programs, well-suited for tracking walking activity.	Suitable for improving physical activity and reducing fatigue, especially for patients undergoing chemotherapy.	Enhances physical activity, reduce fatigue	Improved physical activity, reduced fatigue.
S16 [45]	mHealth app (Smart Aftercare app)	DHI 1.2—Client-targeted (self-monitoring)	Physical activity, intensity tracking	High adherence, feasible for remote monitoring of exercise capacity	Easy to use for tracking physical activity intensity and providing real-time feedback for patients.	Well-suited for increasing physical activity intensity and tracking quality of life improvements.	Tracks PA, HRQoL	Increased physical activity and improved quality of life, especially exercise capacity improvements.

Table 2. *Cont.*

ID.	Technology Type	WHO DHI Classification	Functionality	Feasibility	Usability	Appropriateness/ Suitability	Objective	Key Findings
S17 [46]	Pedometer (ONWALK 100) + Telehealth platform	DHI 1.2—Client-targeted (self-monitoring)	Walking + weekly SMS reminders	Feasible, though fatigue poses challenges to adherence. Technologically accessible and affordable.	Usable for patients needing remote physical activity guidance, but fatigue reduced engagement	Suitable for encouraging physical activity during chemotherapy	Improves physical activity and QoL	Moderate improvements in physical activity and QoL; fatigue limited adherence to the intervention.
S18 [47]	Pedometer-based walking program (SILVA ex connect)	DHI 1.2—Client-targeted (self-monitoring)	Physical activity tracking via pedometer	High adherence, practical for tracking walking-based interventions	Usable for daily step tracking, accessible for home-based implementation	Suitable for maintaining physical activity and improving QoL during chemotherapy	Improves QoL, track daily steps	High adherence, improvements in daily steps and specific symptoms in breast and colorectal cancer patients.
S19 [48]	Pedometer-based walking program	DHI 1.2—Client-targeted (self-monitoring)	Physical activity tracking	Feasible with high adherence, accessible and low-cost, suitable for home use.	Simple and easy to use for tracking daily steps.	Suitable for enhancing physical activity and quality of life during chemotherapy.	Enhances physical activity, improves QoL	Significant improvements in physical activity and quality of life.
S20 [49]	Pedometer (Omron Walking Style Pro) + Multimodal intervention	DHI 1.2—Client-targeted (self-monitoring)	Multimodal rehabilitation (aerobic, strength, nutrition)	Feasible for leukemia patients during consolidation chemotherapy	Usable and practical for comprehensive rehabilitation, including physical activity and dietary support	Suitable for improving physical function, reducing fatigue, and supporting QoL during chemotherapy	Improves physical function, QoL, and reduce fatigue	Significant improvements in physical function, QoL, and reduction in fatigue and anxiety. Emotional well-being was also improved.
S21 [50]	Activity tracker-based PA program	DHI 1.2—Client-targeted (self-monitoring)	Physical activity tracking	Feasible, accessible with affordable technology, adherence varies based on patient motivation.	Easy to use for monitoring and increasing physical activity.	Well-suited for reducing sedentary behavior and improving activity levels during chemotherapy.	Monitors and increases physical activity	Increased physical activity and reduced sitting time.
S22 [51]	SenseWear accelerometer	DHI 1.2—Client-targeted (self-monitoring)	Physical activity, intensity tracking	Feasible for real-time intensity tracking, accessible for most patients, though technical requirements may challenge some users.	Easy to use for tracking activity intensity, providing useful feedback on physical activity levels.	Suitable for promoting moderate-to-vigorous physical activity and improving quality of life.	Tracks PA, provides feedback on intensity	Improved physical activity and quality of life through activity tracking and feedback.

Table 2. *Cont.*

ID.	Technology Type	WHO DHI Classification	Functionality	Feasibility	Usability	Appropriateness/ Suitability	Objective	Key Findings
S23 [52]	Walking program with pedometer	DHI 1.2—Client-targeted (self-monitoring)	Physical activity tracking	Feasible, with high adherence to walking-based programs. Low-cost and accessible, making it practical for patients undergoing chemotherapy.	Simple and easy to use, highly usable for tracking daily steps and improving physical activity.	Well-suited for tracking steps and monitoring fatigue during chemotherapy.	Tracks steps, monitors fatigue	Reduced fatigue and improved quality of life.
S24 [53]	activPAL accelerometer	DHI 1.2—Client-targeted (self-monitoring)	Sedentary behavior tracking	Feasible with good adherence, accessible, though adherence may vary for patients with advanced cancers.	Easy to use for tracking sedentary behavior and motivating patients to increase movement.	Well-suited for advanced cancer patients needing to reduce sedentary behavior.	Tracks sedentary behavior	Improved quality of life and reduced sedentary behavior in advanced cancer patients.
S25 [54]	Misfit Shine activity tracker (eHealth interventions + wearable devices)	DHI 1.2—Client-targeted (self-monitoring)	Physical activity tracking	Feasible with good adherence, affordable, and accessible for daily use; effective for tracking physical activity.	Easy to use, highly usable for monitoring daily activity.	Suitable for improving physical activity and quality of life during chemotherapy or cancer treatment.	Monitors daily physical activity	Improved physical activity and quality of life with daily activity tracking.
S26 [55]	SenseWear Armband	DHI 1.2—Client-targeted (self-monitoring)	Moderate-to-vigorous physical activity tracking	Feasible with high adherence, accessible for tracking MVPA, affordable, and practical for cancer rehabilitation.	Easy to use for real-time physical activity monitoring, providing motivational feedback.	Well-suited for promoting MVPA and reducing cancer-related fatigue.	Tracks MVPA	Reduced fatigue, increased moderate-to-vigorous physical activity.
S27 [56]	Pedometer-based walking program	DHI 1.2—Client-targeted (self-monitoring)	Physical activity promotion	Feasible with high adherence, low-cost, and practical for increasing physical activity through walking.	Easy to use for promoting adherence to walking programs during cancer treatment.	Suitable for encouraging physical activity and adherence to rehabilitation programs during chemotherapy.	Encourages adherence to PA program	High adherence, but no significant difference in physical activity between groups.
S28 [57]	Walking-based outdoor activity (Pedometer)	DHI 1.2—Client-targeted (self-monitoring)	Outdoor activity tracking	Feasible with good adherence, practical for promoting outdoor activity, requires patient motivation.	Usable and simple to implement for increasing outdoor physical activity.	Well-suited for improving quality of life in patients with advanced cancer.	Improves QoL	Increased outdoor activity, improved quality of life in patients with NSCLC and pancreatic cancer.

Table 2. *Cont.*

ID.	Technology Type	WHO DHI Classification	Functionality	Feasibility	Usability	Appropriateness/ Suitability	Objective	Key Findings
S29 [58]	ActiGraph accelerometer	DHI 1.2—Client-targeted (self-monitoring)	Activity tracking for personalized PA	Feasible with high adherence, practical for personalized physical activity interventions.	Easy to use for personalized physical activity tracking.	Suitable for increasing MVPA through personalized interventions in cancer patients.	Monitors activity levels	High adherence, increased MVPA through personalized PA intervention.
S30 [59]	Kinect-based rehabilitation	DHI 1.1—Client-targeted (therapy)	Interactive rehabilitation, fatigue reduction	Feasible for patients with access to gaming systems, high engagement, though some patients may find cost or accessibility a barrier.	Highly usable for interactive rehabilitation, engaging for patients.	Well-suited for reducing fatigue and improving quality of life during cancer treatment.	Improves QoL	Reduced fatigue, improved quality of life through interactive rehabilitation.
S31 [60]	Kinect-based exercise program	DHI 1.1—Client-targeted (therapy)	Shoulder mobility, exercise therapy	Feasible for shoulder mobility improvement, though cost and access to gaming technology may limit feasibility for some patients.	Usable for patients needing rehabilitation of shoulder mobility.	Suitable for improving shoulder mobility, though not as effective for muscle strength improvement.	Improves shoulder mobility, reduces disability	Reduced shoulder disability, no significant changes in muscle strength.
S32 [61]	Wii Fit-based exercise program (exergaming and VR)	DHI 1.1—Client-targeted (therapy)	Physical performance, psychological support	Feasible for patients with access to gaming systems, moderate adherence, practical for psychological support and physical performance maintenance.	Usable and engaging, though adherence varies based on patient condition and technological access.	Suitable for maintaining physical performance and supporting mental health during chemotherapy.	Maintains physical performance, improves mental health	Maintained physical performance, improved anxiety and depression in hematologic malignancy patients.

WHO DHI: World Health Organization Digital Health Intervention; PA: physical activity; MVPA: moderate-to-vigorous physical activity; QoL: quality of life; 6MWT: Six-Minute Walk Test; BMI: Body Mass Index; HRQoL: health-related quality of life; NSCLC: non-small cell lung cancer.

3. Results

A total of 624 articles were retrieved from the initial search across various databases. After removing duplicates, 572 articles remained for the initial screening based on title and abstract. Forty-five articles were selected for full-text review, including those identified through backward citation searching. Ultimately, 32 studies met the inclusion criteria for analysis (Figure 1) [28].

A detailed summary of the included studies, including information on the authors, year and country of publication, study design, objective, population characteristics, technology type, objectives, interventions, measurement tools, and outcomes, is presented in Table 1.

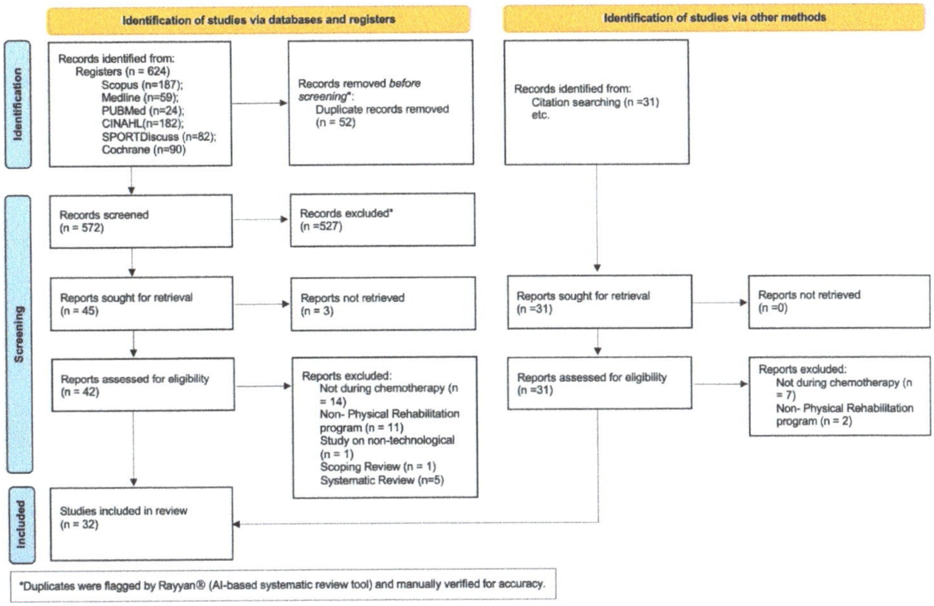

Figure 1. Article identification and inclusion process—PRISMA diagram flow (2020).

3.1. Characteristics of the Included Studies

Although there was no time limit set, the included studies span from 2013 to 2024 [27–58], with the majority published between 2018 and 2024 (S01, S03, S04, S05, S08, S09, S10, S11, S12, S13, S14, S16, S21, S22, S23, S26, S27, S29, and S31). The studies were conducted in various countries, highlighting the global interest in technological interventions for cancer rehabilitation. The most represented countries are the USA (S01, S09, S12, S13, S15, S19, and S29), Canada (S08, S10, S11, S24, and S27), and Germany (S04, S07, S12, and S17), with additional studies from every part of the globe (Brazil, Republic of Korea, China, Australia, Japan, France, Denmark, Sweden, Norway, and Turkey).

The study designs varied, with randomized controlled trials (RCTs) being the most common, used in nine studies (S04, S06, S09, S18, S19, S20, S22, S27, S31). This was followed by single-arm interventional studies, featured in eight studies (S01, S03, S09, S10, S12, S23, S29, S32). Pilot studies were conducted in five studies (S05, S08, S09, S10, S17), while feasibility studies appeared in four studies (S08, S11, S21, S32). Additionally, non-randomized controlled trials were used in two studies (S23, S30), and qualitative studies were included in two studies (S13, S14). The review also included one case report (S07) and two longitudinal observational studies (S15, S24).

The studies included in this review encompassed a diverse range of cancer patients, with populations varying in size, cancer type, and treatment phase. Most studies focused on patients undergoing chemotherapy at various stages of their treatment. A significant number of studies specifically targeted patients actively undergoing chemotherapy, including S01, S02, S04, S06, S08, S10, S11, S13, S15, S17, S18, and S19. Other studies included patients receiving multiple treatments, such as chemotherapy combined with other modalities (S03, S05, S07, S09, S12, S16, S20, S21, S23, and S32). A few studies focused on other treatment phases, such as cancer survivorship (S14, S24, S25). Sample sizes varied across the studies. The smallest study involved a single patient (S07), while the largest primary study included 112 participants (S25). Common cancer types were well-represented, including breast cancer (S01, S04, S05, S06, S12, S15, S18, S19, S21, S23, S27), colorectal cancer (S02, S09, S14, S23), lung cancer (S03, S08, S10, S13, S16, S22), multiple myeloma (S11, S13), and hematologic malignancies (S20, S32).

3.2. Characteristics of Technological Resources

Each technology in the reviewed studies was carefully implemented to address specific rehabilitation goals, including the promotion of physical activity, improvement of mental health, reduction in fatigue, and enhancement of quality of life for cancer patients during and after chemotherapy. The wide array of technological resources used in these interventions, such as wearable devices, mHealth applications, telerehabilitation platforms, VR, and AVGs, reflects the diverse approaches to supporting cancer rehabilitation. These resources can be systematically classified using the WHO Digital Health Intervention (DHI) v1.0 framework [29], which organizes interventions based on the target group—clients (e.g., self-monitoring and coaching), healthcare providers, or health systems. The majority of the interventions targeted clients, focusing on promoting physical activity, monitoring health parameters, and managing symptoms (DHI 1.1–1.4), as outlined in Table 1 [29].

Wearable devices emerged as one of the most widely used tools, particularly for monitoring physical activity, vital signs, and sleep patterns. According to the WHO DHI classification, these devices fall under DHI 1.2: Client-targeted monitoring interventions (S02, S07, S09, S15, S17-S24, S26-S29) [26]. For example, wearables like Fitbit (S09, S15) were commonly used to track steps and physical activity, while accelerometers such as the SenseWear (S22, S26) and ActiGraph (S29) provided continuous monitoring of physical activity and physiological metrics like heart rate and step count. Additionally, sports watches like the Polar V800 (S07) played a role in tracking exercise intensity during high-intensity training programs.

In conjunction with wearables, mHealth applications (apps) were frequently deployed to offer additional functionalities such as feedback, progress monitoring, and tailored rehabilitation programs. In studies like S02, S03, S04, S12, S13, and S16, these applications facilitated physical activity tracking and often included components such as dietary guidance, symptom management, and mental health support. These mHealth apps are categorized under DHI 1.1: Client-targeted digital interventions [29]. Notable examples include the PINK! app (S04, S12), which supported physical activity and provided nutritional and mental health guidance. Similarly, apps like GO-EXCAP (S13) and other smartphone-based applications (S16) facilitated exercise capacity tracking while offering psychological support to patients.

In addition to wearables and mobile apps, digital platforms (S01, S06, S08, S10, S11, S14, S25) enabled patients to participate in home-based rehabilitation programs, with real-time supervision and monitoring of physical exercises. These platforms, classified under DHI 1.4: Client-targeted support for rehabilitation and management, allowed healthcare providers to engage with patients remotely, offering interactive components that enhanced patient engagement and adherence to their rehabilitation programs [29].

Technologies also extended beyond monitoring and feedback into immersive environments such as VR-based interventions (S03, S32), which fall under DHI 1.4 [29]. These VR-based tools combined physical therapy with psychological support to improve both physical and mental well-being during cancer treatment.

AVGs were another innovative approach used in studies such as S05, S30, S31 and S32. Through exergames like Xbox Kinect and Nintendo Wii, patients engaged in gamified exercise programs aimed at improving endurance, strength, and functionality. These interventions are categorized under DHI 1.3: Client-targeted digital health education and training [29].

Furthermore, web-based platforms like the e-CuidateChemo platform (S08) and the Exercise Planning and Tracking (EPT) tool (S01) provided structured exercise programs for patients at home, mitigating physical decline associated with chemotherapy. These systems are classified as DHI 1.1: Client-targeted digital interventions for self-management [29], emphasizing their role in empowering patients to take control of their rehabilitation.

In summary, most of the studies (n = 13) focused on client-targeted interventions (DHI 1.0), with the primary goal of promoting physical activity, monitoring symptoms, and managing rehabilitation remotely [29]. Table 2 provides a comprehensive overview of the technological resources used in these studies, their WHO DHI classifications, functionalities, and key findings.

3.3. *Technological Functionalities*

The technological resources employed across the studies served a wide range of functionalities, categorized according to the WHO's DHI v1.0 classification [29]. A graphical representation of the technological resources and their functionalities is provided in Figure 2, illustrating the distribution of technologies across different categories, including physical activity tracking, exercise programs, symptom management, and mental health support.

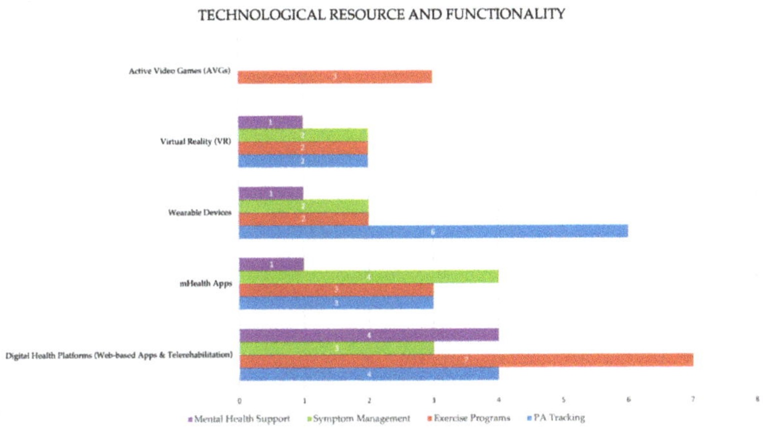

Figure 2. Distribution of technology types and functionalities.

A primary functionality observed was "client-targeted tools for self-monitoring" of physical activity (DHI 1.2), predominantly using wearables. These devices, including Fitbits, accelerometers, and pedometers, were widely used to monitor exercise intensity, track steps, and assess physical activity levels across studies like S02, S03, S09, S11, S13, S16, S22, S23, S25, and S29. Increased adherence to physical activity guidelines was commonly reported with these tools. For instance, the use of Fitbits in S09 was associated with improved step counts and walking distance. Similarly, pedometers and activity trackers in S21, S23, and S25 were linked to enhanced physical activity levels and reductions in sedentary behavior.

Beyond monitoring, several technologies also supported structured exercise programs, classified under "client-targeted therapy" (DHI 1.1). Mobile Health applications (e.g., S02, S05) and telerehabilitation platforms (e.g., S08, S10, S13) allowed patients to engage in structured exercise regimens incorporating both strength and aerobic training. Notably, studies like S01, S06, S12, S18, S20, S30, and S31 demonstrated how web-based or interactive rehabilitation tools contributed to improvements in physical function, endurance, and muscle strength. Furthermore, exergaming technologies in studies such as S20, S30, and S31 provided engaging, interactive exercises, enhancing upper extremity functionality and shoulder mobility.

In addition to physical rehabilitation, several technological resources extended their functionalities to include symptom management and mental health support. For example, wearables in studies like S03 and S13 helped monitor symptoms such as fatigue and psychological distress, enabling patients to manage both the physical and emotional impacts of their treatment. Similarly, VR-based interventions (e.g., S03, S30) contributed not only to physical rehabilitation but also to the improvement of mental health outcomes, reducing anxiety and depression. The PINK! app (e.g., S04, S12) effectively supported mental well-being by reducing psychological distress and fatigue in breast cancer patients.

4. Discussion

This scoping review highlights the potential of technological tools to enhance physical rehabilitation in cancer patients undergoing chemotherapy. The 32 studies analyzed employed a variety of technologies, including wearable devices, mHealth apps, digital platforms (web-based apps and telerehabilitation), VR, and exergaming systems, with a predominant focus on client-targeted functionalities. These tools were found to address critical rehabilitation needs, such as improving adherence to physical activity protocols, enhancing functional capacity, and managing chemotherapy-related side effects.

Wearable devices, such as Fitbits and accelerometers (such as SenseWear, ActiGraph and sports watches), emerged as the most frequently used technology [31,38,44,45]. Primarily serving as self-monitoring tools (DHI 1.2), wearables tracked metrics like steps, heart rate, and sleep patterns. Real-time feedback provided by these devices was shown to improve adherence to physical activity guidelines. For instance, a study in 2022 [38] demonstrated that using Fitbit increased step count and walking distance in colorectal cancer patients during chemotherapy. Similarly, research conducted in 2019 [45] showed the effectiveness of SenseWear in tracking physical performance among advanced lung cancer patients. The feasibility and usability of wearables were consistently high across studies, with patients successfully integrating these tools into their daily lives. A 2017 study [44] found that the Fitbit Zip effectively supported real-time feedback on physical activity, helping patients meet recommended activity levels during breast cancer treatment. Patients showed strong adherence to wearable devices, finding them easy to use even during demanding chemotherapy cycles, as demonstrated in studies [31,44]. These wearables, particularly Fitbit and accelerometers, proved effective in promoting adherence to physical activity, which is essential for maintaining functionality during chemotherapy.

Similarly, mHealth applications and telerehabilitation platforms also demonstrated high usability. Platforms such as eChez-Soi and GO-EXCAP provided real-time feedback and personalized interventions, which patients found intuitive and motivating [37,42]. These tools helped sustain engagement and adherence, particularly when real-time feedback was incorporated into their functionality. However, advanced technologies like VR presented challenges, as access to devices and technological literacy posed barriers for some patients, as noted in studies [32,61].

The technologies evaluated in this review were largely suitable for cancer rehabilitation. Wearable devices were particularly effective in tracking physical activity, a critical component of rehabilitation during chemotherapy [31,44]. Telerehabilitation platforms provided a valuable solution for patients with limited mobility or those living far from treatment centers, as highlighted in studies [37,39]. These platforms enabled remote supervision and interaction with healthcare providers, allowing patients to participate in structured exercise programs from home. However, more complex technologies, such as VR and exergaming, proved more beneficial for younger or tech-savvy patients who were more familiar with gaming systems, as seen in studies [46,60].

Mobile health applications were widely used across studies to support structured exercise programs and symptom management. For instance, the PINK! app was particularly effective in reducing psychological distress and fatigue among breast cancer patients, while GO-EXCAP provided tailored, home-based exercise programs that promoted patient autonomy [41,42]. These applications, categorized as client-targeted interventions for self-management (DHI 1.1), addressed areas such as physical activity, nutrition, and mental health coaching, with high feasibility and engagement, even when patients experienced treatment-related fatigue [42].

Telerehabilitation platforms and web-based applications, as demonstrated in studies such as [36,37], enabled patients to receive remote supervision for their rehabilitation exercises. These platforms, classified under remote care interventions (DHI 1.1), allowed for real-time monitoring and provided feedback, which improved functional capacity and endurance. For example, the eChez-Soi platform [37] achieved high patient satisfaction and notable functional improvements, particularly among lung cancer patients who found it difficult to attend in-person rehabilitation sessions [39].

Virtual reality and exergaming systems were explored in four studies [32,46], offering a more interactive and engaging approach to rehabilitation. Virtual reality was shown to improve body composition and reduce fatigue, as demonstrated in one study [32], while exergaming systems (e.g., Xbox Kinect) used in [46] engaged patients in gamified exercises to enhance muscle function and increase physical activity levels. Although these technologies provided high levels of engagement, their adoption was limited by patient access and familiarity with the devices.

Across the studies, the feasibility of these technologies was consistently rated as high. Wearables like Fitbits and accelerometers demonstrated strong usability and adherence, while telerehabilitation platforms provided an accessible and flexible alternative to in-person rehabilitation. However, advanced technologies like VR faced challenges related to technological literacy and access, limiting their widespread adoption.

The findings of this scoping review align with previous studies that underscore the increasing role of digital health interventions in cancer rehabilitation. Wearable devices and mHealth applications, such as those used to monitor physical activity and manage symptoms, have demonstrated significant potential in improving patient adherence to rehabilitation protocols [17,18]. These technologies not only offer real-time feedback but also facilitate self-management, resulting in improved patient outcomes and satisfaction. However, the integration of more advanced technologies like VR poses challenges, including technological literacy and access [19]. Despite these barriers, VR has been effective in reducing symptoms such as anxiety, pain, and fatigue, emphasizing its potential in cancer rehabilitation. Furthermore, a study [62] has highlighted the importance of balancing the benefits of exercise programs with the potential risks, especially for patients undergoing systemic treatments. Addressing barriers and facilitators, as identified in another study [63], is crucial for ensuring broader adoption and success of digital health tools in oncology care.

Challenges and Limitations

This scoping review identified several challenges when analyzing technological resources for physical rehabilitation in cancer patients undergoing chemotherapy. A significant challenge was the diversity of technologies across the 32 included studies. Interventions ranged from simple wearables like pedometers and accelerometers [31,44,47] to advanced systems like VR and exergaming [32,59], as well as telerehabilitation platforms [37,39]. This diversity made it challenging to categorize and analyze the technologies due to differences in technological complexity and functionality. The technologies were classified using the WHO DHI framework to streamline the analysis.

Another challenge was the inconsistency in study designs, outcomes, and reporting. Some studies were large-scale trials [39,42], while others were smaller pilot studies or case reports [36,38], making direct comparisons difficult. Moreover, few studies provided detailed long-term adherence data, limiting insights into the sustainability of interventions. Although some studies [31,44] reported high adherence to wearables and mHealth apps, the lack of longitudinal data restricted a comprehensive understanding of their long-term impact.

Access to technology and digital literacy were also significant barriers. Advanced interventions, such as VR and telerehabilitation [32,46], posed challenges for older patients or those with limited technological experience. Additionally, telerehabilitation platforms [37] required reliable internet access, which was not always available for patients in rural or low-resource settings, further contributing to disparities in access.

Moreover, there was a lack of personalized interventions. Most technologies followed a standardized approach, which may not have addressed the individual needs of cancer patients. Only a few studies [38] offered tailored interventions based on patient preferences or abilities, and this lack of customization may have impacted patient engagement and outcomes.

Finally, limited evidence exists on the cost-effectiveness of these technological interventions. While the studies demonstrated the feasibility and usability of wearables and mHealth apps [33,41], none provided a comprehensive cost analysis. This absence of cost-effectiveness data raises concerns about the scalability and equitable application of these interventions in broader clinical practice.

5. Conclusions

This scoping review mapped various technological resources used for physical rehabilitation in cancer patients undergoing chemotherapy, including wearables, mobile-based applications, telerehabilitation, web-based platforms, virtual reality, and exergames. These technologies may have the potential to improve physical function, manage symptoms, and enhance quality of life. However, despite the positive outcomes in the short term, their long-term effectiveness remains uncertain and requires further validation through clinical trials. The diversity of tools such as mHealth apps (e.g., the PINK! app) and wearables like Fitbit illustrates the broad range of options available for cancer rehabilitation, though personalization and sustained engagement are areas that need enhancement. A key challenge identified was patient adherence, particularly due to factors such as fatigue and low motivation, which are common in patients undergoing chemotherapy. However, technologies that provided real-time feedback, such as wearables and specific mHealth apps, showed promise in improving engagement with rehabilitation programs. Future research should prioritize the development of more personalized interventions tailored to patients' individual needs and preferences, which can improve adherence and optimize rehabilitation outcomes.

Additionally, evaluating the cost-effectiveness and accessibility of these technologies is crucial, especially for underserved and low-resource populations. Overcoming barriers to access, including digital exclusion, is essential to ensure that these technological resources are equitably available to all cancer patients, thus maximizing their rehabilitation potential.

Author Contributions: Conceptualization, A.A. and C.S.F.; methodology, A.A. and C.S.F.; software, A.A. and C.S.F.; validation, M.M., B.A., and M.C.F.; formal analysis, A.A. and C.S.F.; data curation, A.A. and C.S.F.; writing—original draft preparation, A.A.; writing—review and editing, C.S.F. All authors have read and agreed to the published version of the manuscript.

Funding: This research received no external funding.

Conflicts of Interest: The authors are solely responsible for the content and writing of the paper. The authors report no conflicts of interest.

Appendix A

Table A1. Research strategies according to the database.

Database	Research Strategy
Medline	(((MH "Neoplasms") OR ("Cancer patients") OR (MH "Cancer Survivors") OR (MH "Chemotherapy, Adjuvant") OR (MH "Antineoplastic Agents") OR ("Chemotherapy")) AND ((MH "Technology") OR (MH "Health Resources") OR (MH "Digital Technology") OR (MH "Biomedical Technology") OR (MH "Digital Health") OR (MH "Wearable Electronic Devices") OR ("technological resources")) AND ((MH "Rehabilitation") OR (MH "Physical Therapists") OR (MH "Rehabilitation Nursing") OR (MH "Physical and Rehabilitation Medicine") OR ("physical rehabilitation") OR (MH "Physical Education and Training") OR (MH "Exercise") OR (MH "Telerehabilitation") OR (MH "Exercise Therapy") OR ("Exercise")))

Table A1. *Cont.*

Database	Research Strategy
CINAHL	(((MM "Cancer Patients") OR (MH "Antineoplastic Agents") OR (MH "Chemotherapy, Cancer") OR (MH "Chemotherapy, Adjuvant") OR ("Cancer patients") OR ("Cancer Survivors") OR ("Chemotherapy")) AND ((MH "Health Resource Utilization") OR (MH "Assistive Technology Services") OR (MH "Telerehabilitation") OR (MH "Digital Technology") OR ("Technology") OR ("Health Resources") OR ("Digital Technology") OR ("Biomedical Technology") OR ("Digital Health") OR ("Wearable Electronic Devices") OR ("technological resources") OR ("eHealth")) AND ((MH "Rehabilitation") OR (MH "Rehabilitation, Cancer") OR (MH "Therapeutic Exercise") OR (MH "Aerobic Exercises") OR (MH "Muscle Strengthening") OR (MH "Physical and Rehabilitation Medicine") OR (MM "Exercise Therapy") OR ("Physical Therapists") OR ("Rehabilitation Nursing") OR ("Physical and Rehabilitation Medicine") OR ("Physical Rehabilitation") OR ("Physical Education and Training") OR ("Exercise") OR ("Telerehabilitation") OR ("Exercise Therapy")))
Sport Discus	(((DE "CANCER chemotherapy") OR (DE "CANCER patients") OR ("Cancer patients") OR ("Chemotherapy")) AND ((DE "SPORTS & technology") OR ("Digital Health") OR ("Technological Resources") OR ("Technology") OR ("Health Resources") OR ("Digital Technology") OR ("Biomedical Technology") OR ("Wearable Electronic Devices")) AND ((DE "PHYSICAL therapy") OR (DE "EXERCISE") OR (DE "EXERCISE therapy") OR ("Rehabilitation") OR ("Physical Therapists") OR ("Rehabilitation Nursing") OR ("Physical and Rehabilitation Medicine") OR ("physical rehabilitation") OR ("Physical Education and Training") OR ("Exercise") OR ("Telerehabilitation") OR ("Exercise Therapy")))
Scopus	(TITLE-ABS-KEY (("Chemotherapy Cancer") OR ("Chemotherapy") OR ("Antineoplastic Agents")) AND TITLE-ABS-KEY (("Technology") OR ("Health Resources") OR ("Digital Technology") OR ("Biomedical Technology") OR ("Digital Health") OR ("Wearable Electronic Devices") OR ("technological resources")) AND TITLE-ABS-KEY (("Exercise") OR ("Exercise Therapy") OR ("Rehabilitation") OR ("physical rehabilitation") OR ("Rehabilitation Cancer")))
Cochrane	(((MH "Neoplasms") OR ("Cancer patients") OR (MH "Cancer Survivors") OR (MH "Chemotherapy, Adjuvant") OR (MH "Antineoplastic Agents") OR ("Chemotherapy")) AND ((MH "Technology") OR (MH "Health Resources") OR (MH "Digital Technology") OR (MH "Biomedical Technology") OR (MH "Digital Health") OR (MH "Wearable Electronic Devices") OR ("technological resources")) AND ((MH "Rehabilitation") OR (MH "Physical Therapists") OR (MH "Rehabilitation Nursing") OR (MH "Physical and Rehabilitation Medicine") OR ("physical rehabilitation") OR (MH "Physical Education and Training") OR (MH "Exercise") OR (MH "Telerehabilitation") OR (MH "Exercise Therapy") OR ("Exercise")))

References

1. Siegel, R.L.; Giaquinto, A.N.; Jemal, A. Cancer statistics, 2024. *CA Cancer J. Clin.* **2024**, *74*, 12–49. [CrossRef] [PubMed]
2. Jokhadze, N.; Arunangshu, D.; Dizon, D.S. Global cancer statistics: A healthy population relies on population health. *CA Cancer J. Clin.* **2024**, *74*, 224–226. [CrossRef] [PubMed]
3. World Health Organization. *Cancer [Internet]*; World Health Organization: Geneva, Switzerland, 2020. Available online: https://www.who.int/news-room/fact-sheets/detail/cancer (accessed on 1 October 2024).
4. The Global Cancer Observatory. Cancer Incidence and Mortality Worldwide: *GLOBOCAN* 2022 [Internet]. 2022. Available online: https://gco.iarc.fr/ (accessed on 1 October 2024).
5. International Agency for Research on Cancer (IARC). Cancer Tomorrow [Internet]. *GLOBOCAN*. 2022. (Version 1.1). Available online: https://gco.iarc.who.int/tomorrow/en/about (accessed on 1 October 2024).
6. Anand, U.; Dey, A.; Chandel, A.K.S.; Sanyal, R.; Mishra, A.; Pandey, D.K.; De Falco, V.; Upadhyay, A.; Kandimalla, R.; Chaudhary, A.; et al. Cancer chemotherapy and beyond: Current status, drug candidates, associated risks and progress in targeted therapeutics. *Genes Dis.* **2022**, *10*, 1367–1401. [CrossRef] [PubMed]
7. Lustberg, M.B.; Kuderer, N.M.; Desai, A.; Bergerot, C.; Lyman, G.H. Mitigating long-term and delayed adverse events associated with cancer treatment: Implications for survivorship. *Nat. Rev. Clin. Oncol.* **2023**, *20*, 527–542. [CrossRef] [PubMed]
8. Brianna; Lee, S.H. Chemotherapy: How to reduce its adverse effects while maintaining the potency? *Med. Oncol.* **2023**, *40*, 88. [CrossRef]
9. Penna, G.B.; Otto, D.M.; da Silva, T.C.; Pedroni, A.S.; Macagnan, F.E. Physical rehabilitation for the management of cancer-related fatigue during cytotoxic treatment: A systematic review with meta-analysis. *Support. Care Cancer Off. J. Multinatl. Assoc. Support. Care Cancer* **2023**, *31*, 129. [CrossRef]
10. Alhinai, H. *Supportive Exercises For Cancer Patients*; IntechOpen: London, UK, 2024. [CrossRef]

11. Herranz-Gómez, A.; Suso-Martí, L.; Varangot-Reille, C.; Barrachina-Gauchia, L.; Casaña, J.; López-Bueno, L.; Calatayud, J.; Cuenca-Martínez, F. The Benefit of Exercise in Patients With Cancer Who Are Receiving Chemotherapy: A Systematic Review and Network Meta-Analysis. *Phys. Ther.* **2024**, *104*, pzad132. [CrossRef]
12. Qiu, L.; Ye, M.; Tong, Y.; Jin, Y. Promoting physical activity among cancer survivors: An umbrella review of systematic reviews. *Support. Care Cancer* **2023**, *31*, 301. [CrossRef]
13. Elshahat, S.; Treanor, C.; Donnelly, M. Factors influencing physical activity participation among people living with or beyond cancer: A systematic scoping review. *Int. J. Behav. Nutr. Phys. Act.* **2021**, *18*, 50. [CrossRef]
14. Collado-Mateo, D.; Lavín-Pérez, A.M.; Peñacoba, C.; Del Coso, J.; Leyton-Román, M.; Luque-Casado, A.; Gasque, P.; Fernández-Del-Olmo, M.Á.; Amado-Alonso, D. Key Factors Associated with Adherence to Physical Exercise in Patients with Chronic Diseases and Older Adults: An Umbrella Review. *Int. J. Environ. Res. Public Health* **2021**, *18*, 2023. [CrossRef]
15. Winstein, C.; Requejo, P. Innovative technologies for rehabilitation and health promotion: What is the evidence? *Phys. Ther.* **2015**, *95*, 294–298. [CrossRef] [PubMed]
16. Szabo, D.A.; Neagu, N.; Teodorescu, S.; Apostu, M.; Predescu, C.; Pârvu, C.; Veres, C. The Role and Importance of Using Sensor-Based Devices in Medical Rehabilitation: A Literature Review on the New Therapeutic Approaches. *Sensors* **2023**, *23*, 8950. [CrossRef] [PubMed]
17. Magalhães, B.; Fernandes, C.; Martinez-Galiano, J.M.; Santos, C. Exploring the use of Mobile applications by cancer patients undergoing chemotherapy: A scoping review. *Int. J. Med. Inform.* **2020**, *144*, 104293. [CrossRef] [PubMed]
18. Parikh, R.B.; Basen-Enquist, K.M.; Bradley, C.; Estrin, D.; Levy, M.; Lichtenfeld, J.L.; Malin, B.; McGraw, D.; Meropol, N.J.; Oyer, R.A.; et al. Digital Health Applications in Oncology: An Opportunity to Seize. *J. Natl. Cancer Inst.* **2022**, *114*, 1338–1339. [CrossRef]
19. Fereidooni, M.; Toni, E.; Toni, E.; Ayatollahi, H. Application of virtual reality for supportive care in cancer patients: A systematic review. *Support. Care Cancer* **2024**, *32*, 570. [CrossRef] [PubMed]
20. Haemmerle, R.; Paludo, J.; Haddad, T.C.; Pritchett, J.C. The Growing Role of Digital Health Tools in the Care of Patients with Cancer: Current Use, Future Opportunities, and Barriers to Effective Implementation. *Curr. Oncol. Rep.* **2024**, *26*, 593–600. [CrossRef]
21. Shi, N.; Wong, A.K.C.; Wong, F.K.Y.; Sha, L. Mobile Health Application-Based Interventions to Improve Self-management of Chemotherapy-Related Symptoms Among People with Breast Cancer Who Are Undergoing Chemotherapy: A Systematic Review. *Oncologist* **2023**, *28*, e175–e182. [CrossRef]
22. Munn, Z.; Pollock, D.; Khalil, H.; Alexander, L.; Mclnerney, P.; Godfrey, C.M.; Peters, M.; Tricco, A.C. What are scoping reviews? Providing a formal definition of scoping reviews as a type of evidence synthesis. *JBI Evid. Synth.* **2022**, *20*, 950–952. [CrossRef] [PubMed]
23. Peters, M.D.J.; Godfrey, C.; Mclnerney, P.; Munn, Z.; Tricco, A.C.; Khalil, H. Scoping Reviews. In *JBI Manual for Evidence Synthesis*; Aromataris, E., Lockwood, C., Porritt, K., Pilla, B., Jordan, Z., Eds.; JBI: Adelaide, Australia, 2024. [CrossRef]
24. Peters, M.D.J.; Marnie, C.; Colquhoun, H.; Garritty, C.M.; Hempel, S.; Horsley, T.; Langlois, E.V.; Lillie, E.; O'Brien, K.K.; Tunçalp, Ö.; et al. Scoping reviews: Reinforcing and advancing the methodology and application. *Syst. Rev.* **2021**, *10*, 263. [CrossRef]
25. Tricco, A.C.; Lillie, E.; Zarin, W.; O'Brien, K.K.; Colquhoun, H.; Levac, D.; Moher, D.; Peters, M.D.J.; Horsley, T.; Weeks, L.; et al. PRISMA Extension for Scoping Reviews (PRISMA-ScR): Checklist and Explanation. *Ann. Intern. Med.* **2018**, *169*, 467–473. [CrossRef]
26. Hammady, M.; Fedorowicz, Z.; Elmagarmid, A. Rayyan—A web and mobile app for systematic reviews. *Systematic Reviews.* **2016**, *5*, 210. [CrossRef]
27. Pollock, D.; Peters, M.D.J.; Khalil, H.; Mclnerney, P.; Alexander, L.; Tricco, A.C.; Evans, C.; de Moraes, É.B.; Godfrey, C.M.; Pieper, D.; et al. Recommendations for the extraction, analysis, and presentation of results in scoping reviews. *JBI Evid. Synth.* **2023**, *21*, 520–532. [CrossRef] [PubMed]
28. Page, M.J.; McKenzie, J.E.; Bossuyt, P.M.; Boutron, I.; Hoffmann, T.C.; Mulrow, C.D.; Shamseer, L.; Tetzlaff, J.M.; Moher, D. Updating guidance for reporting systematic reviews: Development of the PRISMA 2020 statement. *J. Clin. Epidemiol.* **2021**, *134*, 103–112. [CrossRef] [PubMed]
29. World Health Organization. *Classification of Digital Health Interventions v1.0: A Shared Language to Describe the Uses of Digital Technology for Health [Internet]*; World Health Organization: Geneva, Switzerland, 2018. Available online: https://apps.who.int/iris/handle/10665/260480 (accessed on 1 October 2024).
30. Albrecht, T.; Chen, Y.; Allen, D.; Pastva, A.; Tian, Z.; Lin, Y.; Bold, D.; Hu, X.; Xiao, R. Digital Health Innovations to Promote Physical Activities in Patients with Cancer. *Stud. Health Technol. Inform.* **2024**, *315*, 608–609. [CrossRef] [PubMed]
31. Cheong, I.Y.; An, S.Y.; Cha, W.C.; Rha, M.Y.; Kim, S.T.; Chang, D.K.; Hwang, J.H. Efficacy of Mobile Health Care Application and Wearable Device in Improvement of Physical Performance in Colorectal Cancer Patients Undergoing Chemotherapy. *Clin. Color. Cancer* **2018**, *17*, e353–e362. [CrossRef]
32. Qi, Y.; Wang, M.; Xue, Y.; Yue, J.; Qi, C.; Shang, W.; Meng, W.; Zhu, W.; Pu, X.; Li, D.; et al. Feasibility of an exercise-nutrition-psychology integrated rehabilitation model based on mobile health and virtual reality for cancer patients: A single-center, single-arm, prospective phase II study. *BMC Palliat. Care* **2024**, *23*, 155. [CrossRef]
33. Wolff, J.; Wuelfing, P.; Koenig, A.; Ehrl, B.; Damsch, J.; Smollich, M.; Baumann, F.T.; Harbeck, N.; Wuerstlein, R. App-Based Lifestyle Coaching (PINK!) Accompanying Breast Cancer Patients and Survivors to Reduce Psychological Distress and Fatigue and Improve Physical Activity: A Feasibility Pilot Study. *Breast Care* **2023**, *18*, 354–365. [CrossRef]

34. Feyzioğlu, Ö.; Öztürk, Ö.; Dinçer, S.; Akan, A. Acute effects of video game-based exercises in patients receiving chemotherapy after breast cancer surgery: A pilot study. *Turk. J. Oncol.* **2021**, *36*, 1–6. [CrossRef]
35. Ariza-Garcia, A.; Lozano-Lozano, M.; Galiano-Castillo, N.; Postigo-Martin, P.; Arroyo-Morales, M.; Cantarero-Villanueva, I. A Web-Based Exercise System (e-CuidateChemo) to Counter the Side Effects of Chemotherapy in Patients With Breast Cancer: Randomized Controlled Trial. *J. Med. Internet Res.* **2019**, *21*, e14418. [CrossRef]
36. Troschel, F.M.; Brandt, R.; Wiewrodt, R.; Stummer, W.; Wiewrodt, D. High-Intensity Physical Exercise in a Glioblastoma Patient under Multimodal Treatment. *Med. Sci. Sports Exerc.* **2019**, *51*, 2429–2433. [CrossRef]
37. Coats, V.; Moffet, H.; Vincent, C.; Simard, S.; Tremblay, L.; Maltais, F.; Saey, D. Feasibility of an eight-week telerehabilitation intervention for patients with unresectable thoracic neoplasia receiving chemotherapy: A pilot study. *Can J Respir Crit Care Sleep Med.* **2019**, *4*, 14–24. [CrossRef]
38. Van Blarigan, E.L.; Dhruva, A.; Atreya, C.E.; Kenfield, S.A.; Chan, J.M.; Milloy, A.; Kim, I.; Steiding, P.; Laffan, A.; Zhang, L.; et al. Feasibility and Acceptability of a Physical Activity Tracker and Text Messages to Promote Physical Activity During Chemotherapy for Colorectal Cancer: Pilot Randomized Controlled Trial (Smart Pace II). *JMIR Cancer* **2022**, *8*, e31576. [CrossRef] [PubMed]
39. Moffet, H.; Saey, D.; Coats, V.; Vincent, C.; Choinière, F.; Comeau, F. Reliability and usability of the eChez-Soi in-home telerehabilitation platform: A new internet-based communication and real-time monitoring software solution combined with interactive exercises-Results of a longitudinal pilot study in four patients with lung cancer. In Proceedings of the ICT4AgeingWell 2015, Lisbon, Portugal, 20–22 May 2015; pp. 137–142. [CrossRef]
40. Purdy, G.M.; Venner, C.P.; Tandon, P.; McNeely, M.L. Feasibility of a tailored and virtually supported home exercise program for people with multiple myeloma using a novel eHealth application. *Digit. Health* **2022**, *8*, 20552076221129066. [CrossRef] [PubMed]
41. Wolff, J.; Smollich, M.; Wuelfing, P.; Mitchell, J.; Wuerstlein, R.; Harbeck, N.; Baumann, F. App-Based Lifestyle Intervention (PINK! Coach) in Breast Cancer Patients-A Real-World-Data Analysis. *Cancers* **2024**, *16*, 1020. [CrossRef] [PubMed]
42. Loh, K.P.; Sanapala, C.; Di Giovanni, G.; Klepin, H.D.; Janelsins, M.; Schnall, R.; Culakova, E.; Vertino, P.; Susiarjo, M.; Mendler, J.H.; et al. Developing and adapting a mobile health exercise intervention for older patients with myeloid neoplasms: A qualitative study. *J. Geriatr. Oncol.* **2021**, *12*, 909–914. [CrossRef]
43. Romero-Elías, M.; Gonzalez-Cutre, D.; Ruiz-Casado, A.; Ferriz, R.; Navarro-Espejo, N.; Beltran-Carrillo, V.J. Exploring the perceived benefits of a motivational exercise program (FIT-CANCER) in colorectal cancer patients during chemotherapy treatment: A qualitative study from self-determination theory. *Eur. J. Integr. Med.* **2023**, *65*, 102328. [CrossRef]
44. Nyrop, K.A.; Deal, A.M.; Choi, S.K.; Wagoner, C.W.; Lee, J.T.; Wood, W.A.; Anders, C.; Carey, L.A.; Dees, E.C.; Jolly, T.A.; et al. Measuring and understanding adherence in a home-based exercise intervention during chemotherapy for early breast cancer. *Breast Cancer Res. Treat.* **2018**, *168*, 43–55. [CrossRef]
45. Park, S.; Kim, J.Y.; Lee, J.C.; Kim, H.R.; Song, S.; Kwon, H.; Ji, W.; Choi, C.M. Mobile Phone App-Based Pulmonary Rehabilitation for Chemotherapy-Treated Patients With Advanced Lung Cancer: Pilot Study. *JMIR mHealth uHealth* **2019**, *7*, e11094. [CrossRef]
46. Villaron, C.; Cury, F.; Eisinger, F.; Cappiello, M.A.; Marqueste, T. Telehealth applied to physical activity during cancer treatment: A feasibility, acceptability, and randomized pilot study. *Support. Care Cancer* **2018**, *26*, 3413–3421. [CrossRef]
47. Backman, M.; Wengström, Y.; Johansson, B.; Sköldengen, I.; Börjesson, S.; Tärnbro, S.; Berglund, Å. A randomized pilot study with daily walking during adjuvant chemotherapy for patients with breast and colorectal cancer. *Acta Oncol.* **2014**, *53*, 510–520. [CrossRef]
48. Gokal, K.; Wallis, D.; Ahmed, S.; Boiangiu, I.; Kancherla, K.; Munir, F. Effects of a self-managed home-based walking intervention on psychosocial health outcomes for breast cancer patients receiving chemotherapy: A randomised controlled trial. *Support. Care Cancer Off. J. Multinatl. Assoc. Support. Care Cancer* **2016**, *24*, 1139–1166. [CrossRef] [PubMed]
49. Jarden, M.; Møller, T.; Christensen, K.B.; Kjeldsen, L.; Birgens, H.S.; Adamsen, L. Multimodal intervention integrated into the clinical management of acute leukemia improves physical function and quality of life during consolidation chemotherapy: A randomized trial 'PACE-AL'. *Haematologica* **2016**, *101*, e316–e319. [CrossRef] [PubMed]
50. Delrieu, L.; Pialoux, V.; Pérol, O.; Morelle, M.; Martin, A.; Friedenreich, C.; Febvey-Combes, O.; Pérol, D.; Belladame, E.; Clémençon, M.; et al. Feasibility and Health Benefits of an Individualized Physical Activity Intervention in Women With Metastatic Breast Cancer: Intervention Study. *JMIR mHealth uHealth* **2020**, *8*, e12306. [CrossRef]
51. Edbrooke, L.; Granger, C.L.; Clark, R.A.; Denehy, L. Physical Activity Levels Are Low in Inoperable Lung Cancer: Exploratory Analyses from a Randomised Controlled Trial. *J. Clin. Med.* **2019**, *8*, 1288. [CrossRef]
52. Gandhi, A.; Samuel, S.R.; Kumar, K.V.; Saxena, P.P.; Mithra, P. Effect of a Pedometer-based Exercise Program on Cancer Related Fatigue and Quality of Life amongst Patients with Breast Cancer Receiving Chemotherapy. *Asian Pac. J. Cancer Prev.* **2020**, *21*, 1813–1818. [CrossRef]
53. Lowe, S.S.; Watanabe, S.M.; Baracos, V.E.; Courneya, K.S. Home-based functional walking program for advanced cancer patients receiving palliative care: A case series. *BMC Palliat. Care* **2013**, *12*, 22. [CrossRef]
54. Marthick, M.; Dhillon, H.M.; Alison, J.A.; Cheema, B.S.; Shaw, T. An Interactive Web Portal for Tracking Oncology Patient Physical Activity and Symptoms: Prospective Cohort Study. *JMIR Cancer* **2018**, *4*, e11978. [CrossRef]
55. Nilsson, M.; Arving, C.; Thormodsen, I.; Assmus, J.; Berntsen, S.; Nordin, K. Moderate-to-vigorous intensity physical activity is associated with modified fatigue during and after cancer treatment. *Support. Care Cancer* **2020**, *28*, 3343–3350. [CrossRef] [PubMed]

56. Vallance, J.K.; Friedenreich, C.M.; Lavallee, C.M.; Culos-Reed, N.; Mackey, J.R.; Walley, B.; Courneya, K.S. Exploring the Feasibility of a Broad-Reach Physical Activity Behavior Change Intervention for Women Receiving Chemotherapy for Breast Cancer: A Randomized Trial. *Cancer Epidemiol. Biomark. Prev.* **2016**, *25*, 391–398. [CrossRef]
57. Mouri, T.; Naito, T.; Morikawa, A.; Tatematsu, N.; Miura, S.; Okayama, T.; Omae, K.; Takayama, K. Promotion of Behavioral Change and the Impact on Quality of Life in Elderly Patients with Advanced Cancer: A Physical Activity Intervention of the Multimodal Nutrition and Exercise Treatment for Advanced Cancer Program. *Asia-Pac. J. Oncol. Nurs.* **2018**, *5*, 383–390. [CrossRef]
58. Parker, N.H.; Ngo-Huang, A.; Lee, R.E.; O'Connor, D.P.; Basen-Engquist, K.M.; Petzel MQ, B.; Wang, X.; Xiao, L.; Fogelman, D.R.; Schadler, K.L.; et al. Physical activity and exercise during preoperative pancreatic cancer treatment. *Support. Care Cancer Off. J. Multinatl. Assoc. Support. Care Cancer* **2019**, *27*, 2275–2284. [CrossRef] [PubMed]
59. Oliveira, P.F.; Iunes, D.H.; Alves, R.S.; Carvalho, J.M.; Menezes, F.S.; Carvalho, L.C. Effects of Exergaming in Cancer Related Fatigue in the Quality of Life and Electromyography of the Middle Deltoid of People with Cancer in Treatment: A Controlled Trial. *Asian Pac. J. Cancer Prev. APJCP* **2018**, *19*, 2591–2597. [CrossRef] [PubMed]
60. de Oliveira, P.F.; Alves RD, S.; Iunes, D.H.; de Carvalho, J.M.; Borges JB, C.; Menezes FD, S.; Carvalho, L.C. Effect of Exergaming on Muscle Strength, Pain, and Functionality of Shoulders in Cancer Patients. *Games Health J.* **2020**, *9*, 297–303. [CrossRef] [PubMed]
61. Tsuda, K.; Sudo, K.; Goto, G.; Takai, M.; Itokawa, T.; Isshiki, T.; Takei, N.; Tanimoto, T.; Komatsu, T. A Feasibility Study of Virtual Reality Exercise in Elderly Patients with Hematologic Malignancies Receiving Chemotherapy. *Intern. Med.* **2016**, *55*, 347–352. [CrossRef] [PubMed]
62. Thomsen, S.N.; Lahart, I.M.; Thomsen, L.M.; Fridh, M.K.; Larsen, A.; Mau-Sørensen, M.; Bolam, K.A.; Fairman, C.M.; Christensen, J.F.; Simonsen, C. Harms of exercise training in patients with cancer undergoing systemic treatment: A systematic review and meta-analysis of published and unpublished controlled trials. *eClinicalMedicine* **2023**, *59*, 101937. [CrossRef]
63. Bamgboje-Ayodele, A.; Smith, A.; Short, C.E.; Fardell, J.E.; Shaw, J.; Beatty, L.; Higgins, K.; Tutelman, P.R.; Chambers, C.T.; Girgis, A. Barriers and facilitators to the availability of efficacious self-directed digital health tools for adults living with cancer and their caregivers: A systematic literature review and author survey study. *Patient Educ. Couns.* **2021**, *104*, 2480–2489. [CrossRef]

cancers

MDPI

Systematic Review

Racial and Socioeconomic Disparity in Breast Cancer Mortality: A Systematic Review and Meta-Analysis

Helena Fiats Ribeiro [1,*], Fernando Castilho Pelloso [2], Beatriz Sousa da Fonseca [3], Camila Wohlenberg Camparoto [1], Maria Dalva de Barros Carvalho [1], Vlaudimir Dias Marques [1], Mariá Romanio Bitencourt [1], Kely Paviani Stevanato [1], Pedro Beraldo Borba [4], Deise Helena Pelloso Borghesan [5], Paulo Acácio Egger [1], Ana Carolina Jacinto Alarcão [1], Roberto Kenji Nakamura Cuman [1], Isabella Morais Tavares Huber [6], Márcia Edilaine Lopes Consolaro [7], Constanza Pujals [1], Carlos Laranjeira [8,9,10], Raíssa Bocchi Pedroso [1] and Sandra Marisa Pelloso [1]

1 Health Sciences Center, State University of Maringá-UEM, Maringá 87020-900, Brazil; camila.wsouza1@gmail.com (C.W.C.); mdbcarvalho@gmail.com (M.D.d.B.C.); vdmarques@uem.br (V.D.M.); romanio.maria@gmail.com (M.R.B.); kelystevanato@gmail.com (K.P.S.); pa_egger@hotmail.com (P.A.E.); ana.alarcao@educaadventista.org.br (A.C.J.A.); rkncuman1@gmail.com (R.K.N.C.); constanza.pujals@gmail.com (C.P.); raissap@gmail.com (R.B.P.); smpelloso@uem.br (S.M.P.)
2 Municipal Health Department, Curitiba 80060-130, Brazil; fercaspell@ufpr.br
3 Nurse Center, State University of Maringá—UEM, Maringá 87020-900, Brazil; beatriz.sousa.fonseca@hotmail.com
4 Department of Medicine, UNIMAR—University of Marilia, São Paulo 17525-902, Brazil; bborbapedro@gmail.com
5 Catholic College of Mato Grosso, Várzea Grande 78070-200, Brazil; prof.deisepelloso@uninga.edu.br
6 Department of Medicine, Inga University Center—Uningá, Maringá 87035-510, Brazil; isabellatavares@hotmail.com
7 Department of Biomedicine, State University of Maringá-UEM, Maringá 87020-900, Brazil; melconsolaro@uem.br
8 School of Health Sciences, Polytechnic University of Leiria, Campus 2, Morro do Lena, Alto do Vieiro, Apartado 4137, 2411-901 Leiria, Portugal; carlos.laranjeira@ipleiria.pt
9 Centre for Innovative Care and Health Technology (ciTechCare), Polytechnic University of Leiria, Campus 5, Rua das Olhalvas, 2414-016 Leiria, Portugal
10 Comprehensive Health Research Centre (CHRC), University of Évora, 7000-801 Évora, Portugal
* Correspondence: helenafiats@hotmail.com; Tel.: +55-44998720408

Simple Summary: Breast cancer is a leading cause of death among women worldwide, but survival rates vary significantly depending on race and socioeconomic status. Women from lower-income backgrounds and minority populations often face barriers to early diagnosis and timely treatment, leading to worse clinical outcomes. This study examines racial and socioeconomic disparities in breast cancer mortality and survival, aiming to quantify the impact of these factors through a systematic review and meta-analysis. By analyzing data from multiple studies, we assess how access to healthcare, screening programs, and treatment availability influence survival rates. Our findings highlight the urgent need for policies that improve access to early detection and equitable treatment, particularly for underserved communities. Understanding these disparities can help guide healthcare interventions and research efforts to reduce inequalities in breast cancer outcomes and improve survival rates for vulnerable populations.

Abstract: Background/Objectives: Breast cancer is one of the leading causes of female mortality worldwide, but significant racial and socioeconomic disparities persist in disease outcomes. This review aimed to analyze racial and socioeconomic inequalities in mortality and survival from breast cancer, identifying the impact of social risk factors on access to diagnosis and treatment. **Methods**: A systematic literature review and meta-analysis was performed following PRISMA guidelines. Eighteen studies published between 2014 and 2024 were included, with 11 contributing to the meta-analysis. Random-effect models were used to assess correlations between socioeconomic status, race, and clinical outcomes, including heterogeneity and publication bias analyses. **Results**: The strongest associations were observed between income, race, and breast cancer survival, with survival significantly worse among Black women and low-income populations ($p < 0.001$). Income also showed a strong positive correlation with clinical outcomes. In contrast, the overall effect on mortality was not statistically significant ($p = 0.290$), likely due to high heterogeneity across studies ($I^2 = 100\%$). These findings suggest that structural disparities in access to healthcare and early detection substantially affect survival rates. **Conclusions**: Racial and socioeconomic disparities in breast cancer outcomes remain critical public health challenges. Targeted policies to expand early diagnosis and ensure equitable access to effective treatment are essential to reduce these disparities and improve survival in underserved populations.

Keywords: socioeconomic disparity; culture-specific cancer outcomes; breast cancer

1. Introduction

With over 2.3 million new cases registered in 2022 [1] breast cancer is the most diagnosed cancer worldwide, 99% of which occur in women [2,3]. The World Health Organization (WHO) stated that breast cancer caused 670,000 deaths globally in 2022 [4]. Over 3 million cases and 1 million deaths from breast cancer are projected to occur yearly by 2040, which represents a global public health concern [2].

Several biological, environmental and social variables contribute to the development and progression of breast cancer [5,6]. Genetic factors (specifically family history), unhealthy lifestyle choices (e.g., diet, physical inactivity, smoking, drinking), environmental hazards (e.g., ionizing radiation), and social and psychological issues contribute to its prevalence [7,8]. Research has shown that hereditary factors and mutations account for 5–10% of breast cancer cases, while modifiable risk factors account for 20–30% [9].

Breast cancer mortality is intrinsically linked to racial and social inequities. Unfortunately, there is a significant disparity in mortality rates between different ethnic and socioeconomic groups, which reflects a clear inequality in access to health care and treatment outcomes. These racial inequities play a crucial role in breast cancer mortality. Studies have shown that women belonging to minority ethnic groups, such as Afro-descendants, Hispanics, and indigenous women have higher mortality rates compared to white women [10,11]. For example, in the United States, the five-year survival rate for non-Hispanic white women is approximately 91%, compared to 82% for Black women and 83% for Native American women [12]. Furthermore, Black women are 40% more likely to die from breast cancer than white women, despite having lower incidence rates [13]. These disparities reflect long-standing structural barriers in access to screening and timely treatment.

These inequalities can be attributed to a combination of factors, including differences in access to health services, lower quality of care, lower adherence to treatment, and diagnosis at more advanced stages of the disease. Women from low socioeconomic backgrounds, with lower educational levels and incomes, are more likely to face challenges in accessing health services and receive late diagnosis. These inequalities can be exacerbated by the lack of adequate health insurance, lack of transportation, language barriers, and lower awareness of the importance of early detection and regular follow-up [14].

Reducing disparities in breast cancer outcomes, early detection, and timely treatment depends on making relevant services available to everyone. The programs for reaching the underserved, however, must eliminate existing structural barriers, including but not limited to distance, costs, and poor health information. Available data support that structural factors, i.e., access to education, employment, and the health system, are not equal and have a significant effect on breast cancer outcomes, particularly in low- and middle-income countries [15,16]. Results that have been contrasted in studies across regions depict the ability of women in high-income countries to benefit from better coverage of screenings and access to treatment on time, women in resource-constrained settings often present with the disease at a later stage and few treatment options [16,17].

For instance, the WHO suggests that women in well-resourced areas who are 50 to 69 years old and at average risk for breast cancer undergo organized, population-based mammography screening every two years [18]. When resources are scarce—as they often are in low-resource areas where mammography screening is impractical or too expensive –, attention should instead be directed towards early detection by ensuring that women experiencing symptoms can get a proper diagnosis and treatment for their breast cancer as soon as possible [2].

Researchers have shown the need for breast cancer studies that address variables such as environmental and lifestyle factors; barriers preventing women from being diagnosed and treated, such as cultural taboos, geographic location, socioeconomic issues, and more effective methods of cancer prevention at the populational level, evaluating screening methods and techniques that meet women's needs. In a study carried out by Yedjou et al. (2019), the authors report that racial and economic disparities persist, and one can identify and reduce these disparities. Although several other studies have shown the importance of knowing and verifying the impact of disparities on breast cancer mortality, to our knowledge, no studies have systematically reviewed the scientific literature to identify how these disparities affect the morbidity and mortality of women with breast cancer and, therefore, how to develop interventions to improve quality of life [19].

A solid grasp of the global patterns and variability in disease burden is essential for the success of these endeavors. Yedjou et al. (2019) highlighted that new strategies and approaches are needed to promote prevention, improve survival rates, reduce breast cancer mortality, and improve health outcomes. Understanding whether there is a relationship between breast cancer mortality and socioeconomic and geographical location variables is important to help build preventive strategies to reduce breast cancer mortality rates. Therefore, the primary aims of this systematic literature review and meta-analysis were to (a) summarize the findings of studies examining racial and socioeconomic inequalities in mortality and survival from breast cancer, and (b) determine the magnitude of the overall associations between breast cancer mortality and social risk factors on access to diagnosis and treatment through a meta-analysis. This information may offer direction to women aiming to mitigate their heightened risk of breast cancer.

2. Materials and Methods

2.1. Protocol and Registration

This study is a systematic review conducted according to the methodology of the Joanna Briggs Institute (JBI) [20], recognized for its rigorous and practical approach to reviews in the health area. The review was also conducted using the PRISMA (Preferred Reporting Items for Systematic Reviews and Meta-Analyses) and PRISMA-NMA guidelines [21]. This review is registered in PROSPERO (International Prospective Register of Systematic Reviews) under number CRD42024599149.

2.2. PICO(S) Criteria

The research design was structured based on the PICO(S) model, as follows: Population (P)—Women with breast cancer; Exposure/Indicator (I)—Analysis of mortality associated with breast cancer; Comparison (C)—Racial and social disparities in mortality;

Outcome (O)—Identification of risk factors and impacts of screening strategies; and Type of Study (S)—Cross-sectional and longitudinal observational studies [22].

2.3. Search Strategy

In June 2024, a systematic literature search was conducted with the assistance of a research librarian. The search was conducted in the scientific databases PubMed, Embase, Scopus, Web of Science, Science Direct, SciELO, Biblioteca Virtual em Saúde (BVS), Cochrane Library and LILACS. Grey literature was also explored to broaden the scope of the results. The Medical Subject Heading (MeSH) terms "breast cancer", "mortality", "social health disparity" and "screening" were combined with Boolean operators and the search strategy was adapted to the specificities of each database. The search was conducted independently by two researchers and validated by the main author (Table 1).

Table 1. Search Strategies Conducted in the Databases.

Database	Search Strategy
PUBMED	((((breast cancer) AND (mortality)) AND (screening)) AND (social disparity)) AND (racial disparity)
EMBASE	(mortality), (screening), (breast cancer), (social determinants of health), (disparity)
Virtual Health Library (BVS)	(breast cancer) AND (mortality) AND (screening) AND (social disparity) AND (racial disparity)
LILACS	(breast cancer) AND (mortality) AND (screening) AND (social disparity) AND (racial disparity)
WEB OF SCIENCE	(breast cancer) AND (mortality) AND (screening) AND (social disparity) AND (racial disparity)
MEDLINE	(breast cancer) AND (mortality) AND (screening) AND (social disparity) AND (racial disparity)
SCIENCEDIRECT	(breast cancer) AND (mortality) AND (screening) AND (social disparity) AND (racial disparity)
COCHRANE	(breast cancer) AND (mortality) AND (screening) AND (disparities)

2.4. Eligibility Criteria

The target was cross-sectional and longitudinal population-based observational studies with random sampling, published between 2014 to 2024. The year 2014 marks the publication of the World Health Organization's position paper on mammography screening [23], which provided global guidance for breast cancer early detection strategies. Limiting the inclusion of studies published after this milestone ensures that the findings reflect contemporary practices, technologies, and health policy environments. Only studies with adult participants (≥18 years) and published in English, Portuguese or Spanish were considered. We included cross-sectional and longitudinal population-based studies because these observational designs are the most appropriate for investigating associations between social determinants and cancer outcomes at a population level. Randomized trials on racial and socioeconomic disparities are extremely limited, and other study designs (e.g., qualitative or case studies) do not allow for generalizable, quantitative comparisons of mortality or survival. Cross-sectional studies offered insight into prevalence and disparities, while longitudinal studies allowed evaluation of trends over time and survival estimates.

Studies conducted in specific populations, such as pregnant women and indigenous people, as well as systematic reviews, meta-analyses, dissertations, theses, technical reports, editorials and qualitative studies, were excluded. This decision was made because Indigenous populations often present unique sociocultural, geographic, and health system-related characteristics that distinguish them significantly from the general population. Including such studies in this meta-analysis could introduce substantial heterogeneity, as these groups face specific barriers to healthcare access and have different health outcomes that require a tailored analytical framework. Therefore, we opted to exclude them in order to preserve methodological consistency and comparability across studies.

2.5. Study Selection

The study selection occurred in three stages. Initially, six researchers (Group 1) screened the articles based on title and abstract. In case of disagreements, there was a discussion among the members or a final decision was made by the project coordinator. Subsequently, the selected articles were randomly distributed among the researchers for full reading and data extraction. The final stage involved an independent review by three experts (Group 2), who certified the final selection of studies.

2.6. Data Extraction and Analysis

The search results from each database were imported into Rayyan® software (https://www.rayyan.ai, accessed on 14 August 2024) [24], a web-based tool designed to assist in the systematic review process, to streamline the review process. The extracted data included title, first author, year of publication, language, study objective, methodological design, collection site, sample size, mean age, socioeconomic variables and frequency of mammographic screening by age group and race/color.

The meta-analysis was conducted using a random-effects model, weighting the effects of each study by the inverse of its variance [25]. Heterogeneity was assessed using the I^2 index and Cochran's Q test, with values greater than 50% being considered indicative of moderate to high heterogeneity. Sensitivity analyses were performed using the robust Huber-White estimator and robust weighted variance meta-analysis. Statistical analyses were conducted using RStudio software, version 4.3.0.

Although the included studies differed in design (cross-sectional vs. longitudinal), all provided quantitative estimates of the association between sociodemographic variables and breast cancer mortality or survival. Given the small number of eligible studies and the use of a random-effects model, we chose to analyze the data jointly. Heterogeneity and publication bias were thoroughly assessed to ensure the robustness of the findings.

2.7. Assessment of Methodological Quality and Risk of Bias

Two researchers using the JBI checklist for prevalence studies and Crombie's criteria for cross-sectional studies independently assessed the methodological quality of the studies. Nine items were considered, including sample adequacy, a detailed description of the setting and methodology, and measurement reliability. The risk of bias was analyzed using a funnel plot and Egger's test. The assessment table is provided as Supplementary Materials (Table S1).

3. Results

3.1. General Presentation

The initial search identified 239 articles, of which 54 were duplicates. After screening titles and abstracts, 38 articles were considered relevant for a full-text review. Of these, 16 articles were excluded because they did not meet the inclusion criteria. Therefore, 18 articles were included in the final sample and 11 participated in the meta-analysis (Figure 1).

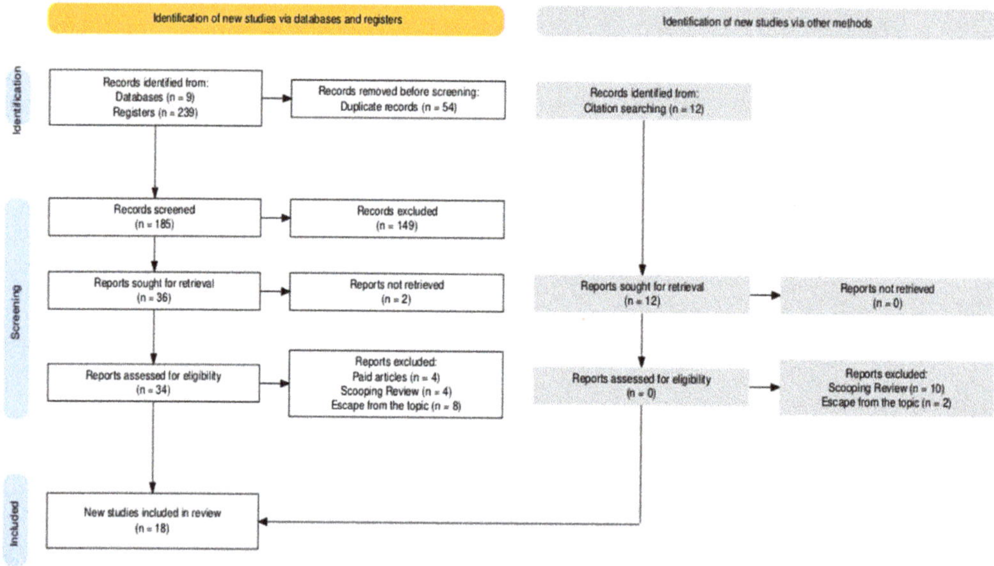

Figure 1. Flow diagram of the systematic review steps.

After analyzing the 18 studies selected for this systematic review, the data were extracted and synthesized according to the research objectives. Regarding the geographical distribution of the studies, the majority (16) were carried out in the United States of America (USA), using large national databases such as SEER and the National Cancer Database [26–41]. Two studies were conducted in Brazil, investigating regional and socioeconomic inequalities in breast cancer outcomes [42,43]. No studies conducted exclusively in Europe or Asia were identified, although some multicenter articles included diverse populations [39,40].

Data for the studies were collected from the early 1990s to the late 2020s. Most reported annual data, while others reported aggregate trends over a decade [29,35]. The studies were cross-sectional analyses for retrospective cohorts and population-based registries based on national health systems [37,38]. One study assessed racial disparities exclusively, and the others assessed an interaction of differences in socioeconomic status, health insurance coverage, and regional disparities in breast cancer outcomes [31].

Methodological approaches varied, with eight studies using large national databases and others employing smaller-scale data from academic hospitals and regional health systems. The studies uniformly observed large heterogeneity in breast cancer mortality rates, diagnostic predictions, and treatment outcomes, highlighting the very complex interplay of biological, socioeconomic, and systemic factors that drive disparities.

Overall, the results of these studies emphasized that there is an urgent need for targeted public health and policy interventions to address the identified inequalities, especially among racial minorities and low-income populations. Table 2 demonstrates the individual characteristics of the studies included in the review.

Table 2. General characteristics of the articles included in the review.

Citation (First Author et al., Year)	Country	Sample Number	Brief Conclusion
Anderson et al., 2023	USA	2.176	Geographic disparities influence breast cancer mortality, with access to treatment a critical determinant.
Chen et al., 2023	USA	415.277	Advanced diagnostic methods reduce disparities, but rural populations still face higher mortality rates.
Azin et al., 2023	USA	382.975	Advanced tumor staging highlights the role of socioeconomic status in breast cancer survival rates.
Fei Wang et al., 2021	USA	78.708	Urban populations have better outcomes due to better access to diagnostic and treatment facilities.
Guan et al., 2019	USA	5.622	Disparities in genetic screening contribute to differential outcomes in minority groups.
Nogueira et al., 2018	Brazil	481	Regional inequalities exacerbate disparities in breast cancer diagnosis stage and mortality.
Li Tao et al., 2016	USA	103.498	Hormone receptor status (ER+/PR+) significantly affects survival, particularly in low socioeconomic status groups.
Boyko et al., 2024	USA	907	Late screening and late-stage diagnosis are associated with higher mortality, even in safety-net hospitals.
Eom et al., 2023	USA	2.284	Targeted interventions in underserved regions reduce late-stage diagnoses and mortality.
Babatunde et al., 2021	USA	3.286	Late diagnosis and limited access to treatment are key factors leading to poor outcomes in low-income settings.
Renna Junior et al., 2021	Brazil	2.045 in Aracaju, 7.872 in Curitiba	Inequalities in access to treatment are important factors in breast cancer mortality in deprived regions.
Feinglass et al., 2015	USA	582.396	Socioeconomic status has a strong impact on mortality, even after adjustment for stage and clinical characteristics.
Sanderson et al., 2015	USA	64.384	Regular mammography reduces mortality by up to 45%, but disparities persist among black women.
Iqbal et al., 2015	USA	373.563	Black women are less likely to be diagnosed at stage I and have higher mortality, even for small tumors.
Akinyemiju et al., 2016	USA	67.084	Black women have higher hospital mortality and post-surgical complications compared to white women.
John et al., 2021	USA	10.366	ER+/PR+ breast cancer mortality is significantly higher in African American women due to socioeconomic status and hospital-type.
Akinyemijua et al., 2015	USA	71.156	Black women face higher hospital mortality and receive fewer mastectomies compared to white women.
Shariff-Marc et al., 2016	USA	9.372	Racial/ethnic disparities in mortality after breast cancer diagnosis highlight the influence of socioeconomic status and race.

3.2. Meta-Analysis

The data presented in Table 3 and Figure 2 indicate that mortality did not exhibit a significant combined effect ($p = 0.290$, coefficient = −0.192), despite high heterogeneity ($I^2 = 100\%$, $p < 0.001$), suggesting substantial variations across studies. These differences may be influenced by factors such as regional disparities, healthcare policies, and population characteristics. Additionally, Egger's test ($p = 0.003$) suggests potential publication bias, supported by the asymmetry in the funnel plot (Figure 2B).

Table 3. Meta-Analysis Results for Mortality, Survival, and Income.

Outcome	Coefficient (Estimate)	Standard Error	z-Value	*p*-Value	CI 95% (Lower Upper)	I^2 (%)	τ^2	Egger's Test (*p*)
Mortality	−0.192	0.181	−1.059	0.29	−0.548 to 0.163	100	195.272	0.003
Survival	5.596	0.622	9.004	<0.001	4.377 to 6.815	98.604	0.032	0.006
Income	5.010	0,129	38.755	<0.001	4.757 to 5.263	84.708	0.001	<0.001

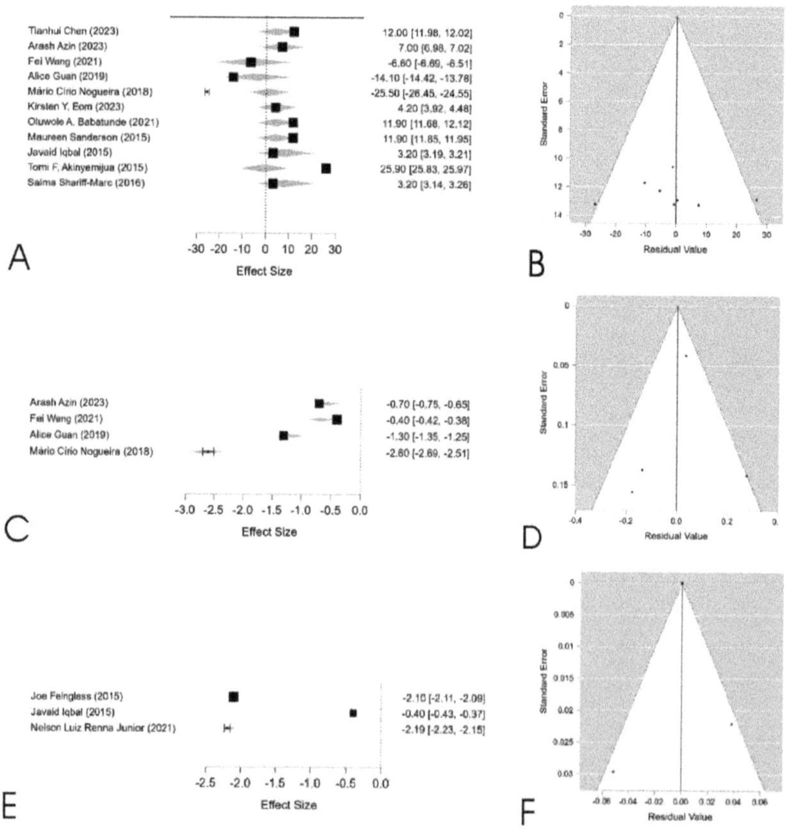

Figure 2. The figure presents the meta-analysis results for mortality (**A**,**B**), survival (**C**,**D**), and income (**E**,**F**). Forest plots (**A**,**C**,**E**) display the effect sizes and confidence intervals for each study, illustrating variability in estimates across different populations. Funnel plots (**B**,**D**,**F**) assess publication bias, where asymmetry suggests potential bias in mortality (**B**) and income (**F**), as confirmed by Egger's test. High heterogeneity is observed in all outcomes, indicating significant variations among studies, which may be influenced by regional, socioeconomic, and methodological differences. Original figure created by the authors based on data included in the present study.

In contrast, the survival analysis revealed a significant positive effect ($p < 0.001$, coefficient = 5.596, 95% CI: 4.377 to 6.815), with high heterogeneity ($I^2 = 98.6\%$, $p < 0.001$). Although the corresponding funnel plot (Figure 2D) appears relatively symmetrical, Egger's test ($p = 0.006$) indicates mild publication bias. Similarly, income showed a significant association with outcomes ($p < 0.001$, coefficient = 5.010, 95% CI: 4.757 to 5.263), with notable heterogeneity ($I^2 = 84.7\%$). The funnel plot (Figure 2F) suggests substantial asymmetry, confirmed by Egger's test ($p < 0.001$). These findings highlight the influence of socioeconomic and demographic factors on the analyzed outcomes and reinforce the need for careful interpretation, particularly in the presence of high heterogeneity and potential bias.

The high heterogeneity observed in the meta-analysis ($I^2 = 100\%$ for mortality, $I^2 = 98.6\%$ for survival) suggests that racial and socioeconomic disparities in breast cancer outcomes vary across different contexts. These variations may be attributed to differences in healthcare systems, screening policies, and population characteristics. Although some studies report survival improvements among Black women, heterogeneity remains high, indicating persistent structural challenges that hinder full equity.

While subgroup analyses could help identify sources of heterogeneity, the limited number of eligible studies (n = 11) reduced the feasibility of stratified meta-analyses. We acknowledge this as a limitation and suggest that future reviews explore larger datasets or focus on specific study designs to enable meta-regression or subgroup comparisons.

In addition to the aggregated effects presented above, Table 4 provides a study-by-study summary of the 11 articles included in the meta-analysis, specifying the outcome assessed, the main sociodemographic variables evaluated, and whether the associations were statistically significant.

Table 4. Summary of key data extracted from the 11 studies included in the Meta-Analysis.

Author (Year)	Country	Sample Size (n)	Outcome Assessed	Effect Size (ES)	SE	Sociodemographic Variables	Statistically Significant?
Tianhui Chen (2023)	USA	415,277	Mortality	12.0	0.0101	Race, income	Yes
Arash Azin (2023)	USA	382,975	Mortality	7.0	0.0083	SES	Yes
Fei Wang (2021)	USA	78,708	Survival	−6.6	0.0458	Urban vs. rural residence	Yes
Alice Guan (2019)	USA	5622	Survival	−14.1	0.1657	Genetic ancestry	Yes
Mário C. Nogueira (2018)	Brazil	481	Mortality	−25.5	0.4858	Region, income	No
Kirsten Y. Eom (2023)	USA	2284	Survival	4.2	0.1438	Race, insurance	Yes
Oluwole A. Babatunde (2021)	USA	3286	Mortality	11.9	0.1143	Insurance, income	Yes
Maureen Sanderson (2015)	USA	64,384	Mortality	11.9	0.0258	Race, mammography	Yes
Javaid Iqbal (2015)	USA	373,563	Mortality	3.2	0.005	Race, stage at diagnosis	Yes
Tomi F. Akinyemijua (2015)	USA	71,156	Mortality	25.9	0.0342	SES, surgical treatment	Yes
Salma Shariff-Marc (2016)	USA	9372	Mortality	3.2	0.0313	Race/ethnicity, SES	Yes

Abbreviations: ES = Effect Size; SE = Standard Error; SES = Socioeconomic Status.

For each study included in the meta-analysis, key information was systematically extracted, including sample size, outcomes assessed, sociodemographic variables analyzed, effect size (ES), standard error (SE), and statistical significance. Effect sizes and corresponding standard errors were directly collected from the results reported by the original authors, considering adjusted estimates (e.g., Odds Ratio, Hazard Ratio, or regression coefficients) whenever available. When the standard error was not explicitly provided, it was calculated based on the confidence intervals reported, following standard statistical procedures. Statistical significance was recorded according to the criteria adopted by each study, with p-values < 0.05 considered significant.

3.3. Methodological Quality Assessment

The studies included in this review were classified according to their methodological design, using the Joanna Briggs Institute's (JBI) criteria applied to prevalence studies and Crombie's criteria used for cross-sectional studies. The methodological assessment indicated that, in most prevalence studies, quality criteria were adequately met, particularly regarding sample representativeness, appropriate recruitment, and the use of validated measures. However, some limitations were identified, especially concerning the detailed description of the study setting and methodology, as well as the lack of control for confounding factors, which may compromise the reliability of the findings.

Overall, the methodological quality of the included studies was classified as moderate to high, with some specific limitations. Nevertheless, the presence of studies with low sample representativeness and insufficient control of confounding variables should be considered when interpreting the findings of this systematic review

3.4. Bias Risk Assessment

To assess the risk of bias, an inverted funnel plot and Egger's test were used [44,45]. The funnel plot (Figure 3) visually suggests a relatively balanced distribution of studies, indicating no strong publication bias. Egger's test ($p = 0.832$) further confirmed the absence of publication bias ($p > 0.05$), suggesting that the findings of this review are robust and reliable.

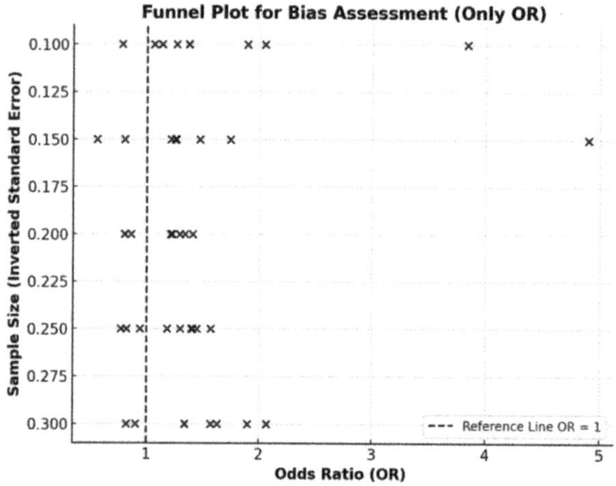

Figure 3. Funnel plot (inverted, or "Christmas tree" shape) assessing potential bias in studies reporting odds ratios (OR). Each "×" denotes a single study. The dashed vertical line represents the null effect (OR = 1).

3.5. Summarized Results

Differences in access to healthcare services and mammographic screening significantly impact clinical outcomes among socioeconomic groups. Patients with private health insurance are more likely to undergo regular mammograms and receive an early diagnosis compared to those with public insurance [39]. However, paradoxically, privately insured patients also exhibit a higher risk of diagnostic delays compared to those in the public healthcare system [35], potentially due to differences in referral protocols, waiting times, and treatment coverage.

Regular mammographic screening is associated with a significant reduction in breast cancer mortality, with studies indicating up to a 45% mortality reduction [40]. Moreover, shorter screening intervals have been linked to reduced overall mortality (adjusted OR = 0.57; 95% CI: 0.36–0.89; p = 0.013) [27]. However, low-income women continue to have reduced access to regular screenings, contributing to delayed diagnoses and increased mortality rates.

Socioeconomic factors such as income, education, and housing conditions strongly influence breast cancer outcomes [43]. Women with lower educational attainment exhibit higher mortality rates even after adjusting for clinical variables (HR = 1.27; 95% CI: 1.24–1.31) [42]. Patients in socioeconomically disadvantaged communities also face barriers such as limited access to advanced medical technologies and reduced social support, directly impacting survival [41]. These findings highlight the need for targeted public policies to ensure equitable access to screening and treatment, minimizing socioeconomic disparities.

Finally, the methodological quality assessment revealed that while most studies employed appropriate statistical methods, approximately 40% did not adequately justify sample size, and 35% had methodological deficiencies that may have influenced results. However, the absence of publication bias, as confirmed by Egger's test (p = 0.832), suggests that the findings of this review are reliable and robust.

4. Discussion

Although breast cancer mortality has been extensively studied worldwide, gaps remain regarding racial and socioeconomic disparities associated with the disease. Our meta-analysis reinforces that socioeconomic and racial factors remain decisive in determining breast cancer outcomes, particularly in relation to survival rates. The high degree of heterogeneity found among the studies analyzed indicates significant variations in demographic characteristics, methodological differences, and access to healthcare systems.

According to Ahmed [46], barriers to accessing mammography screening and early treatment are closely linked to socioeconomic and racial factors. Similarly, a meta-analysis by Silva et al. [15] found that women in low- and middle-income countries experience higher mortality rates due to late diagnosis and a lack of screening infrastructure. These findings suggest that access to healthcare services significantly influences disparities in breast cancer prognosis.

The discrepancies in survival rates among women with breast cancer reflect not only biological tumor behavior but also the impact of social determinants such as access to healthcare services and socioeconomic status. Newman et al. [13] emphasize the importance of public policies aimed at eliminating barriers faced by low-income African-American and Hispanic women, ensuring early screening, appropriate treatments, and strategies tailored to vulnerable populations. Additionally, educational programs, free screenings funded by non-commercial sources, and initiatives promoting equitable distribution of modern evidence-based treatments have been proposed to reduce these disparities.

Targeted intervention programs have demonstrated positive effects on survival among vulnerable groups. According to Grant et al. [47], while such programs improve outcomes, uneven coverage of screening services sustains gaps in late-stage diagnoses. Yedjou et al. [19] further suggest that awareness-raising and social support programs can help reduce inequalities in disadvantaged populations, highlighting the need for more comprehensive interventions.

There is a strong correlation between low income and more advanced clinical stages of breast cancer. Women with lower socioeconomic status have limited access to preventive screenings, early diagnosis, and guideline-recommended drug treatments, which contributes to disease progression and increased mortality. Our meta-analysis confirms these associations, adding pooled statistical support to the literature. Opia [48] observed that economic interventions aimed at expanding access to screening and treatment are associated with reduced inequality. This is supported by Pearson [49], who emphasizes that financial and geographic barriers continue to limit timely access to screening, particularly for women relying on underfunded public health systems.

Study Limitations

The included studies were assessed using different methodological criteria: the JBI Checklist for prevalence studies and Crombie's Criteria for cross-sectional studies. While this approach ensured a systematic and structured analysis, differences in methodological designs may have influenced the findings. Notably, variations in sample size justification and inadequate control of confounding factors in some studies contributed to the observed heterogeneity. One limitation is the combination of different study designs (cross-sectional and longitudinal), which may introduce heterogeneity. However, this was mitigated by the use of a random-effects model and sensitivity analyses. Additionally, the lack of standardization in analyzed variables impacted the consolidated interpretation of findings. Differences in statistical methods, inclusion and exclusion criteria, and outcome measurement approaches pose challenges for generalizing conclusions. Approximately 45% of the studies did not provide clear information on response rates or sample attrition management, potentially introducing bias.

Despite these limitations, the rigorous selection and methodological assessment process—conducted independently and repeatedly—enhances the reliability of this meta-analysis. This comprehensive and methodologically robust approach provides valuable insights into the impact of socioeconomic and racial disparities on breast cancer mortality.

Future research should address these limitations through methodological standardization, more detailed sample size justification, stricter control of confounding factors, and inclusion of grey literature. These efforts will ensure more precise and comparable analyses, further elucidating the impact of inequalities on breast cancer outcomes. Further studies should also consider using mixed-methods approaches, including qualitative analyses, to explore how social, cultural, and psychological dimensions shape access to cancer care and influence outcomes. Such approaches can offer a deeper understanding of the lived experiences behind the statistical disparities. Additionally, there is a need to include evidence from underrepresented regions, particularly in Asia and Africa, where socioeconomic and racial dynamics may differ substantially. Expanding geographic representation will enhance the generalizability of findings and support the development of more globally inclusive health policies.

5. Conclusions

This systematic review and meta-analysis highlighted that racial and socioeconomic disparities continue to play a major role in breast cancer outcomes, especially for African American, Hispanic populations, and those belonging to low-income groups. While such inequalities have been reported in previous studies, few have synthesised comparable quantitative data on death and survival, which indicate high heterogeneity at the population and regional levels. The findings bring out the need for public policies to ensure access and equal rights, to have screening done as early as possible, and to diagnose and treat breast cancer. Actions should include having government-funded programs for screening on a population basis, educating vulnerable communities, and ensuring that there is a fair allocation of evidence-based interventions. On top of this, the current disparities in cancer care show the need for an international collaborative network to cut gaps in equitable access and early detection. Health policies must reinforce health systems with financial support for cancer control programs and ensure that every patient has access to high-quality cancer services. Only through shared world plans can we truly achieve fair results in breast cancer prevention and care.

Supplementary Materials: The following supporting information can be downloaded at: https://www.mdpi.com/article/10.3390/cancers17101641/s1, Table S1: Methodological Quality of Prevalence Studies (JBI Checklist).

Author Contributions: Conceptualization, H.F.R. and S.M.P.; methodology, R.B.P., C.P. and H.F.R.; software, C.P.; validation, H.F.R., B.S.d.F. and C.W.C.; formal analysis, R.B.P., C.P. and H.F.R.; investigation, H.F.R., B.S.d.F. and C.W.C.; resources, H.F.R.; data curation, H.F.R., B.S.d.F. and C.W.C.; writing—original draft preparation, H.F.R., F.C.P., B.S.d.F., C.W.C., M.D.d.B.C., V.D.M., M.R.B., K.P.S., P.B.B., D.H.P.B., P.A.E., A.C.J.A., R.K.N.C., I.M.T.H., M.E.L.C., C.P., C.L., R.B.P. and S.M.P.; writing—review and editing, H.F.R., R.B.P., C.L. and S.M.P.; visualization, H.F.R., R.B.P., S.M.P. and C.L.; supervision, S.M.P.; project administration, H.F.R. and S.M.P.; funding acquisition, H.F.R. and C.L. All authors have read and agreed to the published version of the manuscript.

Funding: This work was supported by the Coordination for the Improvement of Higher Education Personnel (CAPES) (financial code 001). This work is also supported by national funds through FCT—Fundação para a Ciência e a Tecnologia, I.P. (UIDB/05704/2020 and UIDP/05704/2020) and under the Scientific Employment Stimulus-Institutional Call (https://doi.org/10.54499/CEECINST/00051/2018/CP1566/CT0012, accessed on 19 April 2025).

Institutional Review Board Statement: Not applicable.

Informed Consent Statement: Not applicable.

Data Availability Statement: This study is based on a systematic review and meta-analysis of previously published research. All data used were extracted from peer-reviewed articles indexed in databases such as PubMed, Scopus, and Web of Science. The list of included studies is provided in Table 2 and in the References section.

Conflicts of Interest: The authors declare no conflicts of interest.

References

1. WHO. Breast Cancer Cases and Deaths Are Projected to Rise Globally. 2025. Available online: https://www.iarc.who.int/wp-content/uploads/2025/02/pr361_E.pdf (accessed on 25 February 2025).
2. Arnold, M.; Morgan, E.; Rumgay, H.; Mafra, A.; Singh, D.; Laversanne, M.; Vignat, J.; Gralow, J.R.; Cardoso, F.; Siesling, S.; et al. Current and future burden of breast cancer: Global statistics for 2020 and 2040. *Breast* **2022**, *66*, 15–23. [CrossRef] [PubMed]
3. Sung, H.; Ferlay, J.; Siegel, R.L.; Laversanne, M.; Soerjomataram, I.; Jemal, A. Global cancer statistics 2020: GLOBOCAN estimates of incidence and mortality worldwide for 36 cancers in 185 countries. *CA Cancer J. Clin.* **2021**, *71*, 209–249. [CrossRef] [PubMed]
4. WHO. Breast Cancer. 2024. Available online: https://www.who.int/news-room/fact-sheets/detail/breast-cancer (accessed on 20 February 2025).
5. Aizaz, M.; Khan, M.; Khan, F.I.; Ahmad, S.; Obeagu, E.I. Burden of breast cancer: Developing countries perspective. *Int. J. Innov. Appl. Res.* **2023**, *11*, 31–37.
6. Obeagu, E.I.; Babar, Q.; Vincent, C.C.; Udenze, C.L.; Eze, R.; Okafor, C.J.; Ifionu, B.I.; Amaeze, A.A.; Amaeze, F.N. Therapeutic targets in breast cancer signaling: A review. *J. Pharm. Res. Int.* **2021**, *33*, 82–99. [CrossRef]
7. Løyland, B.; Sandbekken, I.H.; Grov, E.K.; Utne, I. Causes and Risk Factors of Breast Cancer, What Do We Know for Sure? An Evidence Synthesis of Systematic Reviews and Meta-Analyses. *Cancers* **2024**, *16*, 1583. [CrossRef]
8. Cohen, S.Y.; Stoll, C.R.; Anandarajah, A.; Doering, M.; Colditz, G.A. Modifiable risk factors in women at high risk of breast cancer: A systematic review. *Breast Cancer Res.* **2023**, *25*, 45. [CrossRef] [PubMed]
9. Sun, Y.S.; Zhao, Z.; Yang, Z.N.; Xu, F.; Lu, H.J.; Zhu, Z.Y.; Shi, W.; Jiang, J.; Yao, P.P.; Zhu, H.P. Risk factors and preventions of breast cancer. *Int. J. Biol. Sci.* **2017**, *13*, 1387–1397. [CrossRef]

10. Hines, R.B.; Johnson, A.M.; Lee, E.; Erickson, S.; Rahman, S.M.M. Trends in breast cancer survival by race-ethnicity in Florida, 1990–2015. *Cancer Epidemiol. Biomark. Prev.* **2021**, *30*, 1408–1415. [CrossRef]
11. Miller, B.C.; Bowers, J.M.; Payne, J.B.; Moyer, A. Barriers to mammography screening among racial and ethnic minority women. *Soc. Sci. Med.* **2019**, *239*, 112494. [CrossRef]
12. DeSantis, C.E.; Ma, J.; Gaudet, M.M.; Newman, L.A.; Miller, K.D.; Sauer, A.G.; Jemal, A.; Siegel, R.L. Breast cancer statistics, 2019. *CA Cancer J. Clin.* **2019**, *69*, 438–451. [CrossRef]
13. Newman, L.A. Disparities in breast cancer and African ancestry: A global perspective. *Breast J.* **2015**, *21*, 133–139. [CrossRef]
14. Ribeiro, H.F.; Carvalho, M.D.d.B.; Pelloso, F.C.; Santos, L.d.; Silva, M.d.A.P.; Stevanato, K.P.; Borghesan, D.H.P.; Romani, I.; Marques, V.D.; de Freitas, K.M.S.; et al. Maternal Risk Factors Associated with Negative COVID-19 Outcomes and Their Relation to Socioeconomic Indicators in Brazil. *Healthcare* **2023**, *11*, 2072. [CrossRef]
15. E Silva, J.D.D.; Pedroso, R.B.; Pelloso, F.C.; Carvalho, M.D.B.; Santos, T.D.S.; Dutra, A.C.; Stevanato, K.P.; Marques, V.D.; De Andrade, L.; Araújo, D.C.M.; et al. Mortality of Young Women due to Breast Cancer in Low, Middle and High-Income Countries: Systematic Literature Review and Meta-Analysis. *Asian Pac. J. Cancer Prev.* **2024**, *25*, 2219–2227. [CrossRef]
16. Anampa-Guzmán, A.; Acevedo, F.; Partridge, A.H.; Alfano, C.M.; Nekhlyudov, L. Cancer Survivorship in Latin America: Current Status and Opportunities. *JCO Glob. Oncol.* **2021**, *7*, 1472–1479. [CrossRef]
17. Unger-Saldaña, K. Challenges to the early diagnosis and treatment of breast cancer in developing countries. *World J. Clin. Oncol.* **2014**, *5*, 465–477. [CrossRef]
18. WHO. Position Paper on Mammography Screening. 2014. Available online: https://www.who.int/publications/i/item/9789241507936 (accessed on 25 February 2025).
19. Yedjou, C.G.; Sims, J.N.; Miele, L.; Abusamaan, M.S.; Payton, M.; Tchounwou, P.B. Health and racial disparity in breast cancer. *Adv. Exp. Med. Biol.* **2019**, *1152*, 31–49. [CrossRef]
20. Joanna Briggs Institute. *Annual Report 2018*; Joanna Briggs Institute: Adelaide, Australia, 2018; Available online: https://jbi.global/sites/default/files/2019-10/31a_Annual_Report_2018.pdf (accessed on 5 March 2024).
21. Page, M.J.; McKenzie, J.E.; Bossuyt, P.M.; Boutron, I.; Hoffmann, T.C.; Mulrow, C.D.; Moher, D.; Shamseer, L.; Tetzlaff, J.M.; Akl, E.A.; et al. The PRISMA 2020 statement: An updated guideline for reporting systematic reviews. *BMJ* **2021**, *372*, n71. [CrossRef]
22. Schardt, C.; Adams, M.B.; Owens, T.; Keitz, S.; Fontelo, P. Utilization of the PICO framework to improve searching PubMed for clinical questions. *BMC Med. Inform. Decis. Mak.* **2007**, *7*, 16. [CrossRef]
23. World Health Organization. *WHO Position Paper on Mammography Screening*; World Health Organization: Geneva, Switzerland, 2014; Available online: https://iris.who.int/handle/10665/137339 (accessed on 17 April 2025).
24. Hammady, M.; Fedorowicz, Z.; Elmagarmid, A. Rayyan—A web and mobile app for systematic reviews. *Syst. Rev.* **2016**, *5*, 210.
25. Borenstein, M.; Hedges, L.V.; Higgins, J.P.T.; Rothstein, H.R. *Introduction to Meta-Analysis*; Wiley: Chichester, UK, 2009; Available online: https://www.agropustaka.id/wp-content/uploads/2020/04/agropustaka.id_buku_Introduction-to-Meta-Analysis.pdf (accessed on 17 April 2025).
26. Anderson, T.; Herrera, D.; Mireku, F.; Barner, K.; Kokkinakis, A.; Dao, H.; Webber, A.; Merida, A.D.; Gallo, T.; Pierobon, M. Geographical variation in social determinants of female breast cancer mortality across US counties. *JAMA Netw. Open* **2023**, *6*, e2333618. [CrossRef]
27. Akinyemiju, T.; Sakhuja, S.; Vin Raviv, N. Racial and socio-economic disparities in breast cancer hospitalization outcomes by insurance status. *Ethn. Health* **2018**, *23*, 499–511. [CrossRef]
28. Feinglass, J.; Rydzewski, N.; Yang, A. The socioeconomic gradient in all-cause mortality for women with breast cancer: Findings from the 1998 to 2006 National Cancer Data Base with follow-up through 2011. *Ann. Epidemiol.* **2015**, *25*, 574–579. [CrossRef]
29. John, E.M.; McGuire, V.; Kurian, A.W.; Koo, J.; Shariff-Marco, S.; Gomez, S.L.; Cheng, I.; Keegan, T.H.M.; Kwan, M.L.; Bernstein, L.; et al. Racial/ethnic disparities in survival after breast cancer diagnosis by estrogen and progesterone receptor status: A pooled analysis. *Cancer Epidemiol. Biomark. Prev.* **2021**, *30*, 531–540. [CrossRef]
30. Boyko, A.; Qureshi, M.M.; Fishman, M.D.C.; Slanetz, P.J. Predictors of breast cancer outcome in a cohort of women seeking care at a safety net hospital. *Acad. Radiol.* **2024**, *31*, 663–670. [CrossRef]
31. Guan, A.; Lichtensztajn, D.; Oh, D.; Jain, J.; Tao, L.; Hiatt, R.A.; Gomez, S.L.; Fejerman, L. Breast cancer in San Francisco: Disentangling disparities at the neighborhood level. *Cancer Epidemiol. Biomark. Prev.* **2020**, *29*, 56–65. [CrossRef]
32. Azin, A.; Tahmasebi, H.; Brar, A.; Azin, S.; Ko, G.; Covelli, A.; Cil, T. Racial, ethnic and socioeconomic disparities in diagnosis, treatment, and survival of patients with breast cancer. *Am. J. Surg.* **2023**, *225*, 123–130. [CrossRef]
33. Tao, L.; Gomez, S.L.; Keegan, T.H.M.; Kurian, A.W.; Clarke, C.A. Breast cancer mortality in African-American and non-Hispanic white women by molecular subtype and stage at diagnosis: A population-based study. *Cancer Epidemiol. Biomark. Prev.* **2015**, *24*, 1039–1045. [CrossRef]
34. Shariff-Marco, S.; Yang, J.; John, E.M.; Kurian, A.W.; Cheng, I.; Leung, R.; Koo, J.; Monroe, K.R.; Henderson, B.E.; Bernstein, L.; et al. Intersection of race/ethnicity and socioeconomic status in mortality after breast cancer. *J. Community Health* **2015**, *40*, 1287–1299. [CrossRef]

35. Babatunde, O.A.; Eberth, J.M.; Felder, T.; Moran, R.; Truman, S.; Hebert, J.R.; Zhang, J.; Adams, S.A. Social determinants of racial disparities in breast cancer mortality among Black and White women. *J. Racial Ethn. Health Disparities* **2021**, *8*, 147–156. [CrossRef]
36. Wang, F.; Zheng, W.; Bailey, C.E.; Mayer, I.A.; Pietenpol, J.A.; Shu, X.O. Racial/ethnic disparities in all-cause mortality among patients diagnosed with triple-negative breast cancer. *Cancer Res.* **2021**, *81*, 1163–1170. [CrossRef]
37. Iqbal, J.; Ginsburg, O.; Rochon, P.A.; Sun, P.; Narod, S.A. Differences in breast cancer stage at diagnosis and cancer-specific survival by race and ethnicity in the United States. *JAMA* **2015**, *313*, 165–173. [CrossRef]
38. Sanderson, M.; Levine, R.S.; Fadden, M.K.; Kilbourne, B.; Pisu, M.; Cain, V.; Husaini, B.A.; Langston, M.; Gittner, L.; Zoorob, R.; et al. Mammography screening among the elderly: A research challenge. *Am. J. Med.* **2015**, *128*, 1362.e7–1362.e14. [CrossRef]
39. Chen, T.; Kharazmi, E.; Fallah, M. Race and ethnicity-adjusted age recommendation for initiating breast cancer screening. *JAMA Netw. Open* **2023**, *6*, e238893. [CrossRef]
40. Eom, K.Y.; Berg, K.A.; Joseph, N.E.; Runner, K.; Tarabichi, Y.; Khiyami, A.; Perzynski, A.T.; Sossey-Alaoui, K. Neighborhood and racial influences on triple negative breast cancer: Evidence from Northeast Ohio. *Breast Cancer Res. Treat.* **2023**, *198*, 369–381. [CrossRef]
41. Akinyemiju, T.F.; Vin-Raviv, N.; Chavez-Yenter, D.; Zhao, X.; Budhwani, H. Race/ethnicity and socio-economic differences in breast cancer surgery outcomes. *Cancer Epidemiol.* **2015**, *39*, 745–751. [CrossRef]
42. Nogueira, M.C.; Guerra, M.R.; Cintra, J.R.D.; Corrêa, C.S.L.; Fayer, V.A.; Bustamante-Teixeira, M.T. Disparidade racial na sobrevida de 10 anos no câncer de mama: Uma análise de mediação usando abordagem de respostas potenciais. *Cad. Saúde Pública.* **2018**, *34*, e00211717. [CrossRef]
43. Junior, N.L.R.; Lima, C.A.; Laporte, C.A.; Coleman, M.P.; Silva, G.A.E. Ethnic, racial and socioeconomic disparities in breast cancer survival in two Brazilian capitals between 1996 and 2012. *Cancer Epidemiol.* **2021**, *75*, 102048. [CrossRef]
44. Egger, M.; Smith, G.D.; Schneider, M.; Minder, C. Bias in meta-analysis detected by a simple, graphical test. *BMJ* **1997**, *315*, 629–634. [CrossRef]
45. Zhou, Y.; Huang, A.; Hattori, S. A likelihood-based sensitivity analysis for publication bias on the summary receiver operating characteristic in meta-analysis of diagnostic test accuracy. *Stat. Med.* **2023**, *42*, 781–798. [CrossRef]
46. Ahmed, A.T.; Welch, B.T.; Brinjikji, W.; Farah, W.H.; Henrichsen, T.L.; Murad, M.H.; Knudsen, J.M. Racial disparities in screening mammography in the United States: A systematic review and meta-analysis. *J. Am. Coll. Radiol.* **2017**, *14*, 157–165.e9. [CrossRef]
47. Grant, S.J.; Yanguela, J.; Odebunmi, O.; Grimshaw, A.A.; Giri, S.; Wheeler, S.B. Systematic review of interventions addressing racial and ethnic disparities in cancer care and health outcomes. *J. Clin. Oncol.* **2024**, *42*, 109–121. [CrossRef] [PubMed]
48. Opia, F.N.; Matthew, K.A. Socioeconomic disparities in breast cancer care: Addressing global challenges in oncology outcomes. *Int. J. Comput. Appl. Technol. Res.* **2025**, *14*, 1003. [CrossRef]
49. Pearson, S.A.; Taylor, S.; Marsden, A.; Zdenkowski, N.; Bates, N.; McNeil, C.; Nair, B.; Wyld, D.; Stockler, M.R.; Kiely, B.E.; et al. Geographic and sociodemographic access to systemic anticancer therapies for secondary breast cancer: A systematic review. *Syst. Rev.* **2024**, *13*, 35. [CrossRef]

MDPI AG
Grosspeteranlage 5
4052 Basel
Switzerland
Tel.: +41 61 683 77 34

Cancers Editorial Office
E-mail: cancers@mdpi.com
www.mdpi.com/journal/cancers